Integrated Clinical Science

Musculoskeletal Disease

Integrated Clinical Science

Other titles:

Cardiovascular Disease
Professor JR Hampton

Psychiatry
Professor JL Gibbons

Nephro-urology
Professor AW Asscher
Professor DB Moffat

Respiratory Disease
GM Sterling

Haematology
JC Cawley

Gastroenterology
P Jones, P Brunt,
NAG Mowat

Neurology
RW Ross Russell
CM Wiles

Endocrinology
Professor CRW Edwards

Human Health and the Environment
Professor R Weir, C Smith

Projected

Reproduction and Development

Integrated Clinical Science

Musculoskeletal Disease

Edited by

Robert A. Dickson, MA, ChM, FRCS, FRCSE

Professor of Orthopaedic Surgery, University of Leeds

and

Verna Wright, MD, FRCP

Professor of Rheumatology, University of Leeds

Series Editor

George P McNicol, MD, PhD, FRCP

(Lond, Edin, Glasg), FRCPath, Hon FACP

Principal and Vice Chancellor, University of Aberdeen. Lately Professor of Medicine, The University of Leeds, and Head, The University Department of Medicine, The General Infirmary, Leeds

William Heinemann Medical Books Ltd
London

ISBN 0-433-16603-7

© 1984 William Heinemann Medical Books Ltd,
   23 Bedford Square,
   London WC1B 3HH

First published 1984
Reprinted 1985

Printed and bound in Great Britain by the
Alden Press, Oxford

Contents

Preface

It is clearly desirable on educational grounds to adopt and teach a rational approach to the management of patients, whereby the basic scientific knowledge, the applied science and the art of clinical practice are brought together in an integrated way. Progress has been made in this direction, but after twenty-five years of good intentions, teaching in many medical schools is still split up into three large compartments, preclinical, paraclinical and clinical, and further subdivided on a disciplinary basis. Lip-service is paid to integration, but what emerges is often at best a coordinated rather than an integrated curriculum. Publication of the INTE-GRATED CLINICAL SCIENCE series reflects the need felt in many quarters for a truly integrated textbook series, and is also intended as a stimulus to further reform of the curriculum.

The complete series will cover the core of clinical teaching, each volume dealing with a particular body system. Revision material in the basic sciences of anatomy, physiology biochemistry and pharmacology is presented at the level of detail appropriate for Final MB examinations, and subsequently for rational clinical practice. Integration between the volumes ensures complete and consistent coverage of these areas, and similar principles govern the treatment of the clinical disciplines of medicine, surgery, pathology, microbiology, immunology and epidemiology.

The series is planned to give a reasoned rather than a purely descriptive account of clinical practice and its scientific basis.

Clinical manifestations are described in relation to the disorders of structure and function which occur in a disease process. Illustrations are used extensively, and are an integral part of the text.

The editors for each volume, well-known as authorities and teachers in their fields, have been recruited from medical schools throughout the UK. Chapter contributors are even more widely distributed, and coordination between the volumes has been supervised by a distinguished team of specialists.

Each volume in the series represents a component in an overall plan of approach to clinical teaching. It is intended, nevertheless, that every volume should be self-sufficient as an account of its own subject area, and all the basic and clinical science with which an undergraduate could reasonably be expected to be familiar is presented in the appropriate volume. It is expected that, whether studied individually or as a series, the volumes of INTEGRATED CLINICAL SCIENCE will meet a major need, assisting teachers and students to adopt a more rational and holistic approach in learning to care for the sick.

George P McNicol
Series Editor

Introduction

As undergraduate teaching becomes more integrated, so it is desirable to teach together subjects which are integrated. Orthopaedic surgery, trauma, rheumatology, and rehabilitation all have the musculoskeletal system as their common denominator, and many medical schools now teach these subjects in combinations. The undergraduate, however, has to seek the basic factual requirements for all these subjects from different sources, and thus an integrated musculoskeletal textbook for the student is long overdue. Furthermore, with the relatively limited teaching time for the musculoskeletal system in the average curriculum it is quite unrealistic to expect students to read and assimilate the available separate accounts of these subjects. Accordingly we have produced a size of text appropriate to curriculum time. To this factual basis, the student should add by clinical exposure to musculoskeletal patients.

Contributors

CE Ackroyd
Consultant Orthopaedic Surgeon
Bristol Royal Infirmary

IA Archer
Lecturer in Orthopaedic Surgery
University of Leeds

P Bliss
Consultant Orthopaedic Surgeon
Bath and Wessex Orthopaedic Hospital
Bath

NJ Blockey
Consultant Orthopaedic Surgeon
Royal Hospital for Sick Children
Glasgow

RF Brown
Consultant Orthopaedic Surgeon
St. James's University Hospital
Leeds

MA Chamberlain
Clinical Lecturer
University Department of Medicine
Leeds General Infirmary

HLF Currey
Professor of Rheumatology
The London Hospital Medical College

RA Dickson
Professor of Orthopaedic Surgery
University of Leeds

JM Fitton
Formerly, Consultant Orthopaedic Surgeon
St. James's University Hospital
Leeds

CSB Galasko
Professor of Orthopaedic Surgery
University of Manchester

AGS Hill
Formerly, Consultant Physician
Stoke Mandeville Hospital
Aylesbury

SPF Hughes
Professor of Orthopaedic Surgery
University of Edinburgh

MIV Jayson
Professor of Rheumatology
University of Manchester

RN Maini
Professor, and Head of Department of
    Immunology of Rheumatic Diseases
Charing Cross Hospital Medical School
London
and Division of Clinical Immunology
Kennedy Institute of Rheumatology
London

B McKibbin
Professor of Orthopaedic Surgery
Welsh National School of Medicine
Cardiff

TE McSweeney
Director, Spinal Injuries Unit
The Robert Jones and Agnes Hunt
   Orthopaedic Hospital
Oswestry

R Smith
Consultant Physician
Nuffield Orthopaedic Centre
Oxford

EA Williams
Lecturer
Department of Orthopaedic Surgery
University of Manchester

DH Wilson
Consultant Surgeon
Leeds General Infirmary

V Wright
Professor of Rheumatology
University of Leeds

Advisory Editors

Professor AS Douglas
Department of Medicine, University of Aberdeen

Pathology: Professor CC Bird
          Institute of Pathology
          University of Leeds

Physiology: Professor PH Fentem
          Department of Physiology and
             Pharmacology
          Nottingham University

Biochemistry: Dr RM Denton
          Reader in Biochemistry
          University of Bristol

Anatomy: Professor RL Holmes
          Department of Anatomy
          University of Leeds

Pharmacology: Professor AM Breckenridge
          Department of Clinical
             Pharmacology
          Liverpool University

1

Approach to the Patient

DETAILED HISTORY

The appropriate treatment for a particular patient depends upon the clinical assessment of that particular individual. Each patient is therefore unique, and in no area is this more evident than in the musculoskeletal system. It is not necessarily the diagnosis which leads to a particular form of management, but how that diagnosis affects that patient. The clinical examination, backed up by any necessary radiographic evaluation and special investigations, may clinch a diagnosis, but the history is of far greater importance; it not only points the clinician in the right diagnostic direction but is the only phase of assessment which highlights the patient's view of his problem.

The skill of a busy general practitioner is the experience that enables him to be selective in history taking. The complexity of many of the problems that face a newly-qualified doctor dictates that he or she should take a detailed history without cutting corners.

In the majority of instances, patients with musculoskeletal problems are not systemically unwell; their pain, deformity or disability occurs in a person who is otherwise fit. It is this interference with what has become a standard way of life that brings the patient to seek a medical opinion. The presenting event may have occurred instantaneously, as in the sudden dissipation of force giving rise to a fracture or internal joint derangement. In this case, the problem, though not the specific diagnosis, is therefore as abundantly clear to the patient as it is to the doctor and such a patient will readily accept the disadvantages of short-term immobilisation or a minor operation for the benefits of an early return to normal activities. On the other hand, a patient presenting with a more insidious condition such

as arthritis, again being perfectly aware of the underlying process, may already have adapted his way of life significantly; his ambition is not normality (and neither is it the aim of the doctor) but rather the attainment of a way of life which is once again acceptable even if only in the medium term. In progressive conditions, halting or even reducing the rate of deterioration may be the only realistic possibility (Fig. 1.1). Therefore it is essential to know the personal, social, family and occupational background to the specific problem. This aspect of history-taking must be conducted with the utmost sensitivity, and may affect the complete age spectrum from the problems of unexpected congenital abnormalities in the newborn to the difficulties of severe disability in the elderly.

The sex of the patient may give a guide to diagnosis. For instance, Reiter's syndrome is rarely seen in women, ankylosing spondylitis and scaphoid fracture are four times as common in men as in women, and systemic lupus erythematosus and Colles' fracture are commoner in women. The age of onset may also be important. Polymyalgia rheumatica is usually found in elderly women, whereas ankylosing spondylitis commonly begins in young men.

The common presenting complaints are pain, swelling, deformity, stiffness and limitation of movement, often in combination (Fig. 1.2).

SYMPTOMS

Local, referred and radicular pain

The patient is always asked to point with one finger to where he feels the maximum discomfort and then to indicate the area of radiation. This is particularly

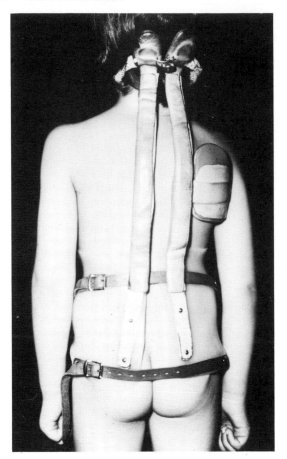

Fig. 1.1 *The Milwaukee brace for scoliosis. It may reduce the rate of deterioration of the curve or even halt progression but never has any corrective effect.*

important in junctional areas, e.g. neck and shoulder, or pelvis and hip (Fig. 1.3). Shoulder pain is felt locally, often just under the tip of the acromion, and radiates no further than the deltoid insertion. Cervical spine discomfort is also felt locally but may be referred across the triangles of the neck, the shoulder, and down to but not distal to the elbow. These are examples of 'local' and 'referred' pains. In addition, lesions of the vertebral column may give rise to nerve root pressure, in which case a more severe discomfort may radiate throughout the distribution of that nerve root, often to the distal end of the affected extremity. The term 'radicular' is applied to this type of discomfort.

Similarly, hip pain is characteristically felt in the groin and may be referred down the anteromedial aspect of

the thigh to the knee. Typically in children, discomfort in the knee may be the sole presenting symptom of pathology in the hip joint. On the other hand, pain felt laterally or posteriorly in relation to the hip is more frequently referred from the lower lumbar spine or sacroiliac joint. Severe pain travelling from pelvis via thigh to leg and foot in the distribution of a nerve root is also radicular and has its origin in the lower lumbar spine.

Local discomfort varies in character according to the nature of the underlying pathological process and to the site – bone, joint or soft tissue. Severe discomfort localised to bone, increased by movement and relieved by rest, is typical of a fracture or acute infection. Severe discomfort localised in a joint, which is held rigidly in semi-flexion in order to avoid the excruciating discomfort of movement, is typical of acute infective arthritis, gout and rheumatic fever. A less severe discomfort localised in a joint, exacerbated both by prolonged function and rest, is typical of degenerative osteoarthritis.

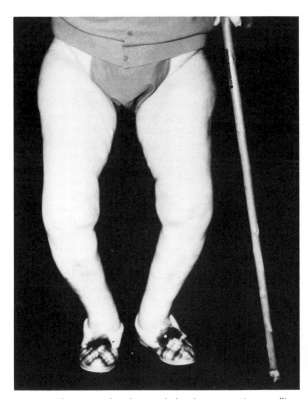

Fig. 1.2 *Rheumatoid arthritis of the knees—pain, swelling, deformity.*

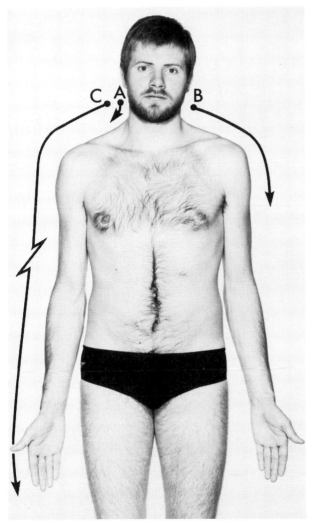

Fig. 1.3 *The site and extent of local, referred and radicular pains from the cervical spine: A, local; B, referred; C, radicular.*

The quality of a referred and a radicular pain is also characteristic. The former is a dull and frequently continuous discomfort, similar to the quality of the local pain and aggravated by the same factors. A radicular pain is a severe, lancinating pain, shooting down the extremity and typically exacerbated by increasing intraspinal pressure, e.g. coughing, sneezing, straining. It is frequently accompanied by neurological symptoms such as paraesthesia in the dermatome distribution of that nerve root.

Factors related to symptoms

In the history of joint disease it is important to determine whether the joint has previously been affected by any traumatic or infective process which would favour an early secondary degenerative process (Fig. 1.4). The presence of similar symptoms coexisting in other joints suggests a generalised arthritic condition. Musculoskeletal pain may also be temporally related. Patients with median nerve compression due to a carpal tunnel syndrome are typically woken with painful paraesthesia in the early hours of the morning, when loss of the normal forearm muscle pump mechanism during sleep has led to a local accumulation of fluid. Similarly, patients with hip arthritis are frequently woken or kept awake by groin and anterior thigh pain which troubled them less when they were more mobile during the day.

The severity of pain may be a diagnostic guide, and a therapeutic indication. The severest pain suffered by rheumatic patients arises from gout, rheumatic fever, and infective arthritis. When the great wit Sidney Smith had an attack of gout, he exclaimed, 'I feel as if I am walking on my eyeballs.'

Aggravating and alleviating factors should also be sought. The back pain of ankylosing spondylitis is characteristically aggravated by rest in bed, whereas that of a protruded intervertebral disc is relieved.

Pronounced morning stiffness is a diagnostic feature of rheumatoid arthritis, and is also characteristic of polymyalgia rheumatica. Its duration reflects the activity of the disease; when rheumatoid arthritis remits, whether naturally or from medication, the morning stiffness ameliorates.

The distribution of affected joints may give a clue to the diagnosis. Rheumatoid arthritis characteristically begins in the metacarpophalangeal joints or wrists, and may go on to affect many joints of the body including the shoulders. The distal interphalangeal joints are characteristically involved in primary generalised osteoarthritis, and sometimes in psoriatic arthritis, but rarely in rheumatoid arthritis. A large joint synovitis involving the knees and ankles is characteristic of Reiter's syndrome and enteropathic arthritis. A flitting polyarthritis is characteristic of rheumatic fever, but may occur in gonococcal and meningococcal arthritis. Symmetry is a diagnostic feature of rheumatoid arthritis.

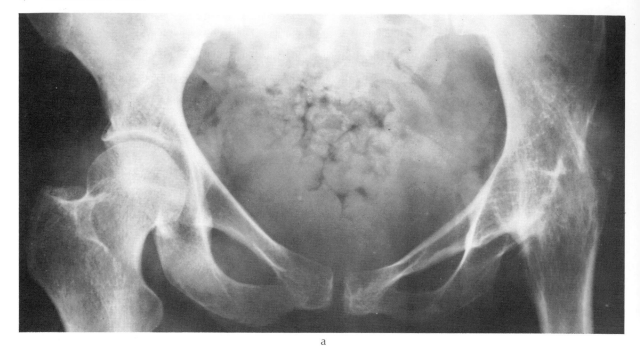

a

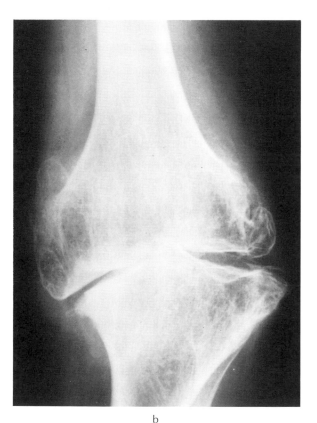

b

Fig. 1.4 (a) *Anteroposterior radiograph of the hip joints: the left hip has fused spontaneously following septic arthritis in childhood. (b) Anteroposterior view of the ipsilateral knee: The joint has worn out because it has taken a much increased load for many years.*

The duration of the arthritis is important in diagnosis. Rheumatoid arthritis can seldom be diagnosed with certainty before three months have elapsed. Rubella synovitis, however, which mimics rheumatoid arthritis, is a self-limiting disease that characteristically disappears within six weeks.

Joint swelling is important in differentiating arthritis from nonarticular rheumatism, and its distribution is even more helpful than the distribution of pain in rheumatoid disorders.

Functional disability

As a result of trauma or arthritis a joint's range of motion may be limited, and this rather than pain may be the major symptom. Patients do not talk of limitation of movement; they talk of stiffness or the consequent inability to perform certain functions. Thus the concept of functional disability is of paramount importance. Patients with severe hip arthritis may no longer be able to flex far enough forward to put on their own shoes and socks, or other clothes, and may come to rely upon their partner for help with dressing. They may adapt to this way of life, and only present when their spouse is invalided or deceased. Before the advent of total joint replacement, the great majority of these patients were relegated to a wheelchair existence in a communal supervised environment. A seemingly insoluble problem may therefore be overcome by the assistance of relatives and friends when the need for reconstructive surgery is denied by the patient's general physical condition.

A history of trauma

An accurate history can help in diagnosing and assessing the effects of trauma. Patients with soft-tissue injuries of the knee, sustained during weekend sporting activities, frequently do not present until two days or so have elapsed from the time of the injury. They often therefore present with a painful swollen knee regardless of the underlying problem. A history of a rotational injury of the flexed knee with the foot firmly on the ground is typical of a cartilage injury (Fig. 1.5). The patient has been unable to continue playing and was usually 'carried off'. He wakes up the following morning with an effusion of the knee joint. Ligamentous injuries of the knee, however, occur from a sideways blow on a straighter weight-bearing knee, and the intra-articular damage to the synovial vasculature causes a haemarthrosis to appear rapidly.

Degree of violence can also be of importance. Whereas the unprotected leg of the motor-cyclist frequently sustains significant injury from severe local forces directly applied, the neck of femur of the elderly postmenopausal female may break in a spiral fashion due to the minimal force of a sudden twisting movement imposed upon unduly soft bone. In this situation, the fracture almost certainly occurred before the fall.

Systematic review

A review of the systems may give important clues to the nature of the condition. General features such as anorexia and weight-loss may indicate the systemic nature of the disease. Sometimes this will be accompanied by pyrexia. The condition of the skin is

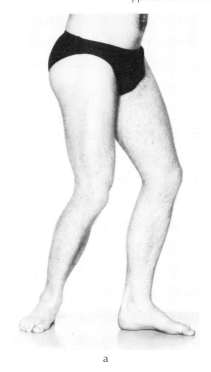

a

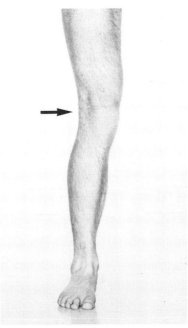

b

Fig. 1.5 *Mechanisms of injury in cartilage and ligament damage to the knee. (a) A rotational injury to the flexed knee causes a cartilage injury. (b) A sideways force to a straighter knee causes a ligament injury.*

important (Fig. 1.6). Psoriasis may be associated with an arthritis, and erythema nodosum often occurs with a large joint synovitis. Systemic lupus erythematosus is characterised by a butterfly rash across the cheeks and bridge of the nose, exacerbated by sunlight. Polyarteritis nodosa may have cutaneous manifestations similar to erythema *ab igne*.

In the cardiovascular system, patients with ischaemic

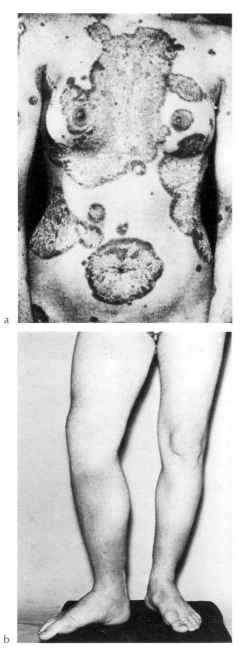

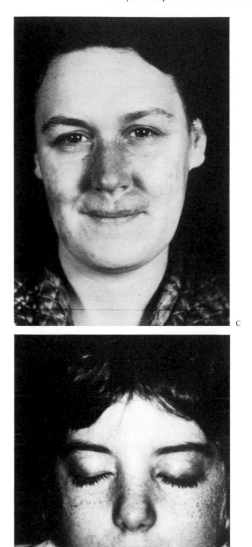

Fig. 1.6 *Four common skin lesions associated with musculoskeletal disorders. (a) Psoriasis. (b) Erythema nodosum. (c) The butterfly rash of systemic lupus. (d) The lilac-coloured rash of dermatomyositis.*

heart disease may develop periarthritis of the shoulder. Several rheumatic disorders affect the heart and blood vessels, e.g. rheumatic fever, rheumatoid arthritis, ankylosing spondylitis, and systemic lupus erythematosus. Where valvular damage gives rise to symptoms, valve replacement may be indicated. Raynaud's phenomenon, in which the fingers go white and blue in the cold, invariably accompanies systemic sclerosis, and commonly precedes it, often by many years. Cardiac decompensation may be a contra-indication to major surgery. There is little point in increasing an arthritic patient's mobility if the cardiovascular system will not allow a greater exercise tolerance. Intermittent claudication is experienced by sufferers of vascular disease and spinal stenosis. Decompressive laminectomy is unlikely to benefit patients with vascular disease.

The same is true in the respiratory system. A number of disorders of connective tissue affect the lungs, such as the fibrosing alveolitis or pleuritis of rheumatoid arthritis, or honeycomb lungs in systemic sclerosis, or pleuritis and lung involvement in systemic lupus erythematosus. A carcinoma of the lung may also produce various types of arthropathy, e.g. hypertrophic pulmonary osteoarthropathy with its characteristic clubbing, aching and swelling at the end of long bones (Fig. 1.7).

In the gastrointestinal system, ulcerative colitis and Crohn's disease are both associated with arthropathy; dysentery may also give a reactive arthritis like Reiter's syndrome. Even more important is the tendency of nonsteroidal anti-inflammatory drugs to cause erosive gastritis. It is important to ascertain, therefore, whether rheumatic sufferers have a hiatus hernia or a peptic ulcer. Steroids may cause a peptic ulcer to bleed or to perforate.

Many rheumatic disorders affect the central nervous system. Peripheral neuropathy may occur with rheumatoid arthritis or with polyarteritis nodosa. Long tract signs can occur as a result of cervical spondylosis (degenerative changes in the cervical spine) or cervical subluxation consequent upon rheumatoid disease (Fig. 1.8). The patient has difficulty in walking or may be

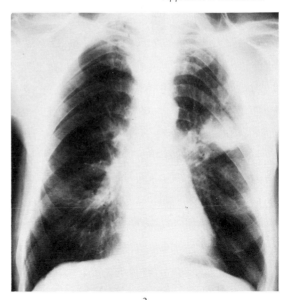

a

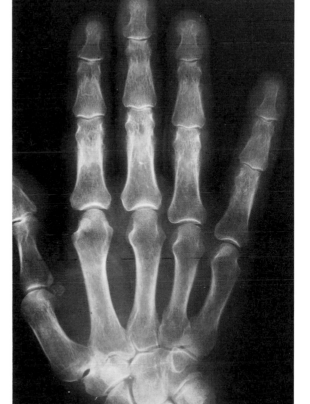

b

Fig. 1.7 *Lung cancer and arthropathy are often associated.* (a) *Posteroanterior chest radiograph showing cancer of the left lung.* (b) *Anteroposterior hand radiograph of the same patient showing hypertrophic pulmonary osteoarthropathy.*

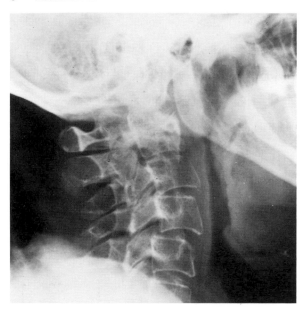

Fig. 1.8 *Lateral radiograph of the cervical spine of a rheumatoid patient: There is upward migration of the odontoid and anterior subluxation of C4.*

paralysed. The characteristic story is of a rheumatoid patient who trips over a step and finds he cannot walk thereafter. This may well be due to an atlanto-axial subluxation which has impinged upon the cervical cord. A neurological history is particularly important in relation to peripheral nerve compression syndromes, but the complaint of numbness in a particular area must be interpreted with caution. Patients seldom mean total loss of sensation and numbness usually implies paraesthesia or hypoaesthesia.

In the genito-urinary system, a mucoid urethral discharge is characteristic of Reiter's syndrome, whereas a purulent urethral discharge may well indicate a gonococcal arthritis.

Previous medical treatment

A careful review of the previous treatment is important. The importance of low back pain increases significantly if it has persisted despite a trial period of bed rest at home. Indeed, no patient should be referred to hospital with low back pain without a trial period of bed rest unless there are objective neurological signs present. Some drugs may cause rheumatic disorders. Gout may be precipitated by diuretics and other drugs, such as pyrazinamide used in the treatment of tuberculosis. A

number of drugs also produce systemic lupus erythematosus. In hospital practice, patients have often received a number of drugs already. It is important to note those that caused side-effects so that the patient is not exposed to these again; and to note those which have produced no benefit, as well as the ones which have.

The previous medical history will often reveal the sort of information obtained in a review of the systems. Quite commonly, moreover, patients will speak of a previous episode of rheumatic disease, such as a 'slipped disc', which they had not linked with their present condition.

Family and social history

The family history is of limited diagnostic help, although gout, psoriatic arthritis and ankylosing spondylitis have a hereditary component. In a careful family history, however, social factors are often revealed. A relative who has had a crippling arthritis may well be the cause of needless worry to a patient with rheumatic symptoms, who fears a similar outcome.

In the social history, the occupation may give an indication of a diagnosis, e.g. bar tenders and brewers are more likely to get gout. Coal miners frequently have degenerative changes in the spine and knee joints. It is important to enquire exactly what the patient does at work. This may reveal the cause of backache, for instance, and it may also show the unsuitability of a particular job for a person with an arthritic disease. The nature of housing is relevant, particularly in patients with multiple joint involvment. A large house with an upstairs toilet may give a clear indication for rehousing a patient with severe rheumatoid arthritis. The responsibilities of a patient at home may aggravate symptoms, or indeed explain them, e.g. a divorced or widowed individual with a number of young children has many pressures to withstand. Smoking and alcohol consumption may be factors in certain rheumatic disorders, e.g. peripheral vascular disease and gout.

EXAMINATION ROUTINE

The examination of the musculoskeletal system is based upon a 'set routine' which is only slightly adapted from part to part. The stages of this routine are inspection, palpation, measurement of range of motion, special tests, and a neurological and general physical examination where indicated.

Inspection

A good exposure is essential. For examination of the upper half of the body, the patient must be stripped to the waist; for examination of the lower half of the body, the patient must be stripped from the waist downwards with the exception of the underpants. For the examination of the spine, all clothes except underpants must be removed. Skin, soft tissue, bones and joints should be inspected, in that order. Skin colour, distribution of hair, and nail quality may indicate a neurological or vascular problem. Muscle wasting is common in musculoskeletal disease, usually secondary to pathology in a nearby joint rather than a primary neuromuscular lesion. The length, alignment and relative size of the long bones should be visually estimated; any local abnormality may suggest a fracture (old or new) or metabolic bone disease, while disproportion may indicate a developmental syndrome.

Enlargement of the ends of long bones may indicate a vitamin deficiency in the younger patient, or the secondary formation of new bone associated with degenerative disease in the elderly. The resting attitude of an extremity may strongly indicate the underlying diagnosis. The shortened, externally-rotated, lower extremity of an elderly female after a fall is diagnostic of a fractured neck of femur. The flexed, shortened and internally-rotated lower extremity of a front seat passenger in a road traffic accident strongly suggests a posteriorly dislocated hip joint (Fig. 1.9). An irritable

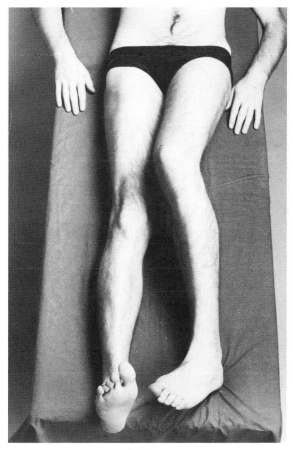

a

b

Fig. 1.9 *The attitude of a limb may be diagnostic.* (a) *The shortened, externally rotated left lower extremity with a fractured neck of femur.* (b) *The shortened, flexed and internally rotated left lower extremity with a posteriorly dislocated hip.*

articulation, such as is found in an acute arthritic process or intra-articular fracture, is characteristically held in a position of semiflexion, often with a component of external rotation providing maximum capsular relaxation. From this resting position the patient is reluctant to move.

Careful inspection of a possibly fractured long bone is essential. The position of the fragments as determined visually and radiographically in the accident department tells nothing of their position at the moment of maximal force dissipation. Thus, a minute penetrating wound visible in the neighbourhood of the fracture may be the only clue to its compound nature (compound from within, when a spike of bone perforated the integument at a time when the fragments may have been at right angles to each other). This markedly alters both initial management and prognosis.

Palpation

The skin, soft tissues, bones and joints should now be palpated with particular reference to temperature, tenderness, crepitus, or the presence of a swelling. Exquisite local bone tenderness with crepitus and mobility is typical of a fracture; the same degree of tenderness in the metaphyseal region, with increased warmth, strongly suggests underlying bone infection. A local bony hard swelling, sometimes with tenderness and warmth, in the younger patient strongly suggests an underlying primary bone neoplasm

Careful joint palpation may be most informative. If a joint appears swollen, and the contiguous bony surfaces do not appear enlarged on palpation, then the swelling must be enlarged synovium, fluid, or both. If the swelling is purely synovium, as frequently occurs in rheumatoid arthritis, then this thickened membrane can be palpated as a distinct entity between finger and thumb. It has a boggy feeling. Synovitis itself seldom gives rise to maximum joint distension. The presence of intra-articular fluid is demonstrated by fluctuation, a fluid impulse transmitted in two planes at right angles. Fluid in the knee joint can be demonstrated by the presence of a patellar tap. The suprapatellar pouch is emptied by manual pressure and the patella is depressed through the main joint fluid, strikes the patellar surface of the femur, and imparts a tap to the palpating digits (Fig. 1.10). Such physical signs are only

attainable in superficial or peripheral joints. The hip joint is a notable exception; its deep-seated anatomical position, surrounded by powerful and bulky muscles, renders palpation extremely unrewarding.

The examination of a painful joint is critical in localising the pathology. The patient having pointed to the painful area, all local sources of tenderness must then be examined. The lesion giving rise to the painful swollen knee in a sports injury can be diagnosed with some degree of certainty by careful palpation. Meniscal tears give rise to local tenderness anteromedially or

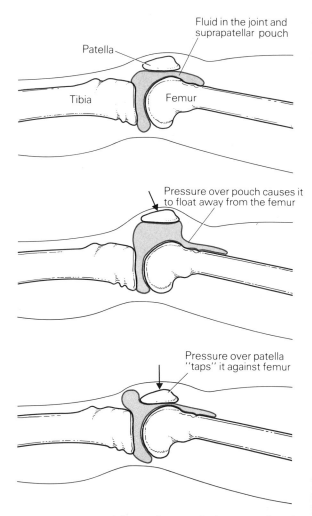

Fig. 1.10 *Diagram of the patellar tap which occurs when the undersurface of the patella strikes the patellar surface of the femur having been depressed through a knee joint containing fluid.*

anterolaterally directly over the joint line. The tenderness associated with a ligament injury of the knee is always above or below the joint line referable to the bony attachment of the collateral ligaments (Fig. 1.11). It is convenient, while palpating, to determine the vascular status of the extremity, particularly if a fracture is present or if major surgery is contemplated on the lower extremity of an elderly patient, in whom a high prevalence of peripheral vascular disease might be expected.

Range of Joint Motion

This should be determined both actively (what the patient can do himself) and passively (what the examiner can achieve). Thus a joint with paralysed muscles or disrupted tendon mechanisms will have little or no active movement but may have a full range of passive movement. The range of motion should wherever possible be measured in degrees from constant starting points. Flexion is thus measured from the position of maximum extension to the position of maximum flexion (Fig. 1.12) while movement in other planes, abduction and adduction, medial and lateral rotation, are measured in each direction from the neutral position. Because there is considerable natural variation from person to person, the joint on the other side should be used as a control wherever possible. In some joints, e.g. elbow and knee, particularly in females and the young, there may be a few degrees of hyperextension. This should be recorded as minus degrees beyond the straight position. Thus a normal

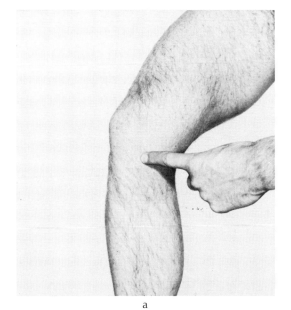

a

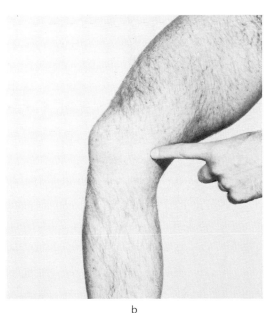

b

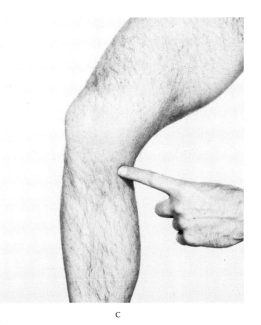

c

Fig. 1.11 *Site of tenderness in soft tissue injuries of the knee: There is tenderness over the joint line with cartilage injuries* (a); *but above* (b) *or below* (c) *with ligament injuries.*

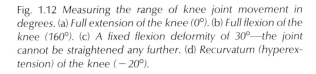

a

c

b

d

Fig. 1.12 *Measuring the range of knee joint movement in degrees. (a) Full extension of the knee (0°). (b) Full flexion of the knee (160°). (c) A fixed flexion deformity of 30°—the joint cannot be straightened any further. (d) Recurvatum (hyperextension) of the knee (− 20°).*

knee joint may have 10° of hyperextension, and flex to 140°, in which case the range of motion is recorded as − 10° to 140°. Sometimes a joint with a long-standing pathological process such as arthritis will not straighten fully, usually due to soft tissue contracture. This is referred to as a fixed flexion deformity. If, therefore, a knee joint will not come straight through the last 20° but flexes to 100°, the range of motion is expressed as flexion from 20° to 100°.

Estimation of the range of motion of joints at junctional areas requires special attention. Thus, in determining the range of hip joint motion, the pelvis must be palpated to ensure that true hip joint movement is being measured. Abduction of the shoulder joint is also a complex movement, involving both the true glenohumeral joint and scapular rotation. The scapula must therefore be observed in order to determine its contribution to movement (Fig. 1.13).

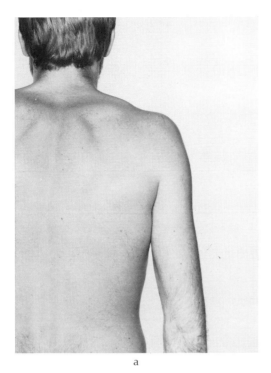

a

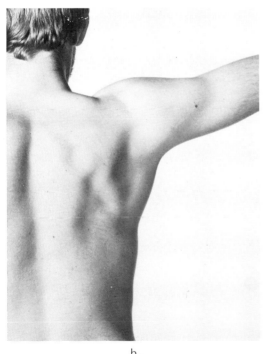

b

Fig. 1.13 (a) *The back of the shoulder with the arm by the side.*
(b) *The back of the shoulder with the arm abducted,*
demonstrating associated scapular rotation.

Indeed, a shoulder joint that is completely stiff may seem to abduct by 90° solely due to scapular rotation.

Determination of range of motion can also be useful diagnostically; there is a general reduction in all planes with arthritis, but a specific reduction in certain movements with mechanical problems. The joint may also impart to the palpating hand a grating sensation, crepitus, or a 'click' or 'clunk' when it is put through its available range. A coarse crepitus typifies a degenerative arthritic condition, while a finer crepitus is more suggestive of an inflammatory lesion. A click or clunk may suggest either an internal mechanical derangement or loss of stability.

In some circumstances it is too pedantic to record movement in degrees, particularly when examining a complex of joints such as the lumbar spine. It is therefore admissible to record the range of movement of the spine in fractions of the 'normal range' (Fig. 1.14). With some pathologies, however, such as ankylosing spondylitis, where movement, treatment and progress have to be titrated, flexion of the spine can be measured as the distance from fingertip to ground, although this is equally influenced by hip movement.

Other Measurements

Measurement is an important part of the examination of the musculoskeletal system. Measurements of leg length, muscle girth, and joint circumference are particularly useful.

Trauma, infection, arthritis and poliomyelitis may cause leg shortening; an increase in leg length may also occur with a local vascular malformation, in hemihypertrophy (where one side of the body is uniformly bigger than the other), and with generalised disorders such as Recklinghausen's disease. Treatment depends upon the extent and anatomical location of the shortening. The first stage in measurement of leg length is to set the pelvis square and to position the legs comparably so that any difference in length observed will be 'real' rather than 'apparent' (Fig. 1.15). If the pelvis is horizontal, but one hip is abducted while the other adducted, then the adducted side will appear shorter. This is exactly the same phenomenon as occurs when the pelvis cannot be put square due to a fixed pelvic obliquity, which therefore is in turn the cause of an apparent leg length inequality.

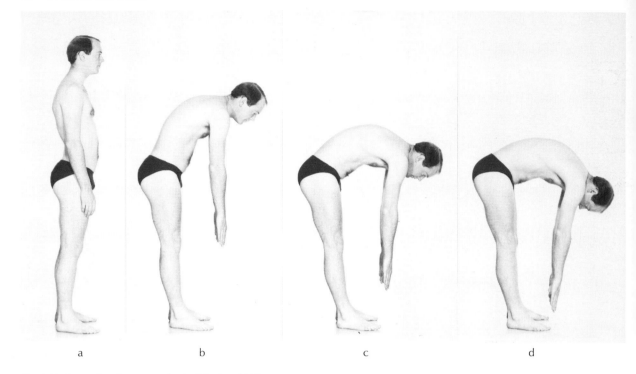

Fig. 1.14 *Recording the range of spinal flexion. (a) The erect or neutral position. (b) Half normal flexion. (c) Three-quarters normal flexion. (d) Full flexion.*

It is frequently said that a fixed pelvic obliquity is not uncommon, and that it is usually caused by a fixed adduction contracture of one hip. Neither of these statements is true, and both are derived from an ignorance of the mechanisms producing pelvic obliquity. There are three types of pelvic obliquity (Fig. 1.16): suprapelvic (a); transpelvic (b); and infrapelvic (c). Suprapelvic pelvic obliquity is caused by a fixed lumbar scoliosis, nearly always in association with a paralytic condition such as spina bifida or cerebral palsy. Transpelvic pelvic obliquity is even less common and is due to unilateral overaction or contracture of the iliopsoas, which is the only muscle to pass across the pelvis from lumbar spine to femur. Again this is usually due to a neuromuscular condition. Infrapelvic pelvic obliquity is most commonly due to a leg-length inequality, or an adduction contracture of one hip commonly caused as a result of arthritis.

Leg length measurements are made with the patient supine, however, and the pelvic obliquity observed when the patient stands or sits can nearly always be readily corrected in the supine position. Indeed, this can always be achieved with infrapelvic pelvic obliquity; a 'fixed' tilted pelvis is only found with marked iliopsoas spasm or contracture, or if a paralytic lumbar scoliosis has been present for many years. If one hip is in a fixed adducted position it has nothing whatever to do with pelvic obliquity and real leg length measurements can readily be made if the other hip is adducted similarly.

With the pelvis set square and the lower extremities in comparable positions, overall lower limb measurements are made from the anterior superior iliac spine to the medial malleolus. If a difference is observed, its anatomical location can be found by measurement from the highest point of the iliac crest to the greater trochanter (shortening across the hip joint), from the greater trochanter to lateral knee joint line (femoral shortening), and from the medial knee joint line to the medial malleolus (tibial shortening). Such measurements are inevitably inaccurate and, once a leg-length inequality has been diagnosed, the exact amount of the discrepancy is best measured on radiographs of the lower limbs calibrated with a grid. On the rare occasions when the pelvis cannot be squared, an overall measurement from xiphisternum to each medial malleolus indicates the amount of apparent discrepancy.

Measurement of muscle girth may be important as an objective neurological measure, and as an index of the severity of a joint problem and its response to treatment. Thus quadriceps wasting is a feature of meniscal lesions, and its return to normality is an index of response to treatment. The quadriceps muscle should always be measured 10 cm above the upper pole of the patella so that the circumference does not include the suprapatellar pouch. Similarly, calf circumference should be measured at a fixed distance below the tibial tuberosity. The contralateral side is used as the control.

Measurement of joint circumference is also useful in assessing the severity of an arthritic process, a traumatic joint derangement, or a haemophilic bleed. Diminution of joint circumference, with eventual return to that of the normal contralateral side, indicates resolution.

Chest expansion is reduced by ankylosing spondylitis, and should always be measured if this diagnosis is being considered. Measurements are made with a tape-measure at the fourth intercostal space. The subject is unclothed to the waist and asked to put his hands behind his head. This obviates the contraction of the subscapularis muscle, which may give spurious results; in women it raises the breasts, facilitating the application of the tape. Measurements are taken in full expiration and inspiration. Male expansion exceeds female expansion and decreases with age after the fourth decade. Chronic obstructive airways disease and

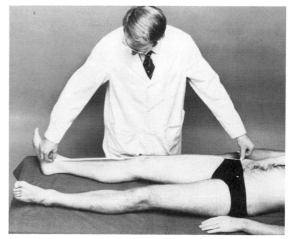

a

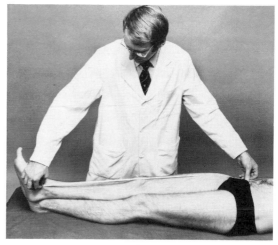

b

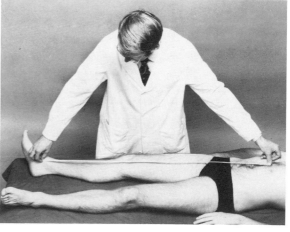

c

Fig. 1.15 *Measurement of leg length.* (a) *With the pelvis square and the legs in a neutral position, measurement is made from the anterior superior spine to the medial malleolus. Any discrepancy represents a true leg length inequality.* (b) *If there is an adduction contracture of one hip, then with the pelvis set square and the legs adducted equally across each other, measurement is again made from the anterior superior spine to the medial malleolus—any discrepancy is again true.* (c) *If there is a fixed pelvic obliquity and the legs cannot be positioned accordingly (a rare situation), measurement is made from the xiphisternum to the medial malleolus—any discrepancy is therefore apparent rather than true.*

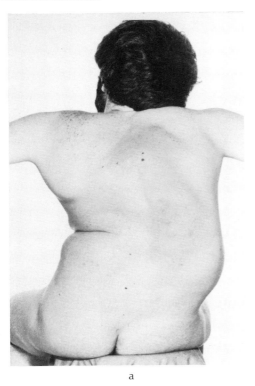

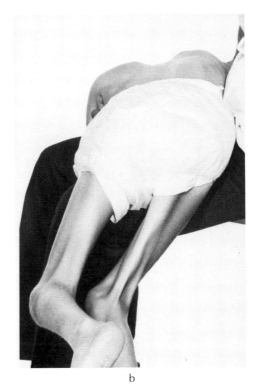

a

b

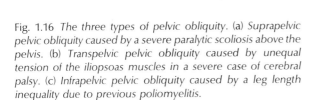

Fig. 1.16 *The three types of pelvic obliquity. (a) Suprapelvic pelvic obliquity caused by a severe paralytic scoliosis above the pelvis. (b) Transpelvic pelvic obliquity caused by unequal tension of the iliopsoas muscles in a severe case of cerebral palsy. (c) Infrapelvic pelvic obliquity caused by a leg length inequality due to previous poliomyelitis.*

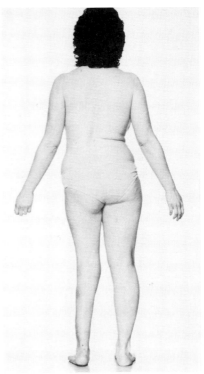

c

obesity will reduce chest expansion, as well as ankylosing spondylitis. In ankylosing spondylitis, however, compensatory diaphragmatic movement produces ballooning of the abdomen.

Stability

In certain situations, examination of the stability of a joint provides the essential information concerning the underlying pathological process. Thus instability of the hip joint of the neonate points to the presence of an underlying hip dislocation. The tests performed are those of Ortolani and Barlow (Fig. 1.17).

Ortolani's test is performed with the child lying supine with hips and knees flexed. The examiner's hands grasp the flexed knees so that the thumbs are medial and the middle finger lateral over the greater trochanter. The hips are now abducted fully and any evidence of instability is felt as a click or clunk. If instability is present, Barlow's test should then be performed.

The starting position for Barlow's test is the same as with Ortolani's test, but only the suspicious side is abducted, to only 45°. At this point pressure of the middle finger over the greater trochanter may cause a dislocated head of femur to slip back into the acetabulum. The sensation imparted to the palpating middle

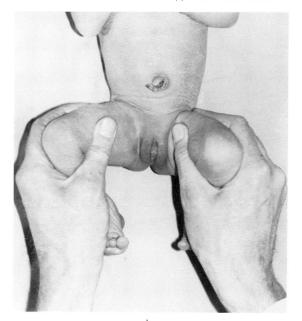

b

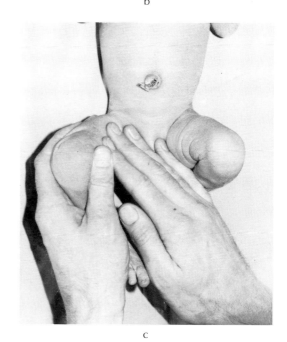

c

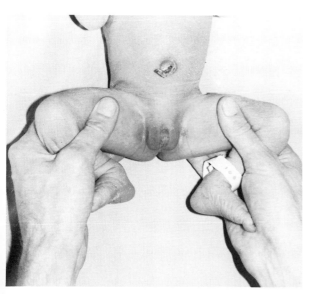

a

Fig. 1.17 (a) Ortolani's test—when the flexed hips are abducted a 'clunk' can be felt as the femoral head slips into the acetabulum. (b) Barlow's test (first stage) for the right hip—in mid abduction, pressure over the greater trochanter pushes the femoral head back into place. (c) Barlow's test (second stage)—superolateral pressure over the upper medial thigh pushes the femoral head out of place.

finger is frequently much more subtle than a click or clunk. This is the first stage of Barlow's test; if it is negative, it indicates that the hip is not dislocated. The second stage should then be performed. With the hip again in 45° of abduction, pressure is exerted by the other hand on the upper medial thigh downwards and outwards. If the hip can thereby be pushed out of joint and returned by pressure from the middle finger over the greater trochanter, then the hip is dislocatable but not dislocated. These tests are very important but they should not be performed within the first two days of birth. Over 90% of hips found to be unstable on the first day of life will spontaneously stabilise by the third day.

Ligamentous injuries of the knee are common in sportsmen, and here tests of ligamentous integrity (Fig. 1.18) are most important. Any abnormal movement in a valgus (lateral) or varus (medial) direction at the knee demonstrates collateral ligament disruption. The posterior capsular complex has a stabilising effect on the knee in full extension, so the test is more accurately performed with the knee in 30° of flexion, when the posterior capsule is relaxed.

With the knee flexed to 90°, and the hamstring musculature relaxed, any abnormal movement in an anterior or posterior direction indicates disruption of the anterior or posterior cruciate ligament respectively. With the tibia in internal or external rotation, the amount of cruciate laxity may change, indicating

associated rotary instability with disruption of a part of the capsule medially or laterally.

In severe arthritic processes, particularly those affecting the knee, there may be an obvious valgus or varus deformity, i.e. an angular deformity with the tibia angled away from the mid-line in valgus, and towards the mid-line in varus. This gives a false impression of laxity of the medial or lateral ligaments respectively.

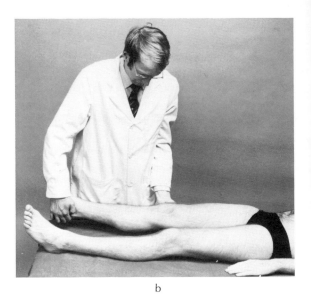

b

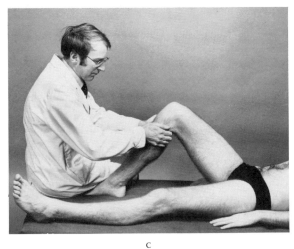

c

Fig. 1.18 *Knee ligament stability tests. (a) A valgus stress in 30° of flexion tests the medial ligament only. (b) A valgus stress in full extension also tests the posterior capsule which is tight in extension. (c) With the knee at 90° of flexion, pulling the tibia forwards or pushing it backwards tests the anterior or posterior cruciate ligament, respectively.*

a

The severity of the arthritic process has eroded bone from one side of the knee, thus giving the appearance of instability in that direction. Indeed the maintenance of integrity of the collateral ligaments, even in the presence of the severest arthritis, is one of the most important factors providing knee stability after artificial joint replacement.

Where mediolateral instability is suspected in other articulations, it can be determined in a similar way to that of the knee joint. In some anatomical areas, e.g. the ankle joint, instability may be difficult to assess because of movement in the same direction provided by a nearby joint, e.g. the subtalar joint. The presence and extent of instability are therefore best determined by the application of valgus and varus stresses under radiographic control. Tilting of the ankle mortice then becomes obvious (Fig. 1.19).

Examination Under Anaesthesia

Unless the patient is particularly cooperative and relaxed and pain is minimal, it is frequently desirable to perform the examination of a joint under general anaesthesia. Indeed, although McMurray's test for a tear of the posterior horn of the meniscus is commonly performed in the outpatient or casualty environment, it has limited value and, in fact, McMurray described this test as performed under general anaesthesia prior to performing arthrotomy and subsequent meniscectomy (Fig. 1.20). In addition, contrary to general belief, the test is only valid from full flexion of the knee to 90° of flexion, and is progressively less useful as a diagnostic test from 90° of flexion to the straight position.

The test is therefore performed with the patient anaesthetised, supine, and with a fully flexed knee. With the patient's heel in the examiner's hand, the examiner's forearm rotates the tibia by pressure on the patient's forefoot. The tibia can thereby be rotated medially or laterally in order to test the integrity of the lateral or medial meniscus respectively. As the rotational movement is taking place, the knee is extended to 90°. If a clunk is palpable to the other hand placed over the knee joint, the test is deemed positive and only indicates a posterior horn tear. By performing this test properly, McMurray was able to diagnose the true nature of meniscal lesions in over 90% of cases, which should be an example to those who neglect the proper

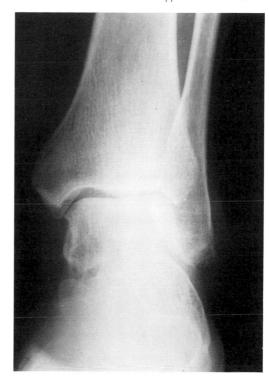

Fig. 1.19 *Anteroposterior x-ray of the ankle with a valgus stress applied, demonstrating mortice asymmetry and therefore instability.*

clinical examination in favour of arthrography or arthroscopy.

Neurological Examination

This is frequently an important part of the examination of the musculoskeletal system with particular reference to disorders of the axial skeleton, the central and peripheral nervous systems, and trauma. Motor examination is particularly important, as the majority of the information provided is truly objective. Power must be tested according to the Medical Research Council (MRC) principles and graded accordingly. Grade 5 is full power; 4 is power against gravity and some resistance; 3 is power against gravity only; 2 is power but not against gravity; 1 is just a flicker; and zero is no discernible power.

It is essential that the muscle under test is simultaneously palpated to avoid trick movements (Fig. 1.21).

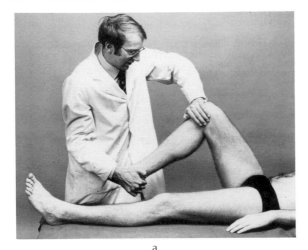

a

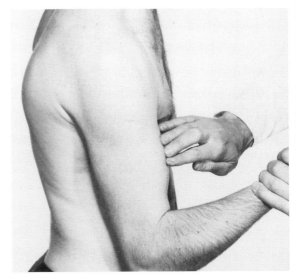

Fig. 1.21 *Testing the power of a muscle properly: Strength is graded by one hand while the muscle belly is palpated by the other.*

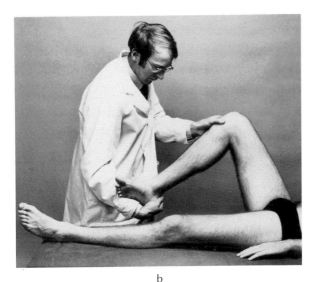

b

Fig. 1.20 *McMurray's test for a tear in the posterior part of the menisci. (a) Testing the integrity of the medial meniscus: In full flexion of the knee the tibia is externally rotated while the knee is straightened to 90° of flexion. If the watching hand detects a 'clunk', the posterior horn of the meniscus is torn. (b) Testing the lateral meniscus: The manoeuvre is reversed with the tibia internally rotated.*

Thus when the biceps is paralysed, elbow flexion is perfectly possible by use of the brachioradialis muscle. Even power is not wholly objective; patients with compensation in mind frequently exaggerate any weakness present. Accordingly, muscle circumference must also be measured since gross weakness is not compatible with normal muscle bulk.

The spinal root values of the major limb muscles must be memorised, and this exercise is facilitated by the fact that muscles with the same action have the same segmental levels, and more distal segmental levels supply more distal muscle groups (Fig. 1.22). Familiarity with this logical sequence can only be consolidated by repeated examination of patients, one's colleagues, or oneself. The segmental levels of the various reflexes are then easily appreciated as they are nothing more than the segmental level corresponding to the muscle whose reflex is being tested.

Sensory examination is also important, but it is much less objective. The dermatome patterns of the extremities with their axial lines should be learned (Fig. 1.23). Axial lines are defined as lines separating discontinuous dermatomes and, when testing sensation, it is important to test across the axial lines. In peripheral nerve lesions it is also important to map out the area of sensory loss according to MRC principles. With particular reference to the hand, determination of two-point discrimination is important in diagnosing peripheral nerve lesions and assessing the efficacy of treatment. Tactile recognition is another variable important in assessing nerve injuries involving the hand. Two-point discrimination and tactile recognition are both markedly impaired in median nerve lesions.

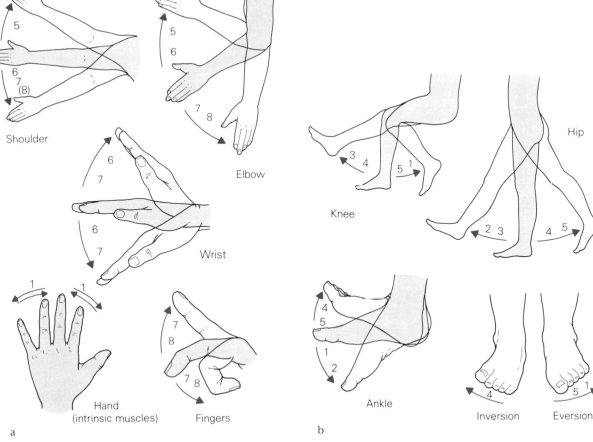

a

b

Fig. 1.22 *The segmental levels of joint movement in the extremities.* (a) *Upper limb.* (b) *Lower limb.* (After Last R.J., Anatomy: Regional and Applied, 4th edn, by courtesy of J. & A. Churchill Ltd, London.)

General Physical Examination

It is often necessary to perform a summary or detailed physical examination of the other systems. The thyroid, breast, abdomen, pelvis and rectum should always be examined when a tumour of the musculoskeletal system is suspected, since secondary bone neoplasms are more than 100 times commoner than primary ones.

Examination of the skin may reveal pallor due to anaemia, associated with diseases such as rheumatoid arthritis or with drugs used in its treatment. Palmar erythema occurs in rheumatoid arthritis, nail fold infarcts in connective tissue disorders, and nail changes in psoriasis. Subcutaneous nodules are pathognomonic of rheumatoid arthritis. Examination of other systems may reveal the clinical findings of the conditions discussed under review of the systems.

REGIONAL EXAMINATION

Cervical Spine

The cervical spine normally has a smooth lordosis; this is obliterated with paravertebral muscle spasm

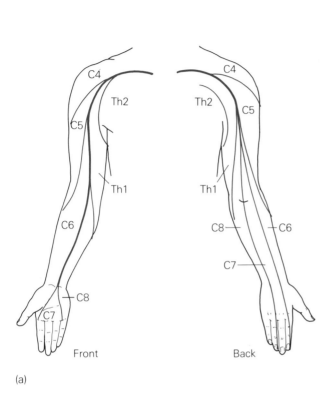

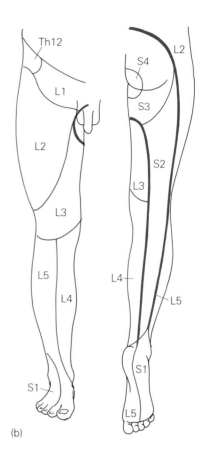

(a)

(b)

Fig. 1.23 *The dermatome patterns of the extremities.* (a) *Upper limb.* (b) *Lower limb.* (After Last R.J., Anatomy: Regional and Applied, 4th edn, by courtesy of J. & A. Churchill Ltd, London.)

secondary to local pain (Fig. 1.24). The spine should be straight when viewed from the front or back. Any lateral deviation (scoliosis) may indicate a structural curve or may be secondary to a tight sternomastoid on one side (torticollis).

Palpation of the posterior elements at each level may yield useful information. In the patient with a suspected cervical spine injury, a gap between successive spinous processes is often felt, which may be filled with haematoma, providing a boggy sensation. With marked displacement, the posterior elements may be felt or seen to be out of alignment. Marked local tenderness at one level is frequently found in osteoarthritis (cervical spondylosis).

The range of movements of the cervical spine (Fig. 1.25) are flexion and extension (mostly occurring at the atlanto-occipital joint), lateral flexion (occurring

throughout the cervical spine), and rotation (mostly occurring at the altanto-axial joint). Reduction of movement in a particular direction may therefore localise the lesion, particularly if it is accompanied by discomfort or crepitus. Pain can be referred to the cervical spine from the ears, nose, throat and shoulders, and these areas should therefore be examined if the cervical spine appears normal.

Thoracolumbar Spine

When viewed from the side, the thoracic spine has a gentle kyphosis and the lumbar spine a gentle lordosis. An increase in the normal thoracic kyphosis is associated with poor posture or, less commonly, Scheuermann's disease (adolescent kyphosis), in which the

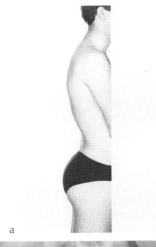

a

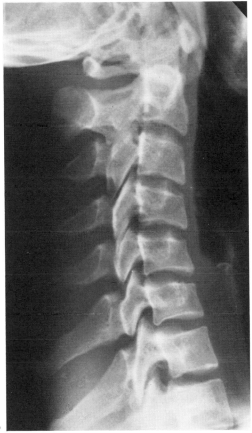

b

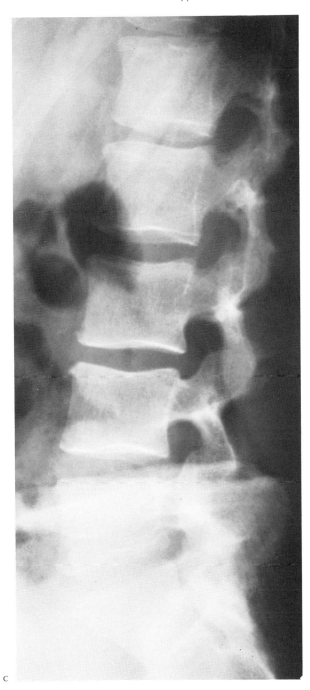

c

Fig. 1.24 (a) *Side view of the body showing the four primary spinal curves—cervical and lumbar lordoses, and thoracic and sacral kyphoses. (b) Lateral x-ray of the cervical spine showing reversal of the normal lordosis due to muscle spasm. (c) Lateral x-ray of the lumbar spine showing a flattened lordosis, again due to muscle spasm.*

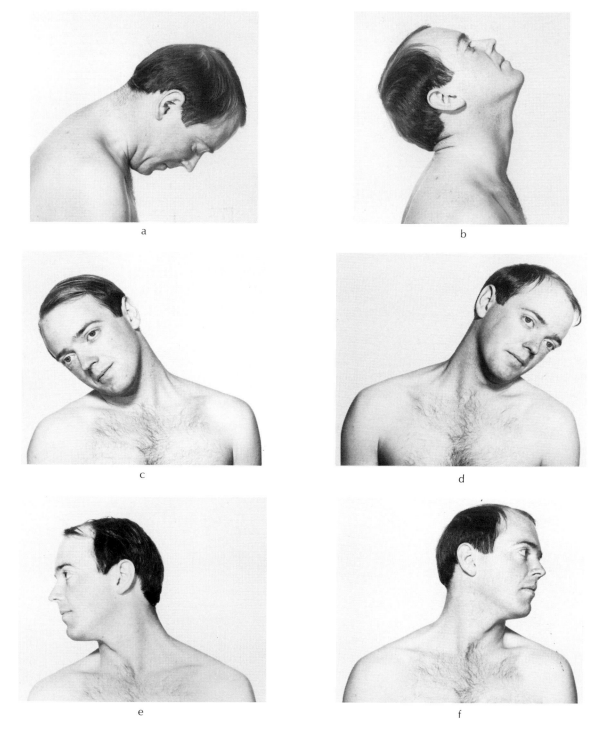

Fig. 1.25 *Range of motion of the cervical spine. (a) Flexion and
(b) extension; lateral flexion right (c) and left (d); rotation right (e)
and left (f).*

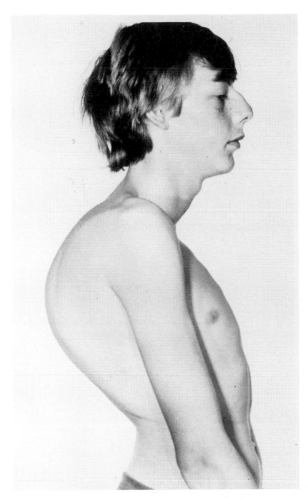

Fig. 1.26 *The increased thoracic kyphosis of Scheuermann's disease.*

deformity is more angular and rigid (Fig. 1.26). When viewed from the back, the spine must be straight. Shoulder asymmetry or a flank recession indicates a scoliosis, which can be confirmed on forward flexion with the appearance of a rotational prominence on the convex side (Fig. 1.27). Inspection of the thoracolumbar spine may indicate the presence of an underlying congenital abnormality. The presence of spina bifida cystica or scarring from previous sac closure are usually associated with paralytic deformities of the lower extremity, but 10% of the so-called normal population have a spina bifida occulta. This is usually at the L5 or S1 level and may be inferred from the presence of a dermal naevus, a patch of hair, lipoma, dimple, sinus or fistula.

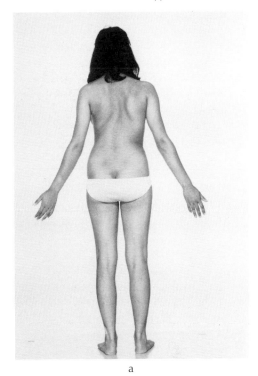

a

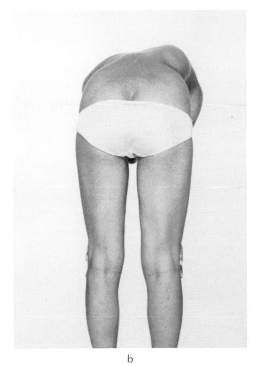

b

Fig. 1.27 *Idiopathic scoliosis.* (a) *Standing erect.* (b) *Leaning forward the rotational prominence becomes obvious.*

Tenderness on palpation or percussion of one segment suggests local degenerative or inflammatory disease. The presence of a step on palpation, usually at the lower lumbar or lumbosacral level, indicates loss of vertebral alignment (spondylolisthesis). The sacro-iliac joint should be palpated and the pelvis stressed in order to localise disease to this articulation.

The movements of the thoracolumbar spine (Fig. 1.14) are flexion, extension, lateral flexion, and rotation. These may be recorded in fractions or percentages of normal. In patients with low back pain, it is important to observe whether the lumbar spine really moves when the patient flexes forwards. With significant paravertebral muscle spasm, the lumbar spine may remain stiff but flexion can occur at the hip joints below and the cervical spine above.

For rotation to be accurately quantified, the pelvis must be held square so that true spinal rotation can be seen. It is important to determine if possible what has caused the particular movement to be limited, whether pain or hamstring tightness. To measure thoracolumbar flexion more accurately, a line is drawn on the skin between the dimples of Venus, thus identifying the lumbosacral junction, and then continued 10 cm up and 5 cm down. The distraction of these skin marks on flexion correlates closely with true angular flexion of the spine. Lateral flexion can be estimated by the approximation of one mark over the iliac crest and another level with the xiphisternum in the coronal plane.

With low back pain and a radicular pain in the lower extremity, the patient should be examined supine, without a pillow under the neck, and each straight leg raised passively (Fig. 1.28). An angle of 90° is normal, but a significant reduction is a constant finding in the presence of lower lumbar nerve root irritation, commonly from an underlying disc protrusion. The limit of straight-leg raising should be recorded in degrees. When straight-leg raising is limited by radicular discomfort (a positive Lasègues's test), and then the leg is lowered slightly so that nerve root tension is diminished, the radicular pain recurs if the ankle is dorsiflexed (a positive 'sciatic stretch test').

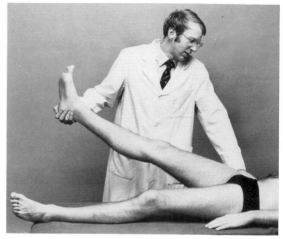

a

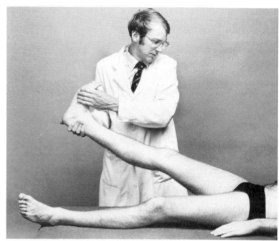

b

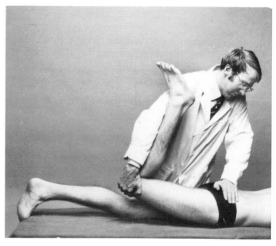

c

Fig. 1.28 *Testing for radicular pressure. (a) The straight leg raising test: This is limited on the right to 40°. (b) The sciatic stretch test: Ankle dorsiflexion causes a radicular pain down the leg. (c) The femoral stretch test: Hip extension and knee flexion cause a radicular pain down the front of the thigh.*

If one of the roots of the femoral nerve is suspected, then the 'femoral stretch test' should be performed with the patient lying prone and the hip extended with the knee fully flexed. Pain is then felt down the anterior thigh to the knee. The sacro-iliac joints are best tested by the 'pump-handle manoeuvre' when the flexed knee of the supine patient is pushed towards the opposite shoulder. Alternatively, a manoeuvre similar to the femoral nerve stretch test, but with the knee straight, stresses the sacro-iliac joint. If a radicular pathology is suspected, a complete neurological examination of the lower extremity is essential.

Shoulder Joint

Derangement of the shoulder joint or its nearby articulations is easily visible. There is a flatness of the deltoid and a bulge antero-inferiorly in an anterior shoulder dislocation; in an acromioclavicular dislocation, the acromion is prominent and the remainder of the upper extremity appears to have sagged.

Each joint in the body takes up a characteristic position of rest when irritable. For the shoulder this is the position of adduction with the elbow flexed. The anterior, posterior and lateral margins of the shoulder joint should be palpated carefully to localise tenderness. Thus the painful arc syndrome and bicipital tendonitis are associated with tenderness localised to the subacromial region and bicipital groove respectively. Flexion and extension, abduction and adduction, internal and external rotation are recorded in degrees (Fig. 1.29). Measurement of rotation is facilitated by flexing the elbow and using the forearm as a pointer. The patient should be viewed from the back while movement is being tested so that both glenohumeral and scapular movement can be seen.

In estimating the power of shoulder movement, it is useful to consider the shoulder muscles as two groups. The scapular muscles give rise to scapular elevation, retraction, protraction and abduction, while the shoulder joint muscles give rise to glenohumeral abduction, adduction, flexion, extension and rotation. Shoulder pain can also be referred from the diaphragm or heart, and if the shoulder appears normal these should be included in the physical examination.

Elbow Joint

It is useful to include the superior radio-ulnar joint in the examination of the elbow. The elbow takes up a position of flexion and pronation when irritable. When the supinated extended elbow is inspected, any medio-lateral angulation (cubitus varus or valgus) can be readily seen. Palpation is useful in localising tenderness to the medial or lateral epicondyles (golfer's or tennis elbow respectively). The ulnar nerve should also be palpated as it passes behind the medial epicondyle. Flexion and extension of the elbow joint are recorded in degrees, as are supination and pronation of the forearm with the elbow flexed by the side of the body (Fig. 1.30).

Wrist and Hand

The painful wrist is held in a position of slight flexion while the painful hand adopts the 'position of rest', in which there is increasing digital flexion from index to little finger. Certain attitudes of the hand are diagnostic (Fig. 1.31). Thus intrinsic muscle wasting in association with the clawing that is more marked on the ulnar side is typical of an ulnar nerve lesion. Wasting of the abductor pollicis brevis indicates a carpal tunnel syndrome. Severe clawing of all fingers indicates a combined median and ulnar nerve lesion.

Tenderness localised to the radial styloid, in association with swelling and crepitus, is diagnostic of de Quervain's tendovaginitis (entrapment of the tendons of abductor pollicis longus and extensor pollicis brevis). Tenderness localised to the mouth of the fibrous flexor sheath with nodule formation suggests a trigger finger (digital stenosing tendovaginitis). The presence of a fibrous band in the palm running longitudinally in association with a flexed digit suggests Dupuytren's contracture. Metacarpophalangeal joint swelling, with ulnar deviation of the fingers, is typical of rheumatoid disease. The first carpometacarpal joint commonly displays bony swelling in generalised osteoarthritis.

Movements of the wrist are flexion, extension, and radial and ulnar deviation, while the lower radio-ulnar joint provides a contribution to forearm supination and pronation (Fig. 1.32). The interphalangeal joints are hinge articulations only allowing flexion and extension. The metacarpophalangeal joints of the fingers, however, allow a few degrees of abduction and adduction.

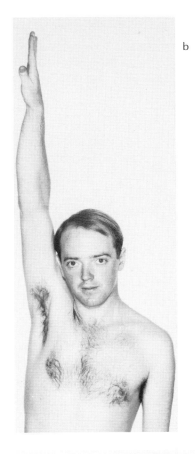

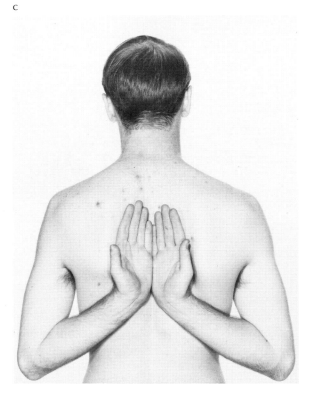

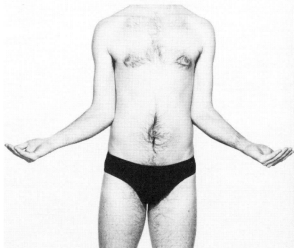

Fig. 1.29 *Range of motion of the shoulder joint.* (a) *Full flexion.* (b) *Full abduction.* (c) *Internal and* (d) *external rotation.*

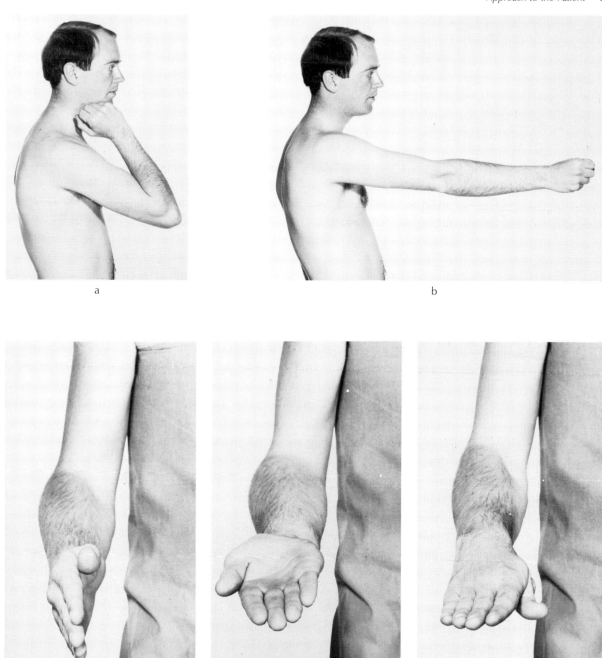

Fig. 1.30 *Range of motion of the elbow joint.* (a) *Flexion.* (b) *Extension.* (c) *Rotation, neutral.* (d) *Rotation, supination.* (e) *Rotation, pronation.*

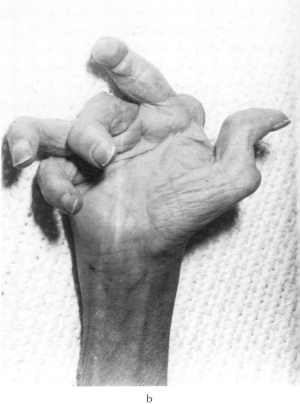

a

b

c

Fig. 1.31 *Characteristic attitudes of the hand.* (a) *The intrinsic muscle wasting of an ulnar nerve palsy.* (b) *The joint contracture and ulnar deviation of rheumatoid disease.* (c) *The swan-neck deformities of intrinsic muscle spasm.*

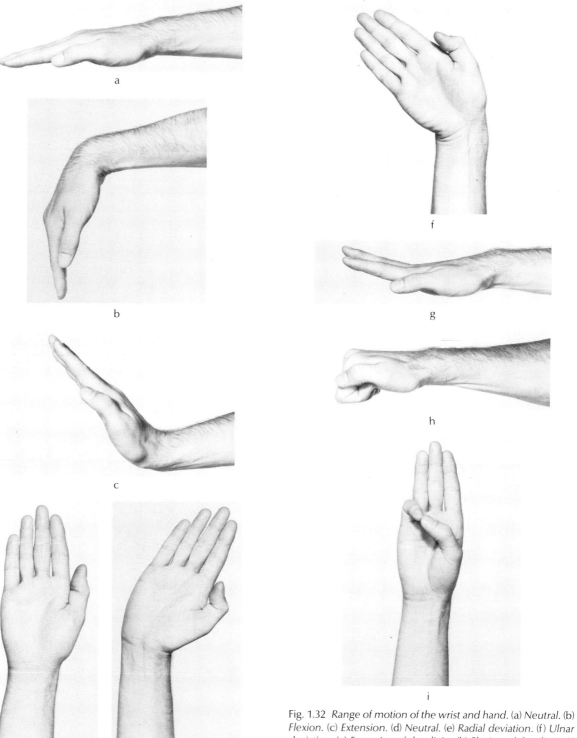

Fig. 1.32 *Range of motion of the wrist and hand.* (a) *Neutral.* (b) *Flexion.* (c) *Extension.* (d) *Neutral.* (e) *Radial deviation.* (f) *Ulnar deviation.* (g) *Extension of the digits.* (h) *Flexion of the digits.* (i) *Opposition of the thumb.*

The carpometacarpal joint of the thumb, a doubly-concave saddle joint, allows flexion, extension, abduction, adduction and rotation, thus facilitating the manoeuvre of opposition. Opposition is measured as the distance of the thumb pulp from the pulp of the little finger. All other movements are measured in degrees.

Hip Joint

The hip joint is a deep-seated joint surrounded by bulky muscles; inspection and palpation are frequently unrewarding, but they may be useful in highlighting an associated condition, such as hernia or lymph node enlargement. Local abscess or sinus formation may indicate a spinal infection that has tracked down the iliopsoas muscle. The presence of a scar may indicate a previous surgical procedure for a childhood hip problem.

The movements available at the hip joint are flexion, extension, abduction, adduction, and internal and external rotation, and all should be measured in degrees (Fig. 1.33). With the patient supine, a fixed flexion deformity can easily be masked by an increase in the lumbar lordosis. Thus it would appear that the affected lower extremity is lying in contact with the examination couch but on close inspection the back is seen to be abnormally arched. In order to unmask a fixed flexion deformity of the hip, Thomas's test is performed. The contralateral hip is flexed until the lumbar spine becomes flattened. A fixed flexion deformity of the hip then becomes apparent as the thigh is lifted from the examination couch.

When measuring movement at the hip in other planes, a hand should be placed on the contralateral anterior superior iliac spine in order to exclude pelvic movement. Hip rotation is best judged using the position of the patella as the reference point. In the neutral position the patella points vertically upwards from the examination couch. With hip arthritis it is common to find the patella externally rotated by about 20°. On attempted internal rotation from this position the pelvis rises on the same side. The hip therefore has a fixed external rotation deformity of 20°. From this position it may be possible to rotate the hip externally by a further 20° and the range of rotation would then be expressed as follows: internal rotation nil, external rotation from 20° to 40°. Leg lengths should then be measured with the patient still supine.

When hip joint pathology is suspected it may be useful to perform Trendelenburg's test (Fig. 1.34). This reveals weakness of hip abduction and was much in vogue when poliomyelitis was prevalent, which gave rise to gluteal paralysis. The patient is asked to stand on the affected leg when, under normal circumstances, the pelvis will rise on the opposite side due to the abductors of the hip elevating the contralateral pelvis. When the gluteal muscles are sufficiently weak, the contralateral pelvis cannot be raised and therefore sags, making the test positive. When the gluteal muscles are normal but their mechanical advantage is sufficiently reduced by shortening across the hip, as in congenital dislocation, then the test again appears positive and is responsible for the waddling gait observed in bilateral untreated cases. The test must, however, be interpreted with caution. A patient with a fixed adducted hip from severe arthritis will appear to have a positive Trendelenburg's sign, but it is in fact the fixed adducted position of the hip which mechanically prevents the contralateral pelvis from rising.

The gait pattern of the patient should now be assessed. An antalgic gait (spending less time on the affected leg) is a feature of discomfort anywhere in that lower extremity, but a stiff hip gait or moment-relieving gait points to hip discomfort. In the former, no flexion occurs at the hip in the swing phase of gait, and movement of the lower extremity forwards is achieved by pelvic rotation. The moment-relieving gait is characterised by the trunk dipping over the affected hip, which has the effect of reducing the lever arm of the femoral neck by placing the centre of gravity of the body as directly as possible over the hip joint itself.

Knee Joint

The irritable knee lies semi-flexed. As the knee is a superficial joint, inspection is frequently rewarding. Swelling confined to the knee joint is characterized by a fullness not spreading higher than four fingers' breadth above the patella (the limits of the suprapatellar synovial pouch) and a fullness on either side of the patella. A posterior fullness suggests a popliteal cyst. In patients with rheumatoid arthritis this may extend into the calf. With a painful lesion of the knee, wasting of the

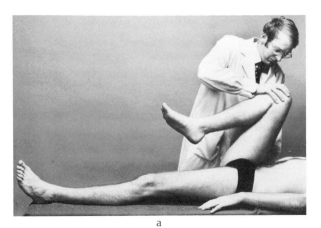

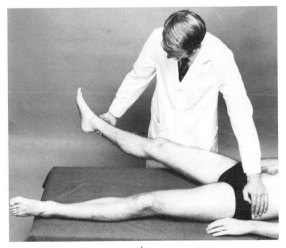

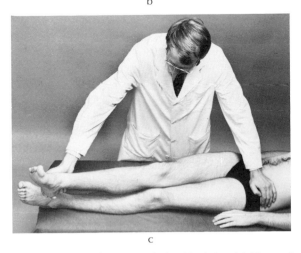

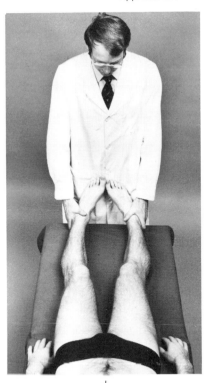

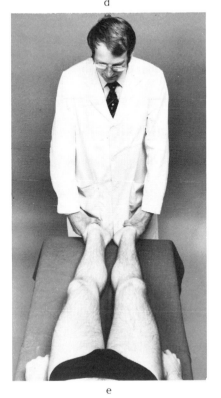

Fig. 1.33 *Range of motion of the hip joint.* (a) *Thomas's test—the other hip is flexed fully to unmask a flexion deformity. Then the hip under test is flexed similarly.* (b) *Abduction and* (c) *adduction.* (d) *Internal and* (e) *external rotation.*

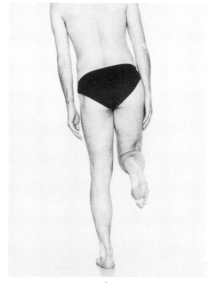

a

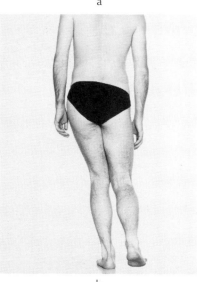

b

Fig. 1.34 *Trendelenberg's test.* (a) *When standing on one leg the contralateral pelvis should rise.* (b) *The pelvis has sagged: Trendelenberg's test is positive.*

quadriceps can be both seen and measured. Tenderness must be accurately localised to the joint line (for a meniscal injury) or to the site of attachment of collateral ligaments (in a ligament tear).

The knee joint flexes and extends in one plane only. This should be recorded (Fig. 1.12) in degrees, and the presence of crepitus in either the main joint or the patellofemoral joint is determined through the range. In the acutely injured knee, the integrity of the collateral and cruciate ligaments should be tested (Fig. 1.18) and the integrity of the menisci (Fig. 1.20) should also be assessed. The snap-extension test and forced flexion tests are most useful in addition to McMurray's test. When a flexed knee is rapidly extended passively, it snaps straight when the posterior capsule suddenly tightens. With a meniscal injury, the patient does not permit full extension, so that when the last few degrees of extension are reached the knee suddenly flexes. When the knee with a cartilage injury is forcibly flexed to the limit, any further attempted flexion causes discomfort localised to the joint line.

Ankle and Foot

The irritable ankle and foot lie flexed and inverted respectively. The presence of a foot deformity should always be assessed with the patient standing, when the deformity tends to become more pronounced. Thus hallux valgus, claw or hammer toes, and flattened or increased arches are more obvious. Most foot deformities are due to wearing shoes of the wrong size or shape. The cavus foot (with an increased longitudinal arch) is prone to flattening or reversal of the horizontal arch; the metatarsal heads are prominent and the toes frequently clawed, with calluses over the dorsum of the interphalangeal joints. These are frequently tender to palpation.

Tender metatarsophalangeal joints are a common feature of rheumatoid arthritis, and indeed may be the presenting sign. Later they become subluxated with overlying callosities and toe deformities that may rub against the shoe and ulcerate. The synovial sheaths of the extensor, flexor and peroneal tendons may also be painful, swollen and tender as a result of mechanical synovitis or rheumatoid disease. Tenderness of the heel or of the plantar fascia should be determined, together with thickening of the tendo Achillis. The ligaments supporting the ankle are frequently sprained, giving rise to local swelling and contusion, most often laterally, where there is also tenderness on palpation.

The ankle joint is a hinge joint allowing only dorsiflexion and plantarflexion (Fig. 1.35). Inversion and eversion take place at the subtalar and midtarsal articulations, each contributing 20° of movement in

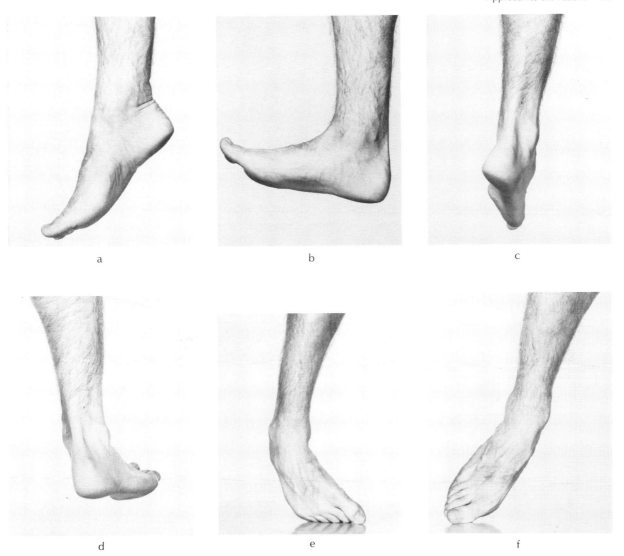

Fig. 1.35 *Range of motion of the ankle and foot.* (a) *Ankle plantar flexion and* (b) *dorsiflexion.* (c) *Subtalar inversion and* (d) *eversion.* (e) *Mid-tarsal inversion and* (f) *eversion.*

each direction. When evaluating movement in the ankle, subtalar and midtarsal joints, these should be examined separately and their movement accurately documented. In determining ankle movement, the mid-foot is grasped and flexed and extended fully, and the movement compared with the contralateral side. To determine movement of the subtalar joint, the heel is grasped with one hand while the lower tibia is held with the other. The heel is then moved inwards and outwards. To assess midtarsal movement, the heel is grasped in one hand and the mid-foot with the other, which is then twisted inwards and outwards.

Ankle joint movement is characteristically reduced in arthritis or after ankle fracture. Subtalar movement is characteristically reduced after a fracture of the os calcis, most usually as a result of a fall from a height. Midtarsal movement is also reduced by arthritis and trauma.

RADIOLOGICAL EXAMINATION

The interpretation of x-rays becomes straightforward with practice, provided a routine is followed. To determine the nature of a pathology radiologically, two views at right angles are required. In describing an x-ray appearance, the direction of the projection and the anatomical part are therefore first identified, together with the name of the patient and the date of the x-ray which should appear on all films. It is frequently taught that the order of assessment should be as follows: bone density; the cortex; the medulla; joints; and then soft tissues. This is quite illogical. Radiographic measurement of bone density is extremely difficult. The apparent radiodensity of bone depends upon exposure, direction of the beam (the heel effect), the variability of domestic voltage, the bulk of the soft tissues, the age and sex of the patient, and a host of other factors. Bones either look dense or they do not, and nothing more can be said.

If there is a radiographically detectable abnormality, then it is usually obvious even to the uninitiated, whose only difficulty is putting it into words. It is usually crying out for description (Fig. 1.36). After this has been completed, then cortex, medulla, soft tissues and bone density can be briefly noted. This is the only logical way of interpreting radiographs and is analogous to the approach of a general surgeon performing a laparotomy for an abdominal mass. He does not palpate the liver for metastases, the mesentery for nodes, or explore the rest of the abdominal cavity until he has identified the site of the mass, its pathology and characteristics.

Fracture

A fracture is a discontinuity in a bone and appears radiographically as a line of lucency (Fig. 1.37). The projection, the bone, and the side of the body should first be identified. Then the site of the fracture should be named, e.g. in the shaft at the junction of the upper two-thirds and lower one-third. If there are more than two fragments the fracture is said to be 'comminuted'. The direction of the fracture is then stated: transverse, oblique, or spiral. If it passes through an important structure, e.g. epiphyseal line or articular surface, this is

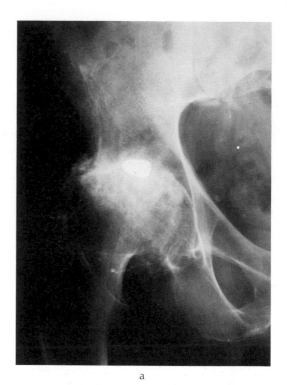

a

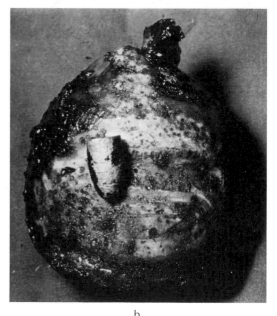

b

Fig. 1.36 (a) *Anteroposterior view of the right hip showing a bullet in the hip joint with secondary osteoarthritis: The patient complained of a 'shooting pain' in the hip. (b) At operation the femoral head had been grooved by the bullet. (Courtesy of the late Professor D. J. Fuller, MS, FRCS.)*

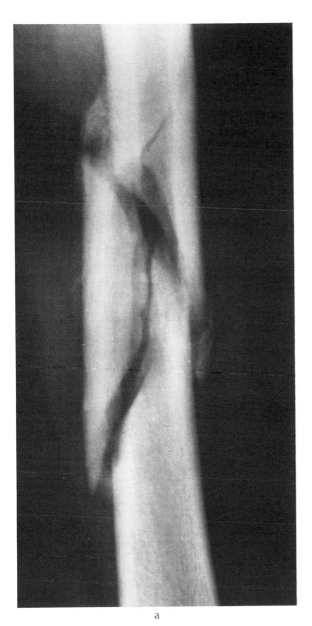
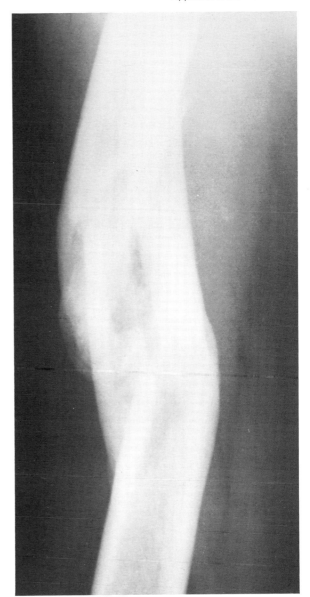

a   b

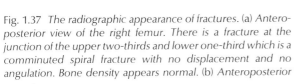

Fig. 1.37 *The radiographic appearance of fractures. (a) Antero-posterior view of the right femur. There is a fracture at the junction of the upper two-thirds and lower one-third which is a comminuted spiral fracture with no displacement and no angulation. Bone density appears normal. (b) Anteroposterior view of the same femur six months later. There is abundant callus formation and trabeculae cross the fracture lines, indicating that union has occurred. The alignment of the proximal and distal main fragments is excellent, but the fracture has united with significant medial displacement.*

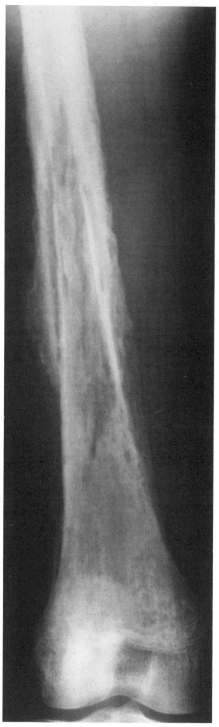

then stated. The position of the two major fragments is then determined, and displacement (minimal, moderate, or complete) is described with reference to the distal fragment. Angulation is described in degrees, again with relation to the distal fragment. Where possible the rotational alignment of the fragments is also described. Only then is a statement made concerning the overall density of the fractured bone. A generalised reduction in density is commonly found in the elderly female when the fracture is pathological due to osteoporosis. Sometimes pathological fractures also occur in bones that appear more dense, as in Paget's disease.

As the fracture proceeds through union to consolidation, it may show up more clearly in the early part of the process when bone is resorbed around the fracture site. Thereafter, periosteal new bone formation produces a local fusiform radio-opacity (callus) which bridges the fracture and gradually obscures its visibility. Union is said to occur when trabeculae are seen to cross the fracture site, and consolidation has occurred when the bone has remodelled to its fullest capacity.

Fig. 1.38 *The radiographic appearance of local bone lesions. (a) Anteroposterior view of the lower femur. There are widespread irregular lucencies in the diaphysis, and the periosteum has produced significant surrounding new bone formation (the involucrum). These are the appearances of chronic osteomyelitis. (b) Anteroposterior view of the pelvis. There is a large irregular area of lucency in the left iliac wing. There is significant cortical loss and no evidence of repair. The appearances are those of a malignant tumour, subsequently, shown to be a fibrosarcoma.*

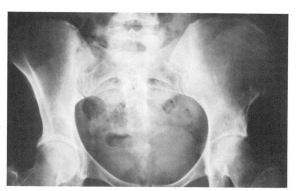

a   b

This may be so complete in children that no radiological evidence is seen of previous fracture, but the ability to remodel fully is seriously curtailed with age.

When there is no radiographic evidence of union by the expected time, delayed union is said to exist. When the fracture line persists, with attenuation of the bony margins which also appear more radio-dense, non-union has occurred. A fracture can thus be simply described, together with its characteristics and natural history. Description may be important, particularly medicolegally or in relation to the diagnosis of child abuse, where a radiological skeletal survey to investigate a new fracture may show up evidence of previous trauma.

Local Bone Lesions

The projection, bone side, and site of the lesion in the bone are first identified. In a local bone lesion there is either too much bone, too little bone, or sometimes both (Fig. 1.38). The shape of the bone may also be altered locally. If there is too little bone (a local area of lucency), then bone has been destroyed. The only two pathological processes which destroy bone are a tumour or tumour-like condition (e.g. cyst or fibrous dysplasia), and infection. Both pathological processes may stimulate periosteal new-bone formation, initially seen as a thin periosteal line parallel to the cortex. Cortical destruction with extra-osseous spread is not a feature of infection; it is diagnostic of malignancy. The radiological appearance, the bone which is involved, and the anatomical site of the lesion in the bone, together with the age of the patient, help in diagnosis.

A local area of sclerosis (new bone formation) may be

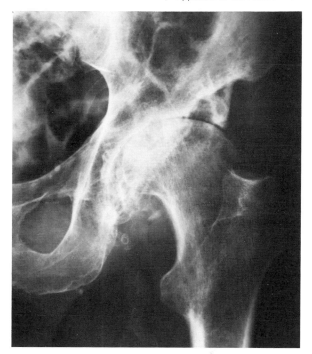

a

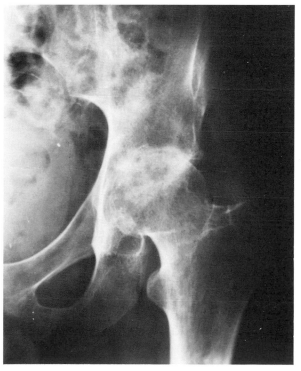

b

Fig. 1.39 *The radiographic appearance of joint lesions. (a) Anteroposterior view of the left hip joint. The joint space is narrowed, particularly in the weightbearing area. The femoral head has lost its sphericity and there is new bone formation inferomedially (an osteophyte). The subchondral bone is sclerotic and there is subchondral cyst formation superiorly. The appearances are those of degenerative osteoarthritis. (b) Anteroposterior view of the left hip joint. There is concentric loss of joint space. There is no evidence of new bone formation and there is mild juxta-articular osteoporosis. The appearances are those of rheumatoid disease.*

an osteogenic metastasis from one of the tumours known to have this potential (e.g. prostate, breast). A larger area of increased density localised to one bone, frequently the pelvis or upper femur, with cortical and trabecular thickening, is typical of Paget's disease of bone.

Joint Lesions

The projection, the joint, and the side of the body should first be stated. Most joint diseases involve the articular cartilage and so the joint space appears narrowed (Fig. 1.39). If active inflammatory disease is present, then the subchondral bone on each side may appear less dense due to a combination of increased vascularity and relative disuse. In rheumatoid disease, the joint margins are eroded by diseased synovium. With degenerative joint disease the stresses normally absorbed by the articular cartilage are passed on to the more labile underlying subchondral bone, which thickens and appears more sclerotic, particularly in weight-bearing areas. The subchondral bone also appears cystic, and the margins of the joint develop osteophytes – marginal spurs of new bone formation surrounding a nidus of effete cartilage cells.

The hip is a common site for an arthritic condition. The standard anteroposterior view also includes most of the pelvis and the hip joint of the other side, which is useful for comparative purposes. Indeed, whenever there is doubt about the radiographic appearance on one side, then a control film of the other side should be taken. Injured joints in children, particularly the elbow, may be difficult to interpret radiographically when only a relatively small portion has ossified and thus become radio-opaque. It is useful to measure a lower extremity deformity on a standing film, since weight-bearing renders the deformity more obvious. The quality of such a film is, however, generally poor.

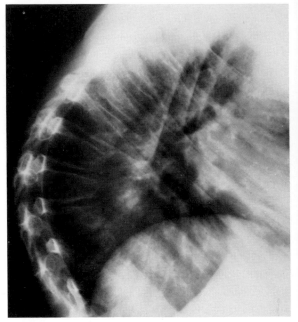

a

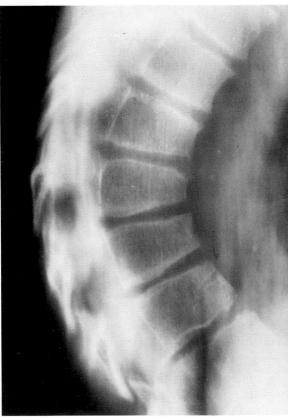

b

Fig. 1.40 *The value of tomography. (a) Lateral view of the thoracic spine of a boy aged 16. There is a significant kyphosis but bone detail is obscured by overlying soft tissue and ribs. (b) Lateral tomogram of the same patient. The beam is focused at one particular depth, so that only the vertebrae are clearly visualised. There is vertebral wedging and endplate irregularity, typical of Scheuermann's disease.*

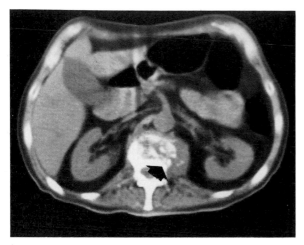

Fig. 1.41 *The value of computerised tomography. Transverse section through the first lumbar vertebra. There is destruction of the vertebral body with a large paravertebral abscess on the right side (arrowed). The appearances are typical of tuberculosis of the spine.*

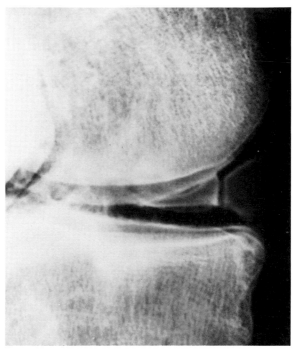

a

Special X-Ray Techniques

Tomography

In some circumstances, routine x-rays do not provide satisfactory definition. This is particularly true in areas where the skeleton is masked by nearby structures, e.g. the thoracic spine (Fig. 1.40). In such cases, the x-ray beam can be focussed at particular planes so that a series of 'cuts' can be made through the depth of the structure under investigation. One particular depth can then be in focus, with the relative exclusion of the others, and this helps to clarify the nature of a pathology which was indistinct on conventional films.

Computerised tomography

This recent innovation is a major advance in the radiographic interpretation of the skeleton. Simul-

Fig. 1.42 *The value of contrast radiography. (a) Arthrography of the knee. Oblique view of the medial joint compartment. Both air and contrast medium fill a vertical tear in the medial meniscus. (b) Myelography. The anteroposterior myelographic appearance shows indentation of the dye column at the L4–5 interspace on the right side, with amputation of the right L5 nerve root. The appearances are those of a posterolateral disc prolapse.*

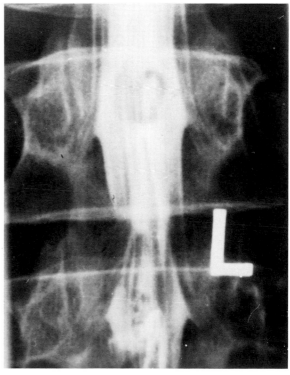

b

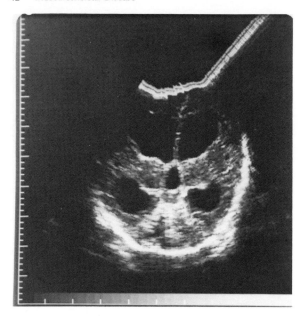

Fig. 1.43 *The value of ultrasound scanning. Coronal section through the anterior fontanelle of a child with spina bifida. There is marked ventricular dilatation, indicating a severe degree of associated hydrocephalus.*

taneous exposures in different directions, processed by computer, produce a sectional radiograph of the trunk, extremity or head (Fig. 1.41). The extent of an intracerebral haematoma, limb neoplasm or intraspinal lesion can be identified in this way with considerable accuracy. The preoperative assessment of these conditions has been revolutionised by this technique, using radiation exposures much smaller than those of more traditional methods.

Contrast radiography

Conventional radiography only detects the calcified parts of the musculoskeletal system. The interior of joints, of the spinal canal or other cavities cannot readily be seen. By the injection of contrast material, sometimes with air as well, the interior of these cavities is well visualised. Thus arthrography will highlight meniscal damage when contrast material, or air, or both, fill the tear in the cartilage (Fig. 1.42). Similarly, myelography can detect a disc prolapse by showing a nerve root distorted by extrinsic pressure.

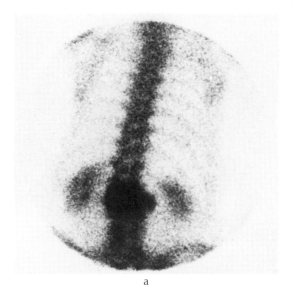

a

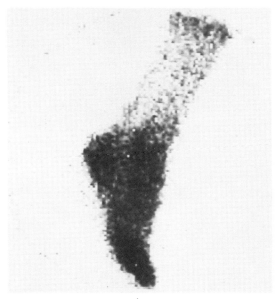

b

Fig. 1.44 *The value of isotope scanning. (a) Technetium scan. There is increased uptake at the L_{2-3} level in this case of spiral osteomyelitis. (b) Gallium scan. This isotope is taken up by white cells. There is a severe infection of the ankle and foot.*

Ultrasound scanning

When ultra-high-velocity sound waves are fired at the body, they bounce back from density interfaces with different characteristics according to the physical properties of the area under investigation. Solid structures promptly rebound the waves, but the contents of hollow cavities offer no resistance to their passage. By this means, solid lesions can be differentiated from cystic ones (Fig. 1.43), thus aiding preoperative diagnosis of tumours and abscesses.

Isotope bone scanning

Bone-seeking isotopes, such as technetium, are taken up by the skeleton and, where bone turnover or vascularity is increased, the density of the scintigraphic appearance is locally increased. Bone-forming tumours, bone infections or fractures appear as 'hot' areas (Fig. 1.44). Isotope scanning is therefore particularly useful in identifying early lesions which are not readily seen on conventional films, and for surveying the skeleton rapidly for secondary areas of pathology. Gallium has a preference for white blood cells; it therefore highlights the inflammatory process and is useful for differentiating between tumour and infection, which both appear 'hot' when scanning is performed with a bone-seeking isotope.

2

Principles of Bone and Soft Tissue Injuries

NATURAL HISTORY OF FRACTURES AND DISLOCATIONS

The stability of a limb may be lost as a result of a fracture or damage to ligaments, and its function or viability impaired by damage to vital structures. It must be remembered that living bone is enclosed within an environment of soft tissue which is also injured as the bone breaks.

Aetiology of Fractures

Traumatic fractures occur when more force is applied than a normal healthy bone can withstand, as in road traffic accidents. Stress fractures occur when repeated stresses on bone cause the cortex to crack. Professional footballers or ballet dancers may suffer in this way. Pathological fractures arise when weakened bone breaks under a relatively minor stress. Osteoporosis in elderly females and secondary deposits of carcinoma are common causes.

Morphology of Fractures

The way in which a bone breaks indicates the magnitude and direction of force which caused the injury (Fig. 2.1). In addition, fractures may be simple (closed) or compound (open). The latter may be compound from within when the jagged bone ends penetrate the skin. They may also be compound from without when the forces disrupt the integument on the way to fracturing the underlying bone.

Greenstick fractures

Because children's bones are pliable they may either buckle (Fig. 2.1a) or bend rather than completely break. The buckle needs no treatment other than protection; the bent bone (Fig. 2.1b) often has to be manipulated and then held straight until it heals.

Transverse fracture (Fig. 2.1c)

This fracture is caused by a force applied transversely to the long axis of the bone. Displacement may be considerable, particularly at the moment of maximal force dissipation, giving rise to compounding from within. The extreme forces required to fracture a healthy bone transversely may also produce severe local soft tissue damage, militating against successful union. The healing process may also be delayed by the very restricted area of the fracture surface. When reduced, however, the horizontal direction of the fracture confers great stability.

Oblique fracture (Fig. 2.1d)

The oblique direction of this fracture makes it unstable. Because the muscles attached to the upper and lower fragments pull to approximate them, there is a tendency for shortening to occur. There is a broader area for healing, however, though traction must be applied to hold the bone to its full length as it heals.

Spiral fracture (Fig. 2.1e)

This injury is caused by a rotational force, such as when a footballer swivels round while his foot is held firmly on the ground. Inherent instability is balanced by a maximal surface area for healing.

Impacted fracture

The fragments are driven together by a compression force. When first examined, the limb may be stable, but within a few days bone resorption at the fracture site tends to produce instability. Immobilisation is therefore necessary.

Comminuted fracture (Fig. 2.1f)

This term describes a fracture in which the bone is broken into more than two pieces. The force has been

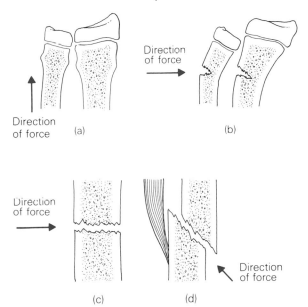

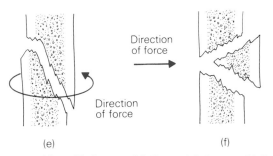

Fig. 2.1 (a) *Buckle fracture.* (b) *Greenstick fracture.* (c) *Transverse fracture.* (d) *Oblique fracture.* (e) *Spiral fracture.* (f) *Comminuted fracture.*

considerable and its dissipation through the bone produces the 'butterfly fragment'.

Epiphyseal injuries (Fig. 2.2)

When the end of a growing bone is fractured, there may be damage to the growth plate. It is important to recognise the pattern of fractures which are particularly dangerous in this respect.

When the fracture line goes through the epiphyseal plate (a slipped epiphysis) it passes through an unimportant layer of non-growing cells (Fig. 2.2a). Growth is therefore not impaired. The most usual fracture in childhood passes along the same layer but then breaks proximally through the metaphysis on one side (Fig. 2.2b). Again, there is no problem with subsequent growth. When the fracture line passes along the epiphyseal plate and then breaks through the epiphysis, again there is no damage to growing cells (Fig. 2.2c). When the fracture passes more vertically through the epiphysis, plate, and metaphysis (Fig. 2.2d), it does not damage growth cells, but unless there is an anatomical reduction the danger of cross-union exists between the bone of the epiphysis and the bone of the metaphysis, which would greatly interfere with subsequent growth. The most severe growth disturbance, and the one most difficult to predict, occurs when there has been compression damage to the growing cells of the plate itself (Fig. 2.2e) leading to premature fusion of the growth plate or asymmetrical growth.

Dislocations

When a joint is dislocated the ligaments and capsule are stretched or torn and the joint cavity fills with blood. The capsule is rich in sensory nerve fibres and the dislocation continues to be painful until it is reduced, unlike a fracture which is relatively pain-free once it is immobilised. The shoulder, the elbow, the finger joints and the patella are the most common sites for dislocations. Usually external manipulation will succeed in reducing the dislocation, but if bone is also broken, open surgical reduction is often necessary. When a joint is not completely dislocated the term subluxation is correct.

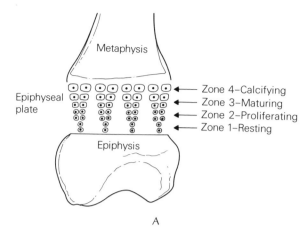

Fig. 2.2A *The epiphyseal growth plate. This provides growth in length of the metaphysis and shaft. Cartilage cells undergo interstitial growth, thus widening the plate while calcification of the cartilage on the metaphyseal side of the plate leads to replacement by bone (endochondral ossification). Fractures occur through the weakest layer which fortunately is the non-growing zone 4 – the calcification layer.*

Fig. 2.2B *Fractures involving the epiphysis and its plate. (a) The epiphysis is separated from the metaphysis through the non-growing portion of the plate. There is, therefore, no growth disturbance. (b) The fracture has gone through the same non-growing layer but at one side has passed through the metaphysis. Again growth is not interrupted. (c) The fracture has passed through the same non-growing layer of the plate and then has passed through the epiphysis itself. Again, growth is not disturbed. (d)i The fracture has split through the plate from the metaphysis to the epiphysis. (d)ii Unless accurately reduced, cross union between epiphysis and metaphysis occurs. (e)i The plate has been crushed more on one side than the other. (e)ii A serious growth disturbance ensues.*

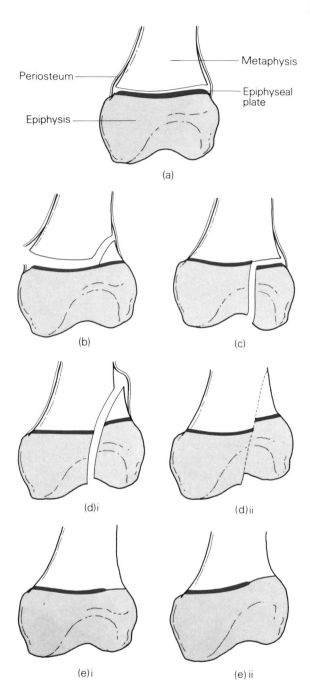

B

NORMAL BONE HEALING

All living bones bleed when they are broken, and blood therefore clots around the fracture. This fracture haematoma is then organised: new capillaries invade it; phagocytes carry away the debris; fibroblasts lay down collagen. By the end of ten days a fairly firm spindle of tissue, procallus, surrounds the fracture (Fig. 2.3).

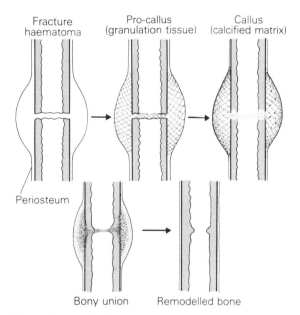

Fig. 2.3 *Fracture healing.*

Calcium salts are deposited in the collagenous matrix, making it stronger and causing a hazy shadow on x-ray. When the cuff of tissue is radiologically opaque it is called callus. This natural splinting of the fracture provides a template in which osteoblasts form new bone, building from the inner layer of the periosteum as well as from between the bone ends, and the subperiosteal and endosteal new bone restores firm continuity. The x-ray appearance of trabeculae crossing the facture, and clinical testing of stability, indicate that the fracture has united. The speed with which this occurs depends on the age of the patient and which limb is injured. An approximate estimate is that a child's upper limb fracture unites in three weeks. A child's lower limb fracture or an adult's upper limb fracture unites in six weeks. A lower limb fracture in an adult takes at least twelve weeks.

There then follows a long process of remodelling, leading to consolidation. As a mature pattern of haversian canals is restored in the cortical bone, the spindle-shaped cuff of extra bone is resorbed. In children, who have great remodelling powers, the appearance of the bone reverts to normal.

There are important clinical implications in the process of fracture healing. The 'primary callus response', a fundamental reaction of bone to injury, appears to occur independently of environmental factors. It is, however, a very brief phenomenon and rapidly subsides if contact between fragments is not soon restored. An amputation stump through bone shows this short-lived phenomenon but proceeds no further because it is, in effect, only one-half of a fracture and quickly regresses. A similar situation pertains if soft tissue keeps the fracture fragments apart. Therefore, not only is reduction of a fracture a desirable thing but also surgical interference at this stage must have overriding indications—failure to achieve reduction by closed means, a compound injury, a fracture through diseased bone, a fracture involving joint or growth plate, or a fracture in the elderly who might otherwise succumb without the more rapid rehabilitation afforded by internal fixation.

As the periosteal blood supply is important in this external callus phase, any dissection should therefore be subperiosteal so that the integrity of vessels entering this important osteogenic layer from neighbouring muscles is not jeopardised. Furthermore, as movement (obviously not excessive), enhances this primary response, there is much to be said for 'immobilising' a limb fracture in the convenient and not too rigid plaster cast. Conversely, rigid internal fixation inhibits the production of external callus, and the fate of the fracture depends solely upon the more longterm phase of 'late medullary callus'. Thus, external callus is nature's way of providing fracture stability so that the secondary medullary callus response can provide union by slowly replacing intervening fibrous tissue with bone. Perhaps the ideal treatment would be the application of semi-rigid internal fixation, which would provide security without inhibiting nature's external efforts.

COMPLICATIONS OF FRACTURES AND DISLOCATIONS

The forces which broke the bone or disrupted the joint were also applied to the surrounding structures, which may have been further damaged by the fractured or displaced bone ends.

Immediate Complications

Blood loss

All fractures bleed and cause local swelling. In an open fracture, with a wound through the skin, bleeding will be more obvious. However, even in closed fractures bleeding into the tissues may remove so much blood from the circulation that the patient will develop oligaemic shock. A fractured femur can lose two litres of blood and fractures of the pelvis often exceed this amount.

Peripheral ischaemia

The arterial blood supply to a limb may be cut off by pressure from the fractured bone ends, as in a supracondylar fracture of the humerus, or a main artery may have been injured in the accident. It is always advisable to feel for the pulse distal to the fracture. If it is not present, restoration of the circulation takes priority over treatment of the fracture. Permanent ischaemic changes result in fibrosis and contracture of muscles, or even loss of the limb.

Damage to nerves

Where peripheral nerves lie in close proximity to a bone they may be damaged at the time of injury.

The radial nerve is frequently damaged where it winds round the middle third of the shaft of the humerus. If there is a fracture at this site, inability to extend the wrist and fingers indicates radial nerve damage.

The ulnar nerve is vulnerable where it lies in the groove behind the medial epicondyle at the elbow. If the patient can spread his fingers then the ulnar nerve, which supplies the interossei, is functioning.

If the median nerve is damaged at the level of the elbow, both long flexors of the index finger will be paralysed. If the ulnar fingers can flex into the palm while the index lags in extension, the median nerve is damaged. When the injury to the median nerve is at wrist level, the long flexors are unaffected. The only motor deficit in the hand is loss of abduction of the thumb. A much more important result is that sensation in the palmar aspect of the radial three and a half digits is lost, with great impairment of hand function (Fig. 2.4).

The sciatic nerve is frequently damaged in posterior dislocation of the hip joint, when it is bowstrung across the displaced femoral head. This renders the patient incapable of flexing or extending the foot. A complication of a fracture at the upper end of the fibula, where the lateral popliteal nerve winds round, is paralysis of foot dorsiflexion – a 'dropped foot'.

The severity of a nerve injury occurs in three grades: neurapraxia, axonotmesis and neurotmesis.

Neurapraxia is a temporary block to conduction in the nerve, due to pressure or bruising. This usually resolves rapidly and is followed by full recovery.

In axonotmesis, trauma damages the axons but the fibrous structure of the nerve remains intact. Wallerian degeneration occurs distally, but proximal regeneration, at a rate of 1–2 mm per day, reestablishes neural continuity. Recovery will eventually be almost complete.

With neurotmesis the whole nerve is divided. Any chance of recovery depends on surgical reconstruction. Early operation, with the use of an operating

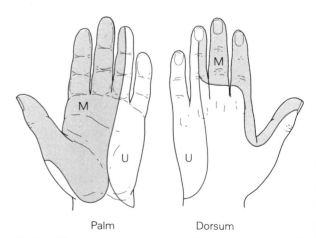

Palm   Dorsum

Fig. 2.4 *The median and ulnar nerve distribution in the hand.*

microscope and appropriate instruments, has greatly improved the prognosis for these injuries. The use of nerve grafts to bridge deficits caused by retraction has made reconstruction of peripheral nerves and the brachial plexus possible.

Intermediate Complications

Fat embolism

Twelve or more hours after injury the patient may become confused and abusive, even after a major injury such as a fractured femur. This is often the first symptom of fat embolism. There may be globules of fat in the sputum or urine and petechial haemorrhages in the warm parts of the skin – the axillae and groin. Examination of the retina may also show local emboli. The patient's confusion is the result of a raised P_{CO_2} and a falling P_{O_2} due to embolisation in the lungs, with shunting of blood, and probably also due to emboli in the brain. In severe cases the patient will become unconscious and may die. Fortunately most cases recover after treatment with oxygen and, if necessary, sedation.

Infection

For patients who have sustained an open fracture there is always the risk of infection. The infecting organisms, which penetrate the wound at the time of injury, may be aerobic or anaerobic. Of the former, *Staphylococcus aureus* is the most common and, if treatment is inadequate, acute pyogenic osteomyelitis may develop. Clostridial organisms are the most important anaerobes. *Clostridium welchii* produces gas infection of muscles which may lead to frank gangrene unless treated immediately by excision of all necrotic tissue, and *C. tetani* may produce tetanus in the non-immune patient. Such disasters are minimised by proper initial wound management.

Deep vein thrombosis

Crushing a limb and then immobilising it in a splint is unfortunately a provocative method for inducing deep vein thrombosis a week to ten days after injury. Persisting thigh or calf pain and tenderness, with increased warmth, swelling and a pyrexia suggest the diagnosis. Early mobilisation diminishes the risk.

Late Complications

Delayed union

This occurs when a bone fails to unite by the expected time. It is not a pathological end-point; union may still take place, although the addition of healthy bone by grafting may expedite the process. Union is often delayed with scaphoid fractures.

Malunion

A bone may heal without correct alignment. The deformity may remodel with growth in children, but in adults it is permanent. In this respect, the varus

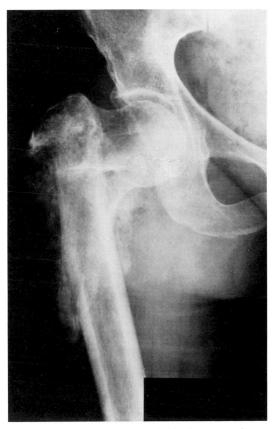

Fig. 2.5 *Anteroposterior view of right hip showing malunion— this unstable trochanteric fracture has collapsed into varus.*

deformity with shortening is notorious in unstable trochanteric fractures (Fig. 2.5).

Non-union

This is a pathological end-point; the fracture will not proceed to union without treatment. The bone ends are rounded and sclerotic and there is no bridging callus. Movement at the fracture site usually persists and is painful, but if there is a firm fibrous union the condition may be asymptomatic. The sclerotic avascular bone ends and intervening fibrous tissue must be excised and replaced by a healthy bone graft if union is to occur. This is aided by rigid internal fixation using a plate and screws. If these measures fail, then locally-applied pulsed electromagnetic energy may achieve union, although its effect has so far defied explanation.

Avascular necrosis

If the fracture disrupts the blood supply to a fragment of bone, this will undergo avascular necrosis (Fig. 2.6). The arterial supply to the head of the femur and humerus and to the proximal part of the scaphoid travels in a distal to proximal direction. Subcapital fractures of the femur and humerus and fractures of the waist of the scaphoid are thus commonly associated with avascular necrosis. The bone becomes sclerotic, collapses, and may be totally resorbed.

Growth disturbances

If the fracture line crosses the epiphyseal plate in a child, and is not anatomically reduced, further growth at the end of the bone may be asymmetrical, leading to an angular deformity, or it may cease completely if the growth plate is crushed. This may result either in a short limb or one in which the deformity becomes more marked as the child grows.

Osteoarthritis

When the fracture line passes into a joint, the subchondral bone heals by forming new bone but the articular cartilage heals by forming scar tissue. Any irregularity of the joint surface may lead to degenerative changes in later years.

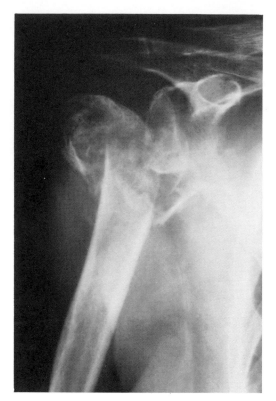

Fig. 2.6 *Anteroposterior view of right shoulder showing avascular necrosis of the humeral head. The head has collapsed following a fracture of the humeral neck.*

SOFT TISSUE INJURIES

With over 60 000 new patients attending an accident department serving a population of 500 000, the great majority of whom have soft tissue injuries, this is a particularly important aspect of medical practice. If the integument is not breached, then the wound presents as a painful local swelling with oedema and contusion. If the skin has been broken, the term open wound is appropriate, and the type of an open wound dictates its management.

Open Wounds

Clean incised wounds (Fig. 2.7a)

These are linear lacerations caused by the cutting surface of a sharp object. The wound needs careful

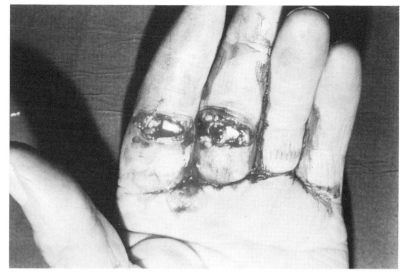

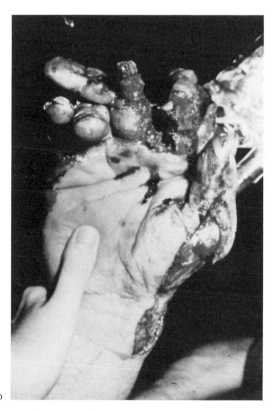

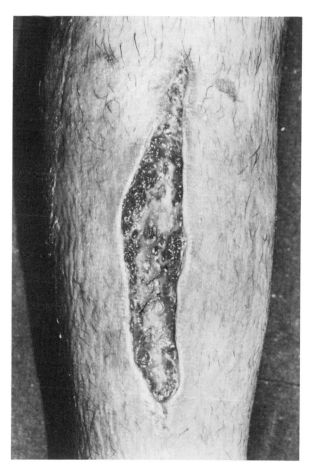

Fig. 2.7 *Three types of wound. (a) Clean—knife lacerations of index and middle fingers dividing the flexor tendons. (b) Untidy—a severe crush injury of the hand caused by an industrial press. (c) Infected—laceration of skin with infected necrotic muscle.*

examination to determine that the integrity of important structures, blood vessels, nerves or tendons has not been jeopardised. This is particularly important with wounds of the hand. In addition, it is essential that the entire depth of the wound should be visualised in order to exclude damage to deeper organs, such as in a penetrating wound of the abdomen. The wound is then dealt with by excision and primary closure. Excision implies removal of the tissue margins of the wound so that the wound then resembles as closely as possible a surgical incision. When the healthy walls have been well coapted primarily, uneventful wound healing can be anticipated. If the wound is more than 24 hours old, then in all probability it has already been colonised by pathogenic bacteria. Excision will then be of no value, since the surrounding soft tissues will harbour organisms, and primary closure is inadvisable as this will seal in potential infection. Such a wound should be left open so that free drainage can occur and then closed secondarily five days after injury.

Untidy wounds (Fig. 2.7b)

Here the wound excision must be generous to ensure that all damaged and devitalised tissue is removed. It will be more difficult to close a widely-excised wound primarily without tension, and it should therefore be left open at first and closed in a delayed primary fashion after three days. If the wound is more than 24 hours old, debridement should be performed. This is not synonymous with wound excision and means that the wound is thoroughly opened and all dirt and foreign materials removed. Such a wound should then be left open and closed secondarily.

Infected wounds

For wounds that are frankly infected at the time of presentation, debridement is the initial treatment of choice; the wound is closed secondarily only when all evidence of infection has settled. Systemic antibiotic treatment is also necessary.

Open fractures

In the management of open fractures, the associated wound takes priority. The skin, subcutaneous tissue and muscle should be treated as if the wound existed in isolation but the excision process should extend to the entire depth of the wound. Any devascularised fragments of cortical bone, or those devoid of nourishing periosteum, must be removed lest they form sequestra and niduses for deep bone infection. No degree of tension is permitted when the wound is closed since the narrowing of local blood vessels occasioned by tension compounds the risk of sepsis. Because of the serious nature of bone infection, prophylactic antibiotics must also be administered.

Skin Loss

When there has been a significant area of skin loss, the integument must be restored. Areas of great skin laxity such as the back of the hand can tolerate surprisingly large areas of skin loss and yet still be repaired primarily without undue tension. Skin in other areas, such as the palm of the hand, is so tightly bound to the underlying tissue that any loss of skin can only be made good by taking skin from elsewhere to replace the deficit.

Principles of skin grafting

When skin is taken from elsewhere (the donor area) to replace an area of skin loss (the recipient area), it is nourished for the first few weeks through the film of extracellular fluid between it and the recipient area until it is fully vascularised by the invasion of new blood vessels from the periphery. This is therefore a critical time for the graft, and its survival depends on four factors: the thickness of the graft; movement; the nature of the recipient area; and infection. The passage of nutriments to the graft is by diffusion and accordingly is subject to Graham's law. This implies that the thickness of graft is related exponentially to the difficulty of sustaining it. Split-thickness skin grafts therefore take much more easily than full-thickness grafts.

The graft is particularly vulnerable to shearing stresses which continually disturb the relationship between graft and recipient area and encourage haematoma formation, further separating the graft from its underlying nourishment. Junctional regions such as the axilla or groin are particularly prone to the adverse effects of shear.

The most important factor governing the survival of

a skin graft is the nature of the recipient area, which is most favourable if it will produce granulations. Subcutaneous fat, muscle, periosteum and paratenon are all favourable areas. Bare cortical bone, bare tendon, and cartilage do not produce granulation tissue and will not sustain a skin graft.

Skin grafts survive and 'take' in the presence of most pathogenic organisms. Infection with *Streptococcus pyogenes* is disastrous, however; the graft is lysed and may disappear in a matter of a few hours.

Split-thickness skin grafts

These thin grafts can be used for most areas of skin loss. The superficial layers of the skin from the donor area, usually the thigh, are shaved off, trimmed to the contour of the defect, and stitched to its boundaries under a compression dressing which prevents movement and haematoma formation. The donor area will produce new superficial layers because its deep regenerative layer has been left undisturbed. The grafted area matures but regains neither full quality nor sensation. Accordingly this method is not suitable for load-bearing areas such as the palms of the hand and soles of the feet, nor is it suitable for areas where skin quality is paramount, such as the face.

Full-thickness skin grafts

When the complete thickness of skin is taken from one area to replace loss in another, the defect in the recipient area must be made good either by primary closure in a lax area or by split skin grafting. Because of the problem of sustaining such a thick piece of skin by diffusion from below, this technique is only suitable for covering small defects in load-bearing areas which need thick and strong cover.

Skin flaps

When a large area of full-thickness cover is required, or when grafting is inappropriate because of the nature of the recipient area, the use of a skin flap (Fig. 2.8) is necessary. The need for sustenance by diffusion from the recipient area is avoided because the skin flap retains its own blood supply until it is vascularised from the periphery. It is therefore left attached by its pedicle to the donor area while the distal part of the flap is first

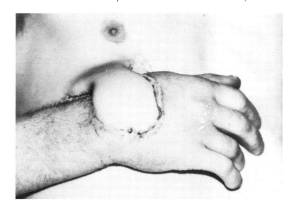

Fig. 2.8 *Skin flap—skin loss on the dorsum of this man's wrist was made good via a flap from the chest wall.*

set into margins of the defect. When revascularisation is complete, the pedicle can be detached. The donor area defect is made good by split skin cover.

If the nature of the blood supply to the flap from its base is haphazard (a random pattern flap) then the length of the flap must not be excessive in proportion to the width of its pedicle, lest peripheral necrosis is incurred. Axial pattern flaps have recently been devised, based upon vessels running predominantly along the length of the flap. The groin flap, based upon the circumflex iliac vessels, is a notable example. Even axial pattern flaps, however, carry the disadvantage of having to retain attachment to the donor area. With the advent of the operating microscope, and the ability to perform small vessel anastomosis, it is now possible to transfer axial pattern flaps freely, by attaching the flap's main vessels to suitably-sized vessels in the recipient area as one microsurgical procedure.

BURNS

The skin may be scalded by hot liquids or burned by dry heat, electricity, friction, chemicals, or radioactivity. In slightly different ways, each of these agents can destroy part or all of the thickness of the skin. Even more dangerous is the inhalation of hot fumes which burn the respiratory mucosa. The increasing use of synthetic foam for padding furniture is now making respiratory burns an even greater threat to life than burns of the skin.

Physiology of the Skin

The skin is the largest single organ in the body. It keeps tissue fluid within the body and keeps out pathogenic bacteria. It is an elastic tissue which expands with respiration and especially in pregnancy. It is a secretory organ for sweat and sebum and plays an important role in temperature regulation. Finally it has a sensory innervation which is highly developed in such important areas as the lips, the finger-tips and the genitalia. All these functions will be lost if the skin is burned so deeply that it cannot regenerate (Fig. 2.9).

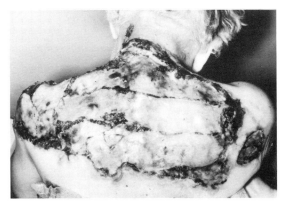

Fig. 2.9 *A significant full thickness burn when this old lady fell backwards into the fire. Immediate skin grafting minimised protein loss and infection and probably saved her life.*

Pathophysiology of the Burn Injury

As soon as the epidermis is burnt, plasma oozes out of the dermis. The body thereby loses water, protein and electrolytes. If the surface area of the burn exceeds 15% of the total body surface in an adult, or 10% in a child or elderly patient, then the loss of fluid will cause circulatory failure.

Whereas healthy skin resists pathogenic bacteria, the warm, raw, moist surface of a burn provides an excellent culture medium. The skin may be sterilised at the moment of burning, but very soon afterwards the burn is colonised by bacteria. If left uncontrolled, the infection may become so extensive as to produce a septicaemia.

A deep circumferential burn may cause such great congestion in the tissues that the circulation is im-

paired. Later, as scar tissue forms, respiratory movements may be restricted if the burn injury passes around the chest, or a subsequent pregnancy may abort because of the inability of a scarred abdomen to contain it. In the acute stage, the pressure in a limb can be released by making deep longitudinal incisions, and the later complications can be eased by excision and grafting of at least some of the scar tissue.

The complication most difficult to mitigate is the destruction of cutaneous sensation. Scarred skin not only fails to serve as a sensory tactile tissue for exploring the environment, it cannot even give warning when it is itself being injured. Consequently this insensitive skin is susceptible to minor injuries or burns. One further aggravation is that the insensitive inelastic scar which forms over a deep burn will subsequently contract, distorting features and limiting the movement of joints.

Assessment and Primary Treatment

Prognosis depends on three factors: the extent of the burn, the depth of the burn, and whether the respiratory tract is affected. Care of the airway is essential if there is respiratory involvement and this may require a tracheostomy.

Calculating the extent of the burn is of critical importance when the patient is first examined. Even if the patient is not in shock, when the percentage area of body surface involved indicates that circulatory collapse is likely or inevitable, then a good intravenous line must be established immediately. It is customary to use plasma to replace the loss of water, protein and electrolytes. The volume and rate of infusion are determined by the extent of the burn calculated by Wallace's rule of nine (Fig. 2.10). An estimate of the volume of colloid required for intravenous infusion during the first 36 hours is provided by the formula

$$\frac{\% \text{ area of burn} \times \text{body weight in kg}}{2}$$

This gives the quantity (in ml) of colloid required during each of six consecutive periods after injury.

For example, a 40% burn in a patient weighing 60 kg requires

$$\frac{40 \times 60}{2} = 1200 \text{ ml for each period}$$

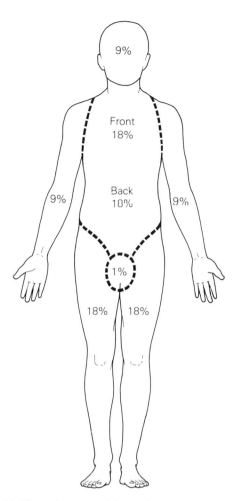

Fig. 2.10 *The surface area of the body in proportions used to calculate the extent of a burn—Wallace's rule of nine.*

This implies a total transfusion of 7200 mls in 36 hours merely to replace what the burned area is losing.

Local Treatment

First aid measures include removing the patient from the source of injury, removing any smouldering clothing, and applying cold water for a heat burn or scald. Small burns can be covered by a sterile first-aid dressing. Large burns will be kept free from contamination if covered by clean linen, e.g. a sheet or tablecloth.

Small blisters should be left intact to form a sterile biological dressing for the wound underneath. Large blisters, which will rupture, can be opened using sterile scissors. A sterile adhesive plastic film is useful for covering superficial burns of the trunk. Burns of the face should be left exposed. Deep burns and burns of the hands are conveniently treated by applying silver sulphadiazine ointment.

Prognosis

This depends on the depth and site of the injury. Burns which affect only the epidermis or superficial dermis, which are red, painful and weeping when first seen, will heal by re-epithelialisation and, provided they do not become infected, should leave no scar. Burns which destroy most or all of the dermis are initially grey or charred and relatively pain-free because the sensory nerve endings have been destroyed. They will heal slowly by the formation of scar tissue unless they are treated surgically by excision and skin grafting.

Deep burns in the region of the face, the hands or the perineum require in-patient treatment because of the special local problems.

TETANUS

Tetanus is a potentially lethal disease caused by the anaerobic organism *Clostridium tetani* which is widely disseminated in soil, manure and faeces. Although the disease is now rare in Great Britain, it is commonplace in other parts of the world and only constant vigilance keeps it at bay in this country.

Symptoms and Treatment

The organism secretes a neurotoxin which acts on the central nervous system. After an incubation period of about 7–10 days, the patient begins to feel stiffness in the jaw or neck and has difficulty in swallowing. Then after a further 2–5 days (the period of onset), muscular spasms develop, which increase in severity and frequency. Death from respiratory or cardiac failure can ensue in 24–48 hours.

Modern treatment for severe cases is by curarizing the patient and maintaining his respiration on a ventilator through a tracheostomy. Excision of the wound, which is the site of toxin production, plus passive immunisation with human antitetanus serum, and antibiotic therapy, together with constant nursing care and physiotherapy usually make it possible to stop the curare after 2–3 weeks. In centres specialising in tetanus treatment, the mortality rate has been brought down from over 70% to under 10% in the last 30 years.

Prophylaxis

Tetanus is almost entirely preventable. Prevention is based on three factors: wound excision, immunisation, and antibiotic therapy. Because the causal organism is anaerobic, it thrives in wounds containing dirt or foreign bodies where oxygen tension is low. Proper surgical care of wounds is the most important factor in preventing tetanus. Antibiotics are only indicated for very dirty wounds with a lot of tissue destruction, or neglected wounds which are already infected.

The following programme is now widely used for active immunisation. The initial programme consists of three intramuscular injections of 0·5 ml of tetanus toxoid, given with 6 weeks between the first two

injections and 5–6 months between the second and third. Ideally, a baby receives this through the Child Welfare Clinic. A booster injection of 0·5 ml is given when the child starts school aged 5 years, and another one before he leaves school aged about 15–16 years. If the subject does not receive treatment for a wound in the meantime, then he should have a further booster injection every 10 years. If he does sustain an open wound then the following alternative procedures are adopted.

1. If the patient has had a complete course of toxoid, or a booster dose within the past 5 years, nothing is required.
2. If it is 5–10 years since the last injection, this occasion is used to renew immunity by a further booster injection.
3. If it is more than 10 years since the last injection, a booster injection should be given and, if the wound is dirty, penetrating, or more than six hours old, one vial of human tetanus immunoglobulin (250 units) is also given.
4. If the patient has not previously been immunised, and has a superficial wound, active immunisation with toxoid is begun. For deeper or dirty wounds, the patient should also be passively immunised.

3

Injuries of the Thorax and Spine

Closed injuries of the chest and spine are usually associated with traffic accidents and with accidents in heavy industry and demolition work. A significant number also occur in the home and in sporting activities. In contrast, penetrating injuries are seen in warfare, and nowadays as a result of inner city violence. Associated injuries must be assessed as these have a bearing on treatment; head injuries and increasing age worsen the prognosis.

THORAX

Isolated Fractures

While these injuries are common, they must be viewed with the suspicion of a more serious accompanying intrathoracic lesion. A direct blow on the chest may cause a fracture of the ribs or sternum in which the fragments are driven inwards. Attendant lacerations of the lung or pleura may lead to pneumothorax, hae-mothorax, or both. The intercostal vessels may be torn, resulting in a massive haemothorax.

It is important to note that fractures of the first or second ribs are often complicated by damage to the subclavian vessels or to the brachial plexus. Similarly, fractures of the floating ribs raise the possibility of renal, hepatic or splenic injury. Fractures of the sternum or forward dislocation of the manubriosternal joint often accompany flexion–compression injuries of the mid thoracic spine.

Multiple Fractures

When the force is applied over a wider area, the ribs break in the middle and often at two levels. They break outwards, so that while local pulmonary injury is unusual, a variety of intrathoracic lesions may be produced, depending on the severity of the compressing force. In young children the rib cage is so flexible that serious visceral damage may occur without evidence of a bony injury.

Multiple rib fractures and fractures of the costal cartilages and sternum lead to 'flail chest' and paradoxical respiratory movement. In this situation, while the intact rib cage expands on inspiration, the flail portion is driven inwards by atmospheric pressure. The reverse effect occurs on expiration, so that intrathoracic pressure is greater than atmospheric pressure, and the floating segment is pushed outwards. This leads to alterations in the intrapleural pressure, additional airway resistance, and increasing respiratory distress.

Complications

The bony injury is usually self evident; the importance of recognising a possible visceral injury cannot be over-stressed. Such injuries vary in severity. Most are potentially lethal and include cardiac contusions and tamponade, rupture of the aorta, oesophageal tears and injuries of the diaphragm. Traumatic asphyxia may follow the sudden rise of pressure in the great veins due to the compressive force. Changes occur in the upper part of the body, where the veins are deficient in valves. The vessels and capillaries are atonic and become engorged with blood. The striking violaceous colour of the skin is due to oxygen desaturation of the stagnant blood.

Pulmonary contusion may compound the problem,

leading to post-traumatic pulmonary insufficiency, sometimes called 'shock lung'.

Clinical Examinations

The four basic procedures of inspection, palpation, percussion and auscultation are employed.

Inspection may demonstrate airway obstruction or paradoxical respiration. Palpation defines the sites of tenderness and may reveal the 'crackling' sensation of air in the subcutaneous tissues (surgical emphysema, Fig. 3.1). Pneumothorax is evidenced by the hyper-resonant note on percussion, diminished air entry and displacement of the apex beat. Haemothorax presents dullness on percussion and a greatly decreased or absent air entry on auscultation (Fig. 3.2).

The response to treatment and the clinical progress should alert the examiner to more subtle intrathoracic injuries. Even on suspicion of complications, these patients should be admitted to an Intensive Care Unit utilising the skills of specialised staff, where frequent blood gas analyses and cardiac enzyme estimations can be performed. High quality radiography will delineate many of the more unusual injuries. For example, widening of the mediastinal shadow accompanying rupture of the great vessels will dictate the need for aortography (Fig. 3.3).

Treatment

The aims of treatment are to secure a good airway and an adequate respiratory exchange, confirmed in the more serious cases by arterial blood gas studies.

The pain of rib fractures inhibits deep breathing and coughing, thus predisposing the patient to chest infections. Analgesics which do not depress respiration, local infiltration with lignocaine hydrochloride, or intercostal nerve blocks are normally effective in reducing pain. The patient is instructed in deep breathing exercises and on the need to support the chest when coughing.

A small haemothorax responds to aspiration; a large haemothorax or pneumothorax demands urgent closed-tube drainage (Fig. 3.4). Immediate respiratory distress rarely requires a tracheostomy. Most patients can be treated successfully by intermittent positive

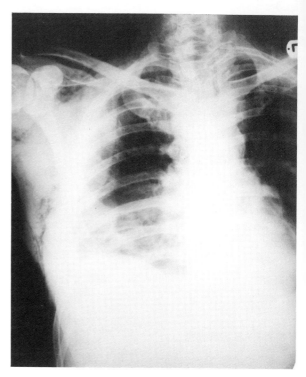

Fig. 3.1 *Posteroanterior view of chest. There is surgical emphysema extending onto the chest wall and root of the neck following minor rib fractures. Note pulmonary contusion and opacification of the right basal area.*

pressure ventilation through an endotracheal tube. The choice of ventilator and monitoring of gas volumes are decided by the anaesthetist, and the skills of a thoracic surgeon are required when there are major intrathoracic injuries.

SPINE

Injuries of the spine are commonly caused by indirect violence applied to the head, shoulders or buttocks. Direct injuries may result in fractures of the posterior arches and shearing forces are sometimes associated with fracture–dislocations.

Flexion, extension, compression and rotation are the main injuring forces. These are usually combined, and the resulting bony or ligamentous injury is further modified by intrinsic factors such as the varying

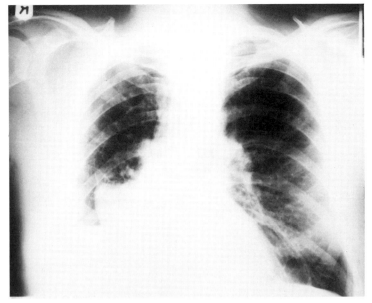

a

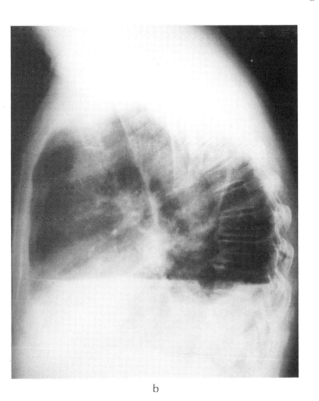

b

Fig. 3.2 (a) *Posteroanterior view of the chest. There is a haemopneumothorax showing a fluid level at the right base.* (b) *The lateral projection confirms a clearly defined fluid level and pulmonary contusion. (Courtesy of Dr E. D. O'Doherty, FFR.)*

strength of ligaments and bones at different ages and whether the muscles are 'on guard' at the time of injury.

The Bony Injury

A distinction is made between those injuries which are stable and unlikely to displace with normal handling, and injuries which are inherently unstable. This is determined to a large extent by the integrity of the ligaments which hold the bones together. Clinical experience and experimental cadaveric studies have shown that ligamentous disruption and dislocations are readily produced when rotation is added to the main injuring force.

In most of the injuries to the spinal column, stability is not affected, including the majority of flexion–compression injuries of the vertebral bodies and injuries of the transverse and spinous processes. When greater forces are involved and where these include rotational or torsional elements, fracture–dislocations are produced, and these are commonly associated with injury to the spinal cord or nerve roots.

It is important to note that ligamentous injuries often heal badly, leading to chronic pain and instability. Even when reduced and well immobilised, ligamentous injuries without significant bony damage remain suspect.

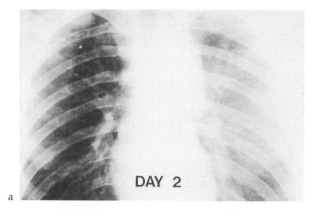

a

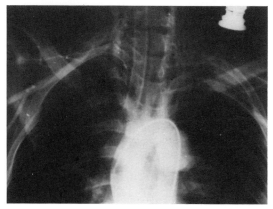

b

Fig. 3.3 (a) *Postero-anterior view of chest with widening of the superior mediastinal shadow and shadowing of the left lung field. The aortic arch is not clearly defined. The radiograph suggests a rupture of the aorta but it is not diagnostic of this condition; further investigation including aortography is required. (b) Postero-anterior view of upper chest. Retrograde arteriography shows a pseudo-aneurysm near the attachment of the ligamentum arteriosum. (Motor cyclist in collision with a tree; a high speed deceleration injury. Recovery followed surgical repair.) (Courtesy of Dr I. W. McCall, FFR.)*

Spinal fusion is often necessary sometime later. In contrast, sound fusion usually follows where the bony injury predominates and where large areas of cancellous bone are exposed. A conservative policy is favoured in the management of these injuries, unless there is gross displacement and assuming that the bony injury can be re-aligned. Certain bony injuries require early surgery.

The Neurological Injury

Great forces are required to produce disruption or

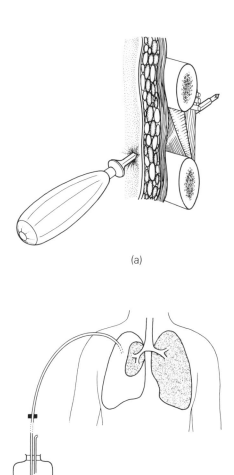

(a)

(b)

Fig. 3.4 *Intercostal drainage for pneumothorax (or haemothorax). (a) An immediate radiograph should confirm the presence of air in the chest. The tube is inserted with the patient inclined upright at 60°. The tissues over the second intercostal space are widely infiltrated with a local anaesthetic to include the pleura. The needle is inserted into the mid-clavicular line and must be passed into the chest to demonstrate that an air space has been entered. A small incision is made at the lower border of the interspace so that the trocar and cannula enter obliquely. The cannula is withdrawn and an Argyle or Malecot catheter is passed into the pleural cavity and secured with a suture. (b) The catheter is connected to a tube leading to a large bottle placed two feet lower than the patient. The bottle is filled to a depth of 8 cm and the tube must remain under water at all times. An extra cannula in the cork permits the excape of air or allows attachment to a suction apparatus. (Drainage of a haemothorax: A similar method is used but the catheter is inserted in the fifth or sixth intercostal space in the mid-axillary line.)*

displacement of the normal spinal column. Once these unusual forces have acted, the parenchymatous tissue of the spinal cord is so poorly supported by its fibrous scaffolding that even minor deformation may cause irreparable nerve damage.

The spinal cord and nerve roots may be crushed by bony displacement, stretched or torn by torsional forces, or compressed by bony fragments as in axial loading fractures which 'explode' the vertebral body (Fig. 3.5). These same forces may tear the meninges and impair the tenuous blood supply to the cord. The oxygen requirements of neural tissue are high, and the vascular supply may be further impaired by swelling of the cord in the spinal canal.

Experimental studies on laminectomised animals, using an impact force, suggest that the primary lesion is in the central grey matter. There is disruption of vessels and capillaries with diapedesis of red cells leading to areas of haemorrhage and necrosis. The process

appears to be self-perpetuating for a time. The white matter is involved by spreading oedema, and later by chromatolysis and disintegration of the long tracts. The clinical stiuation is probably similar, but more severe injuries cause direct damage to the white matter. This is followed by demyelination of the long tracts, ingestion of debris by macrophages, and ultimately by cavitation and cyst formation. Repair is by astrocytic infiltration and the laying down of dense scar tissue.

It should be appreciated that the neural damage varies with the nature and severity of the injuring force. Rarely, there is a transitory paresis (spinal concussion) in which the changes are probably at neuronal level and confined to the synapses. There may be isolated areas of haemorrhagic necrosis and oedema corresponding in clinical terms to the various incomplete syndromes, or extensive infarction of one or more segments may occur resulting in a complete cord lesion.

Diagnosis

The order of responsibilities when examining a patient who has sustained an injury to the spine is: 1, the assessment of respiratory function; 2, evaluation of the vertebral injury and the extent of any neurological impairment; and, 3, a review of associated injuries.

This section is mainly concerned with patients who have sustained damage to the spinal cord or nerves in addition to vertebral injury. Similar principles, appropriately modified, apply to uncomplicated spinal injuries.

A detailed history of the accident from the victim or witnesses often gives a clue as to the nature of the bony injury. It is of the utmost importance to establish whether the patient moved his limbs after the accident, and to enquire about sensory impairment or electric shock-like feelings suggesting neural damage.

Important physical signs

The patient may complain of pain at the site of injury even when paralysed, and there may be a localised spinal deformity. Lacerations and bruise marks of the face or scalp, fractures of the facial bones, and swelling of the neck should suggest an injury to the cervical spine. The trunk is examined for abrasions and bruises, and the whole spine is palpated for localised tender-

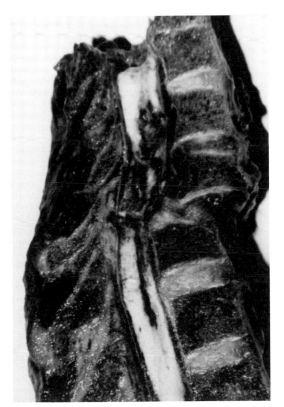

Fig. 3.5 *Bilateral facet dislocation of the cervical spine. Note the longitudinal extent of the lesion and the gross disruption of the spinal cord.*

ness. A gap may be felt between the spinous processes in the thoracic or lumbar regions and this indicates a disruptive injury. On the basis of these findings, preliminary radiographs are requested.

Neurological examination

The general assessment and resuscitation is a continuing process, but the neurological examination is so important that it should be regarded as a distinct procedure. It is repeated every few hours, without causing the patient undue distress and in the light of the initial findings. Each examination is precisely documented. The aim is to determine the level of the cord or nerve-root injury and to establish whether the lesion is complete or incomplete.

Ability to move the limbs and the general posture is noted. At the initial examination it is sufficient to test voluntary contraction of muscle groups (active joint movement) rather than of individual muscles. At this stage, paralysed muscles are flaccid. Later, preservation of muscle power is graded on the 0–5 scale recommended by the Medical Research Council. Familiarity with the myotome arrangements, and with the segmental value of certain key muscles is essential (see Figs 1.22 and 1.23).

The sensory examination records the response to light touch, to pin prick, to vibration, and sense of joint position. Proceeding systematically from the normal to the denervated areas, a zone of hyperaesthesia is usually found. This transitional area is a good guide to the level of the lesion and should be marked with a skin pencil. The sensory examination is not complete without a careful scrutiny of the perineum and sacral area. Appreciation of pin prick over the sacral area or in the perineum is good evidence that the lesion is incomplete. This is of great prognostic significance.

Two cord-mediated reflexes, the bulbocavernous reflex and the anal skin reflex, are usually in abeyance during the stage of spinal shock. This ill-understood state of reflex depression begins to recover within 24 hours of injury, but full reflex automatism may be delayed for many weeks. The return of these reflexes indicates commencing autonomy of the isolated cord.

The bulbocavernous reflex is positive when the anal sphincter or the bulbocavernous muscle can be felt to contract on squeezing the glans penis or the clitoris. The anal skin reflex is elicited by stimulating the perianal skin with a pin; a positive result is indicated by contraction of the external sphincter. The cord lesion is judged complete when there is no sensation or voluntary muscle power below the predetermined level of the injury and when the anal skin and bulbocavernous reflexes are present.

No useful functional recovery may be expected when the paralysis follows immediately after the injury and the signs of a complete lesion remain unchanged for 48 hours. The neurological assessment on admission offers a better prognostic index than the type of bony injury or displacement.

Radiological examination

Preliminary anteroposterior and lateral pictures of suspected areas are essential. It is wise to seek the help of a radiologist when more definite information is required; he can advise on more informative imaging and on the merits of tomography, xeroradiography and other special techniques. Computerised tomography (Fig. 1.41) is especially useful in displaying the spinal canal.

It may be difficult to demonstrate injuries at the cervicothoracic, thoracolumbar and lumbosacral junctional areas. Oblique and posteriorly projected exposures often display unsuspected distortion of the intervertebral foramina and fractures of the laminae, spinous processes, and facet joints (Fig. 3.6).

Standard radiographs of the neck often fail to visualise the odontoid process and the seventh cervical vertebra, injuries which are often missed. Transoral views will display abnormalities at the atlanto-axial level (Fig. 3.7), and sustained traction on the arms will depress the shoulder girdles which often obscure the cervicothoracic junction. Lumbar puncture and myelography are seldom required in the acute stage of injury.

Clinical Course

A complete transverse lesion leads to total motor and sensory paralysis below the level of the cord injury and paralysis of the sphincters. The consequences are less dramatic when the damage is incomplete.

These overt effects should not be regarded as an isolated phenomenon. There are many cardiovascular and metabolic disturbances associated with temporary

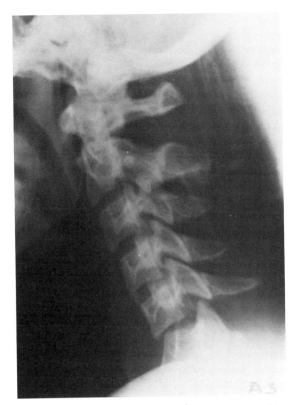

Fig. 3.6 *Lateral view of cervical spine showing unilateral facet dislocation C5 on C6. There is less than half the diameter of the vertebral body displaced forwards: This suggests a unilateral dislocation.*

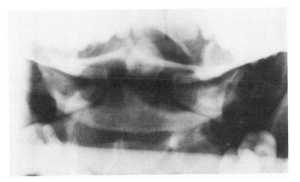

Fig. 3.7 *Transoral radiograph showing displaced fracture through the waist of the odontoid process, an injury destined to non-union. Observe the accompanying subluxation of the atlanto-axial joints.*

imbalance of the autonomic system. The consequences are more marked in complete cervical and upper thoracic lesions, where paralysis of the sympathetic outflow is almost total. They include bradycardia and respiratory depression, hypotension, paralytic ileus, and sodium retention, as well as a number of ill-understood hormonal abnormalities. The autonomic paralysis 'recovers' after a few weeks but, in complete lesions, the fine balance is never regained.

Initially, the paralysis is flaccid; varying degrees of spasticity develop with the return of involuntary muscle tone. The physical signs are then similar to those of an upper motor neurone lesion. The flaccid paralysis may persist when there is extensive longitudinal damage to the anterior columns. The paralysis is of lower motor neurone (flaccid) type in cauda equina lesions, and in isolated nerve root injuries.

Patients who have suffered an incomplete lesion tend to improve slowly, but only a few make a full functional recovery.

Sub-total syndrome

Recovery is often nearly complete when the individual muscle paralysis is partial or otherwise bizarre, and when the initial sensory loss is equivocal.

Central cord syndrome

This is the classical syndrome associated with hyperextension injuries of the neck in older patients. Radiographs of the degenerative cervical spine may show little evidence of a bony injury and a similar situation is encountered in patients with congenital fusions of the vertebrae. As a consequence of the haemorrhage into the grey matter there is a flaccid paresis of the upper limbs and a spastic paresis of the lower limbs. Sphincter control, if lost, is rapidly regained and the lower limbs usually recover. Functional recovery in the hands is often negated by stiffness in the small joints and by the gradual onset of spasticity.

Anterior cord syndrome

Severe compression fractures and axial loading injuries may be accompanied by bony encroachment on the spinal canal and impact damage to the cord. The muscle paralysis is complete, but joint position sense, vibration, and deep-pressure sensations are retained. The prognosis for motor recovery is poor.

Posterior cord syndrome

This may follow any type of spinal injury, notably depressed fractures of the posterior arch. The motor loss may be minimal and deep-pressure sensation as well as proprioception are affected. There is usually some persistent ataxia.

Brown–Séquard syndrome

There is paresis with overlying spasticity on the side of the lesion, with blunting of pain and thermal sensibility on the opposite side. The syndrome is rarely seen in its classical form, but variants occur in high cervical injuries and in open wounds.

Complications

Not many years ago the complications of spinal cord injury included pressure sores, joint contractures, excess spasticity, pathological fractures, and early death from renal failure or amyloid disease. These are minimised in specialist spinal injury centres. To this dreary litany must be added the psychological depression associated with chronic ill-health and social isolation. It is true that some of these complications still occur in neglected or undisciplined patients. A breakdown in domestic arrangements, especially during an intercurrent illness, is probably the commonest cause for emergency readmission to a spinal injury unit.

Treatment

Successful treatment depends upon many factors, notably an understanding of the nature and long-term effects of the injury, and on teamwork and discipline.

General measures

These are particularly applicable to paralysed patients. Respiratory care is essential. Frequent 'chesting' by an experienced physiotherapist will prevent most chest complications and forestall the need for tracheostomy

(Fig. 3.8). One of the essential factors in rehabilitation of these patients, particularly for those who have sustained a complete neurological lesion, is the development of the unparalysed muscles to the highest peak of efficiency, and this is also performed by the physiotherapist.

Gastrointestinal suction is essential in the prevention and treatment of paralytic ileus. Care of the bladder is also essential and aseptic intermittent catheterisation (Fig. 3.9) is the recommended routine. A small silastic

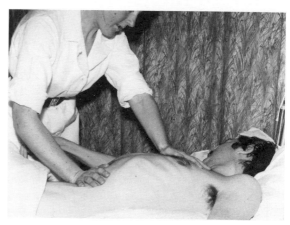

Fig. 3.8 *A physiotherapist must be available round the clock. Manual stabilisation of the lower rib cage and appropriate encouragement will help the patient to cough, and so clear the respiratory passages. Humidification is useful, and a suction apparatus should be to hand. Ward staff and relatives are instructed in respiratory care.*

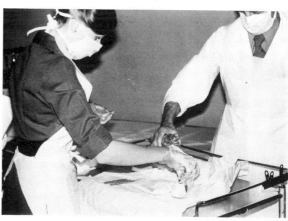

Fig. 3.9 *Intermittent catheterisation requires an aseptic ritual and a full non-touch technique. A disposable silastic catheter is recommended; good lighting and a skilled assistant are essential.*

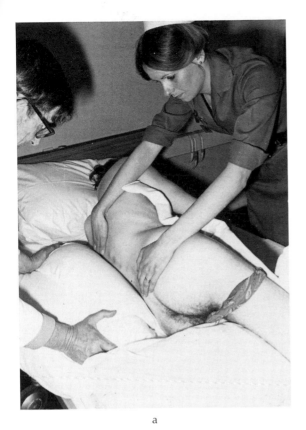

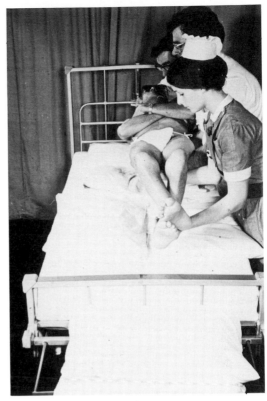

a   b

Fig. 3.10 (a) *A log rolling method is advised for thoracic and lumbar injuries. Cervical injuries are nursed on a mechanical turning bed. (b) At a later stage, the patient may be lifted in one piece. This method is also applicable in the acute phase, when a minimum of four assistants are required.*

catheter is passed, and immediately withdrawn after emptying the bladder. A 6–8-hourly catheterisation routine is then followed until automatic micturition is established.

Care of the skin and joints is critical and the patient should be turned every two hours, manually, by a log-rolling technique (Fig. 3.10) or on a mechanical turning bed. All paralysed joints are put through a full range of passive movement on each turn (Fig. 3.11), and the limbs are pillowed in a functional position.

Cervical spine injury

Minor compression fractures of the vertebral bodies, isolated fractures of the transverse and spinous processes, and hyperextension injuries in older patients are treated by immobilisation in a collar until the pain has disappeared. Dislocations and subluxations must be promptly reduced and then rigidly immobilised. This is facilitated using skull traction via a 'halo' screwed into the diploë of the skull (Fig. 3.12). With the halo attached by uprights to a body cast, the cervical spine is held rigidly while the rest of the body can be mobilised. At three months stability is assessed under radiographic control and fusion is performed if the injury is still unstable.

Thoracic spine injuries

Most of these injuries are stable provided the thoracic cage is intact. They may be treated by postural reduction. Minor compression injuries require immobi-

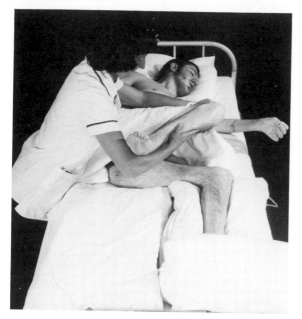

Fig. 3.11 *The paralysed joints are put through a full range of movement every two hours as the patient is turned. Gentleness is essential. Intermittent elevation and compression bandaging of the hand is recommended in cervical injuries. Resistance exercises for the unparalysed muscles are advised at an early stage.*

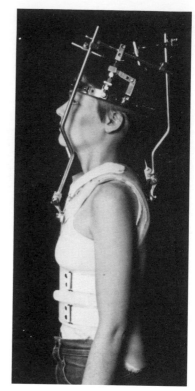

Fig. 3.12 *The halo-vest. The halo is easily applied under local anaesthesia. Four screws hold the halo to the skull. Traction is first applied to reduce the fracture or dislocation. The halo is then attached to a body-vest using uprights so that the fracture is rigidly immobilised while the patient can ambulate.*

lisation until the pain has diminished. More serious injuries usually stabilise after three months' recumbency. Internal fixation is rarely required.

Thoracolumbar injuries

Postural reduction is appropriate for most injuries at this level. Internal fixation using Harrington rods is advisable when satisfactory reduction cannot be achieved or maintained and when there is gross displacement at the site of injury (Fig. 3.13). The spinal cord normally ends at the lower border of the first lumbar vertebra so that, in some of these injuries, the conus and the lumbar and sacral nerve roots may escape serious damage.

Injuries below the second lumbar vertebra

Compression fractures are usually treated conservatively. Fracture–dislocations are best treated by open reduction and internal fixation using Harrington instrumentation.

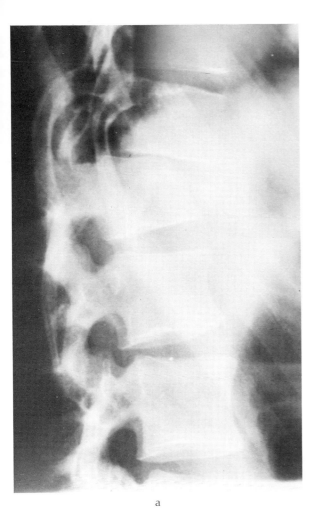

a

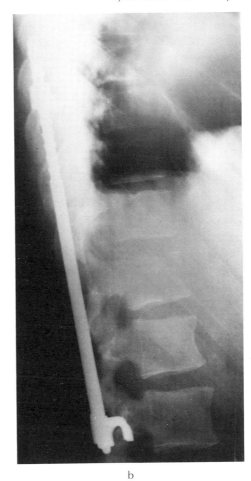

b

Fig. 3.13 (a) *Lateral view of thoraco-lumbar junction showing a fracture–dislocation with significant displacement.* (b) *Lateral view after internal fixation showing reduction.*

4

Injuries of the Upper Limb

An intact and fully functional upper limb is necessary for the purpose of placing the hand in the appropriate position to enable it to perform its vital prehensile activity. Injury to any part of the upper limb impairs this function.

Fractures and dislocations of the upper limb are usually caused by a fall onto the outstretched hand. More severe violence, sustained in road traffic accidents, results in more severe injuries, often with crushing of soft tissues and creation of open wounds with potentially serious complications.

INJURIES OF THE PECTORAL GIRDLE

Fractures of the Clavicle

Mechanism of injury

The clavicle is the only bony strut attaching the upper extremity to the axial skeleton. In a fall on the outstretched hand with the elbow extended, reaction forces from the ground are dissipated by fracturing the mid-shaft of the clavicle. The outer end is fractured much less commonly, by direct violence.

Clinical features and diagnosis

When the clavicle fractures in the middle, gravity causes the remainder of the upper extremity to sag (Fig. 4.1). The medial fragment tents the skin, but only rarely perforates it. The local deformity, pain, and tenderness make the diagnosis easy. The brachial plexus and axillary vessels, which run behind the middle third of the clavicle, are injured only exceptionally.

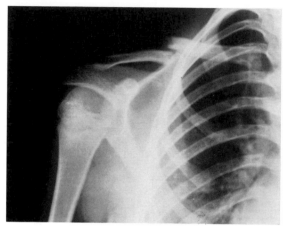

Fig. 4.1 *Anteroposterior radiograph of the shoulder showing a fracture of the mid shaft of the clavicle. The lateral fragment is depressed by the weight of the arm.*

Treatment

The weight of the extremity should be supported in a broad arm sling until local discomfort has subsided. This is the most rapid fracture in the body to unite, and rarely takes as long as three weeks. Slight malunion is inevitable.

Dislocation of the Acromioclavicular Joint

This is caused by the arm being dragged downwards, usually in a contact sport. The conoid and trapezoid ligaments binding the outer clavicle to the scapula are disrupted (Fig. 4.2), and the clavicle and upper extremity drop with gravity, rendering the acromion more prominent.

Treatment is difficult, but a triangular sling is usually

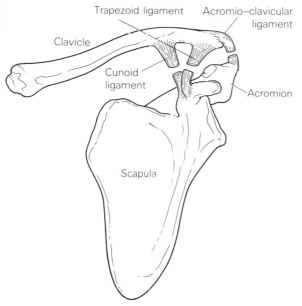

Fig. 4.2 *Diagram showing disruption of the conoid and trapezoid ligaments which allows the arm to sag.*

sufficient to convert a dislocation to a subluxation and thus provide an acceptable long-term result.

Dislocation of the sternoclavicular joint is rare; it follows a forced retraction injury of the shoulder where the sternal end of the clavicle has been levered forward, and is best treated by a sling until symptoms have subsided.

Fractures of the Scapula

These may occur either in the body or the neck. Neck fractures are undisplaced impacted fractures caused by a fall directly onto the shoulder. Fractures of the body of the scapula are caused by direct violence, and the pain, tenderness, swelling and bruising are localised to the supraspinous or infraspinous fossae by firm fascial attachment. Treatment is symptomatic, using a triangular sling.

INJURIES OF THE SHOULDER JOINT

Dislocation of the Shoulder Joint

Anterior dislocation is common; it is caused by a fall on the outstretched hand with the humeral head being levered forwards and (usually) downwards (Fig. 4.3). Inferior dislocations are less common. Posterior dislocations, usually caused by direct violence on the front of the shoulder, are rare.

Clinical features and diagnosis

There is loss of the normal rounded contour of the shoulder, the glenoid fossa is empty on palpation, the humeral head is felt as a separate entity, and the arm is supported by the other hand. Anteroposterior and — more important — lateral radiographs confirm the dislocation and the direction. The circumflex nerve is sometimes stretched by the displaced humeral head, giving rise to deltoid paralysis and hypoaesthesia over the upper outer arm (Fig. 4.4).

Treatment

Anterior and inferior dislocations are best reduced by Kocher's manoeuvre, which involves traction, external rotation, adduction, and internal rotation, in that order. During the phase of adduction, the humeral head is felt to slip back into the glenoid. This should be performed under general anaesthesia to allow muscle relaxation, but in the elderly it can often be accomplished under sedation alone. Posterior dislocations are difficult to stabilise and require careful radiographic control.

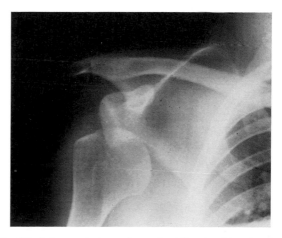

Fig. 4.3 *Anteroposterior radiograph of the shoulder showing the common antero-inferior dislocation.*

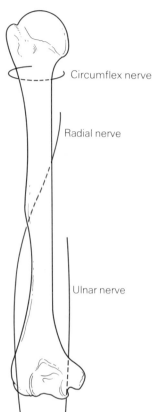

Fig. 4.4 *The humerus has three important nerves close to it. Nearby fractures may damage them.*

Circumflex nerve

Radial nerve

Ulnar nerve

After reduction, the arm is rested in a triangular sling under the clothes for three weeks before active exercises are commenced.

Recurrent Dislocation

Anterior muscular support of the shoulder is weakened by acute anterior dislocation, thus providing a potential space for future dislocation without trauma. This is very common in young adults, and may happen every time the arm is abducted and externally rotated. Reduction by manipulation is easy and can often be accomplished by the patient himself. Treatment of this problem is by surgery to tighten the subscapularis muscle anteriorly (the Putti–Platt procedure) so that the potential space is

eliminated. In the elderly, recurrent dislocation does not occur because the initial dislocation is accompanied either by a capsular tear, which then heals, or by a fracture of the greater tuberosity of the humerus, which then unites.

FRACTURES OF THE HUMERUS

Fractures of the Surgical Neck

These are caused by a fall on the outstretched hand, and are generally undisplaced and impacted. Reduction of displaced fractures is not necessary. Displacement in the young is corrected by bone remodelling; in the elderly patient, restoration of shoulder movement takes priority. Treatment is therefore the same for all patients, i.e. a triangular sling until symptoms have subsided, followed by active exercises.

Fractures of the Shaft

These usually occur in adults from direct violence (Fig. 4.5). Local pain, tenderness, deformity and movement indicate the diagnosis. Involvement of the radial nerve, either initially or later with callus formation, is common, and extensor weakness or a complete wrist drop are frequent. Treatment is by placing the arm in a collar and cuff; when correctly aligned, traction is supplied by gravity. A plaster U-slab is also applied for protection and to add weight. Union often takes 8–10 weeks.

Supracondylar Fractures

These nearly always occur in children and are caused by a fall on the outstretched hand with the elbow flexed so that the lower humerus, elbow and forearm are driven backwards (Fig. 4.6, p. 72). Displacement is often considerable and gross local swelling and extreme tenderness are typical. The brachial artery is frequently compressed and occasionally torn, so that reduction is an absolute emergency if the radial pulse is absent. The median nerve is also commonly involved, giving weakness of finger flexion and diminution in sensation

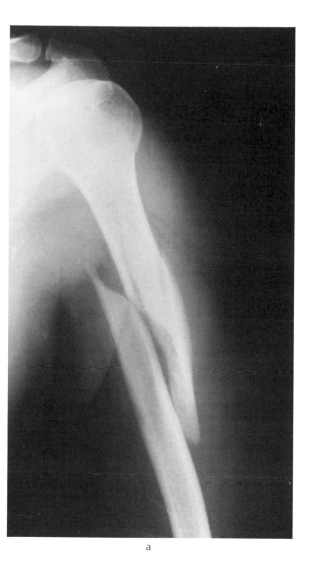

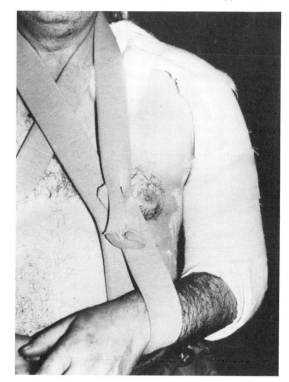

b

a

Fig. 4.5 (a) *Anteroposterior radiograph showing fracture of the humeral shaft.* (b) *Arm with a U-slab and collar and cuff.*

over the lateral three and a half digits on their palmar aspect.

Treatment is by traction and flexion under general anaesthesia. Flexion tightens up the triceps muscle and tendon posteriorly, which stabilises the reduction position. The radial pulse must be palpated immediately after reduction to check on vascular continuity. If the pulse is absent, the elbow must be explored and the brachial artery decompressed or repaired as necessary. After reduction, the arm is immobilised in a collar and cuff; union occurs in three weeks.

Persistent loss of blood supply distally gives rise to Volkmann's ischaemic contracture of the forearm muscles. The muscles are replaced by non-elastic fibrous tissue, causing a contracture of the wrist and fingers (Fig. 8.3). Malunion often occurs with these fractures, giving rise to an ugly varus deformity.

Fracture of the Medial Epicondyle

This is also a fracture occurring in children. Avulsion of a piece of bone at the origin of the flexor forearm muscles occurs when there is a fall on the outstretched

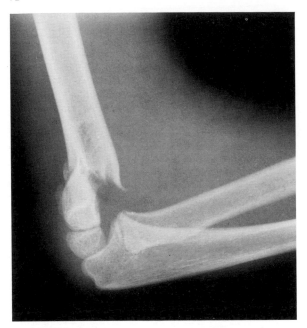

Fig. 4.6 *Lateral radiograph of the elbow showing a supra-condylar fracture.*

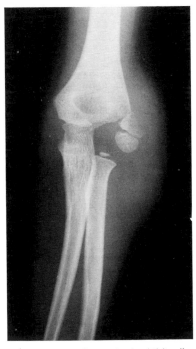

Fig. 4.7 *Anteroposterior radiograph of a child's elbow showing a displaced fracture of the lateral condyle.*

hand and a valgus stress at the elbow. Reduction is usually unnecessary and union occurs rapidly within three weeks while the arm is rested symptomatically in a collar and cuff. Sometimes the medial epicondyle is trapped inside the joint and must be replaced surgically. The ulnar nerve runs directly behind the medial epicondyle and may suffer a compression neurapraxia, giving painful paraesthesia localised to the ulnar one-and-a-half fingers.

Fractures of the Lateral Condyle

Again occurring in children, these injuries (Fig. 4.7) are very important. They occur as a result of a fall on the outstretched hand with a varus stress at the elbow. There is local bony tenderness and swelling, and movement of the elbow joint is restricted by pain. This is an epiphyseal injury, and any displacement must therefore be detected so that no growth asymmetry results. Radiographs should be compared with the normal side. These fractures must always be openly reduced and internally fixed, because they have a high rate of nonunion, and malunion with a valgus deformity is a frequent occurrence.

Condylar Fractures in Adults

These are caused by direct violence on the point of the elbow as a result of a fall. There is local bony tenderness and a restricted range of elbow movement. Radiographs frequently reveal severe comminution but the most usual pattern is a T-shaped fracture involving both condyles. A good reduction is frequently achieved by traction and flexion, but internal fixation is often necessary. Elbow movements should be commenced as early as possible to minimise the residual joint stiffness so common with elbow injuries.

INJURIES OF THE ELBOW REGION

Dislocation of the Elbow Joint

This occurs in both adults and children and is caused by a fall on the outstretched hand with the elbow flexed

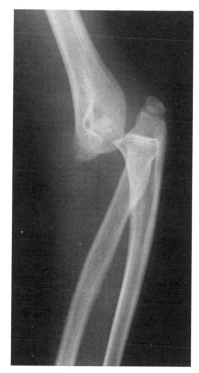

Fig. 4.8 *Lateral radiograph showing a dislocation of the elbow joint.*

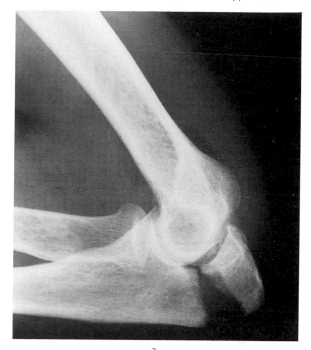

a

and the forearm pronated (Fig. 4.8). The elbow is held flexed, with local pain and swelling, and the olecranon is unduly prominent posteriorly. The injury is best shown on a lateral radiograph, which sometimes also shows a chip fracture of the coronoid process pushed off by the lower humerus. Closed reduction by traction and rest in a collar and cuff for no more than three weeks is followed by active exercises.

Fractures of the Olecranon

These occur in adults, either from a direct blow to the posterior aspect of the elbow or, more commonly, from a fall onto the outstretched hand with the elbow semi-flexed, when the sudden contraction of triceps avulses a large fragment (Fig. 4.9). The fracture is inevitably displaced by the pull of the triceps muscle and therefore a step is palpable along the upper subcutaneous posterior border of the ulna. The fracture always passes into the elbow joint and an anatomical reduction is essential. This can only be achieved by

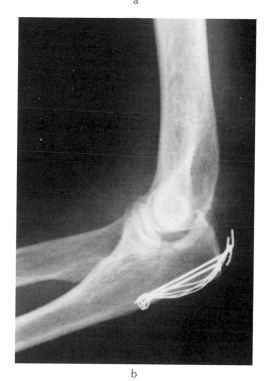

b

Fig. 4.9 (a) *Lateral radiograph of the elbow showing a fracture of the olecranon.* (b) *Internal fixation is necessary to counteract the pull of the triceps.*

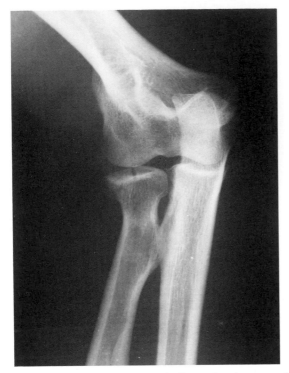

Fig. 4.10 *Anteroposterior view of elbow showing a crack fracture of the radial head.*

open reduction and internal fixation. The elbow is then rested in a collar and cuff for not more than three weeks, when active exercises are commenced.

Fractures of the Head of the Radius

These occur in adults when a fall on the outstretched hand impacts the radial head against the capitellum (Fig. 4.10). Tenderness is felt, particularly posterolaterally over the radial head. Pronation and supination are limited by local discomfort. Radiographs sometimes demonstrate a crack fracture but not displacement; oblique views are sometimes necessary to show this. Treatment is then by rest to the elbow in a collar and cuff until symptoms resolve, usually within two weeks. More usually, however, radiographs demonstrate significant displacement or comminution, in which case the injury is irreparable. Fortunately the radial head plays little part in elbow function and treatment is by radial head excision.

Fractures of the Neck of the Radius

These injuries occur in children by the same mechanism as fractures of the radial head. Displacement is usually minimal but if the angulation exceeds 30° this is beyond the scope of bone remodelling and the deformity is corrected by open reduction and internal fixation using a Kirschner wire. On no account should the radial head be removed in children, for the resulting growth asymmetry will inevitably lead to deformity.

Myositis Ossificans

Elbow injuries are particularly prone to progressive local ossification of soft tissues. Complete stiffness of the elbow may occur as this heterotopic bone matures. Treatment is by resting the elbow in a collar and cuff until reabsorption takes place, which may be several months. Persistent mature bone causing a mechanical block should then be removed.

FRACTURES OF THE FOREARM

Fractures of the Shaft, Radius and Ulna

These occur commonly in both children and adults. They are usually caused by a fall on the outstretched hand, but sometimes occur by direct violence. In children these injuries are frequently angulated but seldom displaced, since the periosteum is intact on one side. Accordingly reduction by closed traction and manipulation is usually successful.

Fractures in adults are nearly always displaced (Fig. 4.11), and reduction by closed means is particularly difficult. Nonetheless, this should be attempted in the first instance by a combination of traction and manipulation. The forearm may need supination or pronation, depending on whether the fractures are distal or proximal. Only an anatomical reduction can be accepted, since any angulation or displacement will lead to malunion, with a mechanical block to full forearm rotation.

Cross-union occasionally takes place between radius and ulna, causing complete loss of forearm rotation.

Open reduction and internal fixation with plates and screws is therefore more commonly needed. Children require immobilisation in an above-elbow cast, with the elbow at a right angle, for only three weeks. Adults usually require immobilisation for up to eight weeks before there is radiological evidence of union.

The Monteggia and Galeazzi Fractures

An undisplaced fracture of the shaft of the radius or ulna may occur in isolation; if there is displacement, however, a dislocation of the other bone must occur either at the elbow or wrist (Fig. 4.12). This is because displacement implies shortening, and the elbow and wrist are thereby approximated while the intact bone maintains its length and thus dislocates. A fracture of the proximal ulna with dislocation of the radial head is called a Monteggia fracture, while a fracture of the distal radius with dislocation of the ulnar head is called a Galeazzi fracture. In children, reduction is possible by closed means due to the intact periosteal hinge; in adults, open reduction and internal fixation of the fracture with a plate and screws is essential. When the fracture is accurately reduced, the dislocation corrects spontaneously.

FRACTURES OF THE LOWER END OF THE RADIUS

The Colles' Fracture

This is the fracture most often seen in clinical practice. It is defined as a fracture of the lower end of the radius within one and a half inches (4 cm) of the wrist joint, which is both displaced and angulated in a dorsal direction (Fig. 4.13, p. 77). It occurs from a fall on the outstretched hand and, in the majority of cases, it is pathological, occurring in the osteoporotic wrist of the elderly. The deformity, when viewed from the side, has been likened to a dinner fork. Treatment, always by closed means, comprises traction to disimpact the fragments, flexion and ulnar deviation to correct the deformity, and pronation to stabilise the reduction position. A below-elbow cast is then applied, which

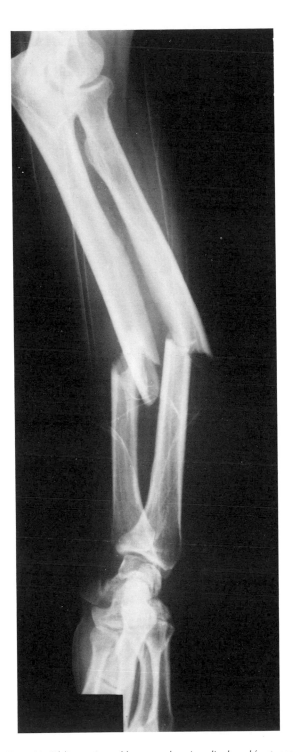

Fig. 4.11 *Oblique view of forearm showing displaced fractures of the mid shaft of both bones of the forearm.*

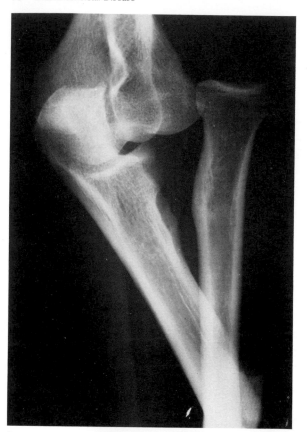

a

should allow full finger and elbow movement, and is retained for not more than six weeks.

Complications are common, including finger and shoulder stiffness which should be minimised by active movements while the forearm is in plaster. One-third of cases go on to malunion, due to an inadequate initial reduction or loss of position within the cast, leaving an ugly deformity. Delayed rupture of the long extensor tendon of the thumb occasionally occurs, due to attrition over the fracture site.

Smith's Fracture

This is the reverse of a Colles' fracture, and occurs by a fall onto the hand tending to flex the lower radius. Reduction, achieved by closed means, comprises traction and extension. The reduction position, which is less stable than with a Colles' fracture, requires an above-elbow cast with the elbow at a right angle. Again, joint stiffness is a common complication and movements of the shoulder and fingers should be commenced immediately.

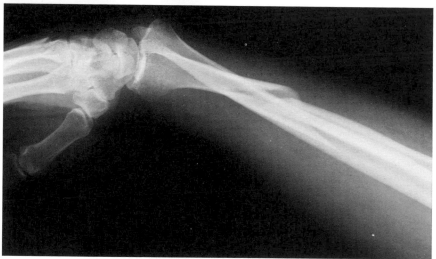

b

Fig. 4.12 (a) *Monteggia fracture–dislocation; anteroposterior view of elbow showing a displaced fracture of the proximal ulnar shaft with anterior dislocation of the radial head.* (b) *Galeazzi fracture–dislocation; lateral view of wrist showing a displaced fracture of the lower radius with dorsal dislocation of the ulnar head.*

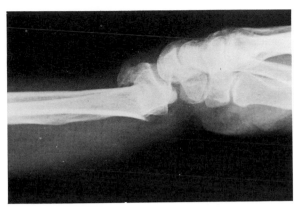

Fig. 4.13 *Lateral radiograph of the wrist showing a fracture of the lower end of the radius, with dorsal displacement and angulation—a Colles' fracture.*

Intra-articular Fractures of the Lower End of the Radius

The mechanism of injury is the same as that producing a Colles' or Smith's fracture, but the forces are dissipated more distally and the fracture involves the wrist joint. Displacement is caused by the wrist subluxating dorsally (Barton's fracture, Fig. 4.14) or anteriorly. Treatment is by traction and manipulation, but these fractures are unstable and always require an above-elbow cast. Often, the reduction position is lost and internal fixation with a plate and screws is

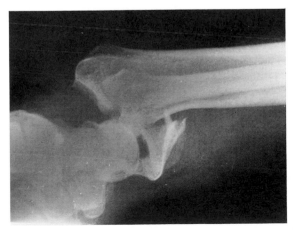

Fig. 4.14 *Lateral radiograph of the wrist showing a fracture of the articular surface of the radius with subluxation of the carpus—Barton's fracture.*

necessary, but because this is an intra-articular injury, there is frequently residual local discomfort and limited wrist movement.

Fractures of the Lower End of the Radius in Children.

Greenstick fractures of the lower end of the radius are common in children as a result of a fall on the outstretched hand. They usually occur about one inch above the wrist joint, with little or no displacement. Such fractures can easily be managed by a protective below-elbow cast and union occurs within three weeks. The occasional significantly-displaced fracture is often difficult to reduce, and should be immobilised in an above-elbow cast with the elbow at a right angle for four weeks.

In adolescence, a separation of the distal radial epiphysis is common. The fracture line passes through the majority of the epiphyseal plate and then takes off a small fragment of the metaphysis (Fig. 2.2b). This fracture is usually displaced in the same fashion as a Colles' fracture, and is reduced similarly without difficulty.

CARPAL INJURIES

Scaphoid Fractures

These are by far the most common injuries to the carpus and are caused by forced hyperextension of the wrist, as the result of a fall on the outstretched hand, or by a force imparted to the first interdigital cleft by a motorcycle handlebar or by the violent kick-back of a crank handle. Tenderness localised to the anatomical snuffbox is diagnostic. Wrist joint movement is restricted, particularly radial and ulnar deviation. Special radiographs of the wrist are required to demonstrate the fracture; four views are traditionally taken – anteroposterior, lateral, semipronated and semisupinated. The lateral view is scrutinised to exclude an associated carpal dislocation, but the fracture itself is best visualised on the anteroposterior or semipronated views, when the scaphoid bone is seen *en face* (Fig. 4.15).

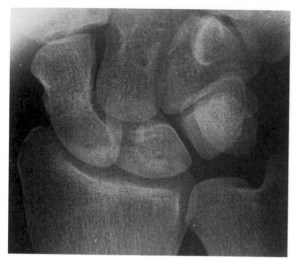

Fig. 4.15 *Anteroposterior view of a transverse fracture of the waist of the scaphoid.*

Fractures may occur through the distal pole, the waist, or the proximal pole. These fractures are rarely displaced, and in any event cannot be reduced by closed means. A below-elbow cast including the thumb is applied until the fracture unites, which may be anything from six to twelve weeks.

The blood supply of the scaphoid resembles that of

the femoral head in direction, passing from distal to proximal. Accordingly, fractures of the distal pole unite without complications but 5% of fractures of the waist and proximal pole fail to unite due to avascular necrosis of the proximal fragment. This is visible radiographically as increased radiodensity, frequently with cystic change. Treatment is by a bone-grafting operation.

Carpal Dislocations

These are usually in the nature of a perilunar dislocation of the carpus or a dislocated lunate bone (Fig. 4.16). Both occur from a fall on the outstretched hand, and the condition usually affects young adults. With a perilunar dislocation of the carpus, the lunate stays in position, articulating with the lower end of the radius, while the capitate and the rest of the wrist and hand dislocate dorsally. The deformity resembles that of a Colles' fracture at the level of the wrist joint. The diagnosis is confirmed radiographically; on the antero-posterior view there is overlap of the proximal and distal row of the carpal bones. The lateral view more clearly demonstrates the dislocation. By traction and extension under anaesthesia the capitate is relocated

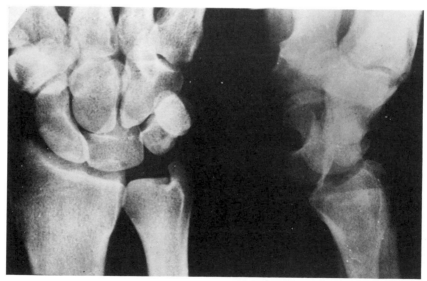

Fig. 4.16 *Anteroposterior and lateral radiographs of the wrist showing a dislocated lunate. The AP view shows carpal overlap (always abnormal). The lateral view shows the lunate turned 90° and lying anteriorly.*

onto the lunate, and a below-elbow plaster is then applied for four weeks.

Sometimes the perilunar dislocation of the carpus moves from its dorsal position back into alignment with the radius and, in the process, pushes the lunate bone anteriorly off the lower end of the radius. The capitate then articulates with the lower radius. The median nerve is often compressed over the displaced lunate, with hypoaesthesia across the palmar aspect of the lateral three-and-a-half digits of the hand. Treatment is by closed manipulation, pushing the capitate backwards off the radius and allowing the lunate bone to be repositioned. Further reduction is then carried out as for a perilunar dislocation of the carpus. These dislocations may disrupt the blood supply to the lunate bone, and avascular necrosis with sclerosis and fragmentation is common. Sometimes these dislocations are accompanied by a displaced fracture to the waist of the scaphoid which, after closed manipulation, must be treated by open operation, the scaphoid fragments being held anatomically by a screw.

FRACTURES OF THE HAND

Fractures of the Metacarpals

These are common and occur as a result of direct violence either applied transversely or in the long axis of the bones. They fall into four main groups: fractures of the base, both transverse and spiral fractures of the shaft; and fractures of the neck. There is localised tenderness and swelling, with limited movement of the joints of the digital ray involved. They are readily visible radiographically (Fig. 4.17).

Fractures at the base are usually stable and only symptomatic treatment is necessary. Union occurs within two to three weeks. Transverse and spiral fractures of the shaft are frequently displaced, and the rotational alignment of the fragments must be accurate otherwise the finger may overlap its neighbour during flexion. The majority can be reduced by traction with the metacarpophalangeal joint flexed, and the hand can be immobilised in that position using a 'boxing glove' bandage, which is also of great symptomatic value as there is usually considerable swelling and contusion. If reduction cannot be achieved by closed

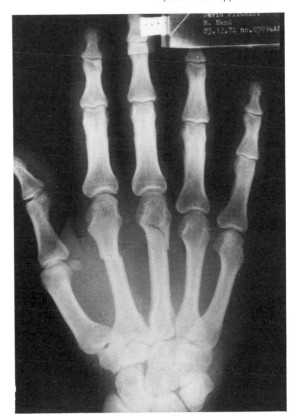

Fig. 4.17 *Anteroposterior radiograph of the hand showing a transverse fracture of the second metacarpal and a spiral fracture of the third.*

means, open reduction is indicated, with fixation by a Kirschner wire or a small plate and screws.

Fractures of the neck are flexion injuries often caused by punching. Although there is usually anterior angulation, they are stable due to the impaction of the injury mechanism and unite with little deformity in three weeks.

Bennett's Fracture–Subluxation

This is a fracture of the base of the first metacarpal with dorsoradial subluxation of the carpometacarpal joint (Fig. 4.18). It is caused by a force on the radial side of the hand with the thumb adducted. The fracture is easily reduced by traction and abduction of the thumb metacarpal, and should be immobilised in this position in a scaphoid plaster for three weeks. The position is

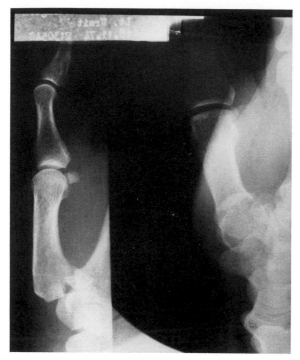

Fig. 4.18 *Anteroposterior and lateral radiographs of the thumb showing a Bennett's fracture–subluxation.*

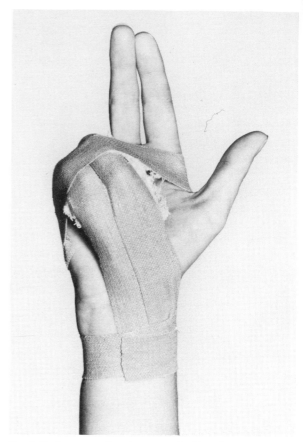

Fig. 4.19 *Fracture splinted over a roll of bandage.*

difficult to maintain, however, and sometimes requires internal fixation with a Kirschner wire before application of the cast.

Fractures of the Phalanges

These are the result of direct injury and may occur in any part of the bone. Local swelling and tenderness render the diagnosis simple and radiographs clearly show the fracture. Treatment depends upon the stability of the fracture. Stable fractures require only symptomatic treatment with the finger strapped to its neighbour for support until symptoms subside, when active mobilisation is commenced.

Unstable fractures require stabilisation in flexion, and the finger can be conveniently taped in the flexed position over a roll of bandage (Fig. 4.19). Fractures involving the condyles are difficult both to reduce and to hold reduced by closed means. Internal fixation is necessary, using a Kirschner wire or small cancellous

screw. With marked comminution, closed treatment should be followed by the earliest possible mobilisation. To minimise joint stiffness, it is essential to mobilise hand fractures as soon as symptoms will allow.

Dislocations

These may occur at any joint in the hand, and are usually caused by an axial force, as when a cricket ball strikes the end of a finger. The dislocation is nearly always dorsal, with the head of the bone riding anteriorly and distally. Reduction, which is easily achieved by traction and manipulation, is often performed on the sports field by the patient or a physiotherapist. There is occasionally a soft-tissue obstruction to reduction, requiring open operation. Instability after reduction is a sign of a concomitant ligamentous tear; the joint should be opened and the ligament repaired surgically.

TENDON INJURIES

These often occur at the level of the wrist, hand and fingers, and may be the direct result of a laceration or indirect by way of avulsion.

Extensor Tendon Injuries

Lacerations of the dorsum of the hand and wrist may be complicated by an injury to the extensor tendons. This may occur spontaneously, due to synovial infiltration, in rheumatoid patients. The finger immediately adopts the semiflexed position and the affected digit cannot be actively extended (Fig. 4.20). Simple primary repair of the tendon, followed by splintage in extension to relieve tension on the suture line for three weeks, gives excellent results.

There are two common closed ruptures of extensor tendons as a result of avulsion, usually caused by stubbing the finger (Fig. 4.21). The extensor tendon of a finger passes across the dorsum of the metacarpopha-

langeal joint, where it divides into three bands. The central slip is inserted into the base of the middle phalanx, thus extending the proximal interphalangeal (PIP) joint. The two lateral bands pass distally, to be inserted into the base of the terminal phalanx, thus extending the distal interphalangeal (DIP) joint.

Rupture of the central slip of the extensor apparatus over the PIP joint leads to a Boutonnière deformity. The PIP joint is held semiflexed and there is loss of active extension. There is concomitant hyperextension of the DIP joint as the lateral bands now pass dorsal to its axis of movement. Rupture of the extensor apparatus over the dorsum of the DIP joint gives rise to a mallet finger deformity. Here there is flexion of the DIP joint, with loss of active extension.

Both are treated by holding the affected joint in extension by small plastic splints. Occasionally a small fragment of bone is avulsed at the insertion of the tendon and this can be replaced openly using a small pin.

Flexor Tendon Injuries

Injuries to flexor tendons are much more disabling because of the presence of the fibrous flexor sheath,

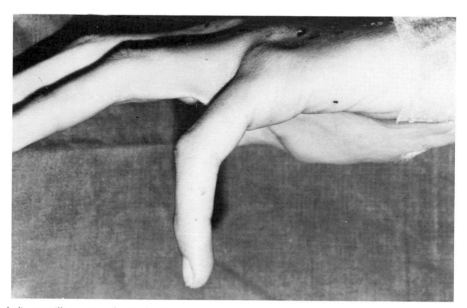

Fig. 4.20 *The little finger will not extend actively. The extensor tendon is therefore damaged.*

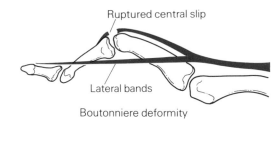

Ruptured central slip

Lateral bands

Boutonniere deformity

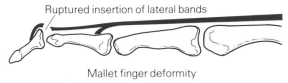

Ruptured insertion of lateral bands

Mallet finger deformity

Fig. 4.21 *Diagram to show Boutonnière and mallet finger deformities.*

which extends from the distal palmar crease to the distal interphalangeal joint of each digit. The profundus and sublimis tendons to each finger are buffered from the indirect trauma of hand function by this sheath but, when they are divided, adhesions occur between tendon and sheath which severely compromise active flexion. The site of the flexor tendon injury thus has great prognostic significance.

There are five zones (Fig. 4.22), of which zone 2, the area of the fibrous flexor sheath, is associated with the worst prognosis. Indeed until recently this zone was referred to as 'no man's land', because direct surgical repair was not recommended and treatment consisted of removing the tendon and substituting a graft to minimise adhesion formation.

Surgical techniques have improved over the past fifteen years, and flexor tendon injuries can be dealt with by primary repair, even though the results in zone 2 are less satisfactory.

HAND INFECTIONS

The palmar aspect of the hand and fingers is a working surface whose integument is frequently penetrated. Hand infections are therefore common and, unless the diagnosis is made early and followed by the appropriate treatment, may have a serious outcome. All but the most trivial hand injuries show the cardinal signs of

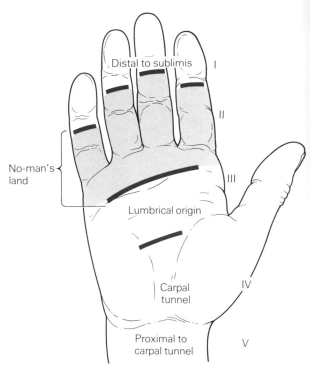

Distal to sublimis   I

II

No-man's land

III

Lumbrical origin

Carpal tunnel   IV

Proximal to carpal tunnel   V

Fig. 4.22 *The five zones of flexor tendon injuries in the hand. Zone II is associated with a bad prognosis and is referred to as 'no-man's land'.*

inflammation tenderness, redness, increased warmth, loss of function, and swelling. The site of maximum swelling is misleadingly on the dorsum of the hand, where venous and lymphatic drainage is directed. The precise location of the infection must be accurately established by careful clinical scrutiny, which includes defining the precise site of maximal tenderness, determination of range of joint movement, and inspection of the lymphatic drainage. In this way the prognosis and potential for spread can be assessed.

Infections of the Digits

Paronychia

This infection commences under the nail fold, often on one side, and then extends under the nail as a subungual abscess. At this stage there is intense pain on nail compression. Pus then tracks to one side of the nail (Fig. 4.23), producing local granulations.

surrounded by loose fibro-fatty tissue. Tenderness and redness are greatest over the web, but the greatest swelling is dorsal, and the digits on either side characteristically move apart (Fig. 4.24). The web spaces communicate distally with the proximal pulp space and proximally with the midpalmar space; in severe or untreated cases, all three areas may be involved.

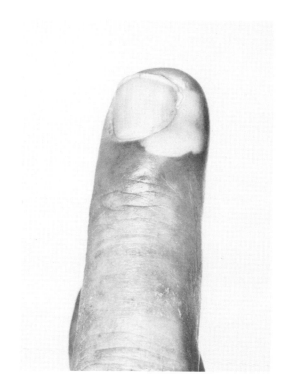

Fig. 4.23 *Paronychia—infection beneath the eponychium points to one side.*

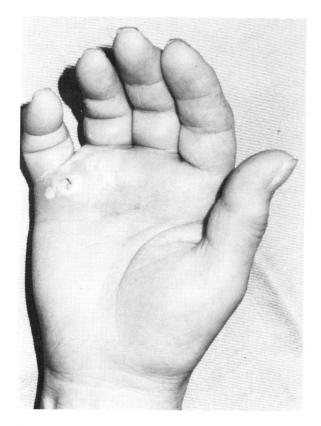

Fig. 4.24 *A web space infection—the adjacent fingers are separated and flexed while pus is pointing in the web.*

Pulp space infection

The palmar aspect of each finger is divided into three segments by skin creases which firmly bind the skin to the deep fascia. The pulp of the distal segment is a completely closed space; infection here gives rise to intense local discomfort and throbbing, particularly at night. The pressure within the pulp may be so severe as to compromise the local arterial supply, giving rise to skin necrosis or even gangrene. The middle space is less confined and the signs of local inflammation are less intense. The proximal space communicates with the adjacent web space, the latter often being involved before the diagnosis is made.

Web space infection

Web spaces lie between the bases of each digit, where the palmar aponeurosis splits into bands passing to the sides of each digit. They contain the neurovascular bundles and the tendons of the intrinsic muscles,

Palmar infections

A deep fibrous septum passes dorsally from the palmar aponeurosis to the third metacarpal, dividing the palm into the thenar space on the radial side and the midpalmar space on the ulnar side (Fig. 4.25). Each space is bounded anteriorly by the flexor tendons and dorsally by the interosseus muscles. Infection occurs either as a result of a penetrating palmar wound or by spread from an adjacent web space. There is intense

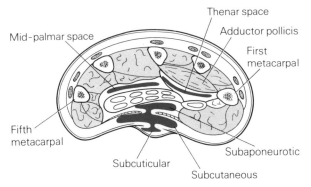

Fig. 4.25 *Cross-sectional diagram of the palm, showing spaces where pus collects.*

local discomfort and often a constitutional reaction. The site of maximum tenderness is directly over the space involved, but again the maximum swelling is dorsal. The fingers whose flexor tendons overlie the space adopt a semiflexed position. With increasing pressure, the abscess may burst through the aponeurosis, giving rise to a collar-stud extension.

Acute suppurative tenosynovitis

This is a very severe condition, involving infection of the synovial sheaths of the flexor tendons. Only the earliest cases, given the most vigorous treatment, escape some limitation of movement. There is usually a penetrating wound at the level of the distal palmar crease, where the mouth of the fibrous flexor sheath is subcutaneous. Infection spreads throughout the sheath, the finger adopts a semiflexed position at all joints (Fig. 4.26), and there is redness and swelling throughout the length of the palmar aspect of the digit involved. Tenderness is greatest over the proximal mouth of the fibrous flexor sheath, and the slightest passive extension of any of the joints gives rise to intense local discomfort.

Principles of Treating Hand Infections

Occasionally, in very early cases, the infective process can be aborted by antibiotic treatment. The great majority of hand infections are caused by staphylococcus, and a combination of penicillin and cloxacillin is most appropriate. If pus is present, however, or if there is evidence of local spread or a constitutional reaction,

the patient must be placed in a hospital. The pus is drained, either over the site of maximal tenderness or directly over where the collection is pointing. The hand is then splinted and elevated in order to reduce inflammation and swelling, and the above antibiotics are prescribed. The position of safety should be adopted for hand splintage, i.e. with the metacarpophalangeal joints flexed and the interphalangeal joints extended. In this position the collateral ligaments are maximally extended so that there is little danger of permanent stiffness as long as the hand is not immobilised for more than three weeks.

Tendon sheath infection requires special treatment. The proximal and distal ends of the sheath are opened so that a small catheter can be passed through, and the sheath is irrigated with saline impregnated with antibiotic.

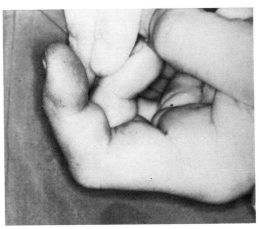

Fig. 4.26 *Acute suppurative tenosynovitis—the finger is held flexed and any passive extension is vigorously opposed due to excruciating pain.*

5

Injuries of the Lower Limb

FRACTURES OF THE PELVIS

Mechanism

The bony pelvis not only protects the organs contained within it but is also a main weight-bearing structure. Its strength is therefore considerable, and great force is required to injure it. Fractures occur either from a fall from a height, or in a road traffic accident, or when the pelvis is crushed between two rigid structures. In elderly people with osteoporosis or osteomalacia, a minor fall is a common cause of a pelvic fracture.

Diagnosis

The patient may be in severe pain and is unable to bear weight on the pelvis. There is seldom marked swelling or bruising initially, and crepitus is only felt if the superficial parts of the ilium are fractured. Hip movements may be restricted due to irritation of the muscles crossing the pelvis, but the most important sign is pain on pelvic compression (Fig. 5.1).

Considerable swelling may develop over the next few days, and bruising tracks along fascial planes appearing in the buttock, thigh and perineum, and spreads up the posterior aspect of the lumbar region.

Complications

Massive haemorrhage

This results from tearing of the thin-walled intrapelvic

veins; it may be difficult to control, and often presents a life-threatening emergency. Such a patient is shocked and requires adequate and rapid blood replacement

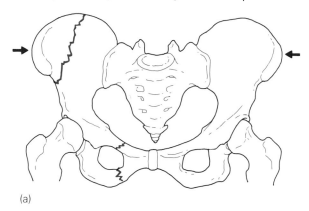

(a)

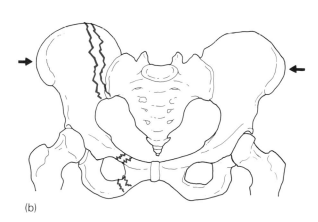

(b)

Fig. 5.1 *Pain on pelvic compression is diagnostic of a pelvic fracture. (a) A stable fracture—the ring is broken in only one place. (b) An unstable fracture—the ring is broken in two places.*

while the pulse, blood pressure, and central venous pressure are monitored.

Injuries to the bladder and urethra

These are common and can present difficulties in diagnosis. Blood at the external urethral meatus, together with inability to pass urine, is a cardinal sign of urethral injury. Absence of a palpable bladder, with evidence of suprapubic tissue extravasation, indicates rupture of the bladder. An intravenous pyelogram should be performed and, if the bladder is palpable, it is advisable to insert a suprapubic catheter. Alternatively a small soft urethral catheter may be inserted, although this has a danger of causing further damage to the urethral epithelium. Surgical repair is the definitive treatment.

Injuries to the rectum and vagina

These are rare. The diagnosis is suggested by fresh bleeding. Treatment is by primary repair and, in the case of the rectum, a defunctioning colostomy is additionally performed.

Injuries to the sciatic nerve

These are not common. Occasionally the nerve is trapped between fracture fragments, but the need for exploration is unusual. Recovery occurs very slowly, and there is usually a considerable persistent neurological deficit.

Treatment

If the fracture is stable, bed-rest and analgesics until symptoms subside are all that is required. If there is displacement with instability, reduction is carried out by skeletal traction through the femur and is maintained until union has occurred. The use of external fixation devices allows primary reduction to be achieved, and rigid stabilisation permits greater comfort and much earlier mobilisation (Fig. 5.2). This method has largely superseded the use of pelvic slings.

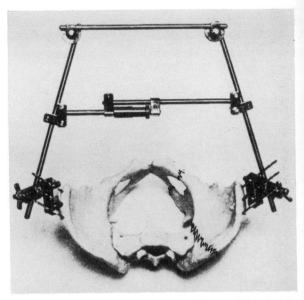

Fig. 5.2 *An unstable pelvic fracture rigidly immobilised in the reduced position by means of external fixation.*

DISLOCATIONS AND FRACTURE-DISLOCATIONS OF THE HIP

Mechanisms

The hip joint is a strong and stable joint; injury results from considerable violence, often in road traffic accidents. The motorcyclist or unrestrained car occupant is particularly at risk when the knee is driven back with the hip flexed, producing a posterior dislocation (Fig. 5.3). Depending on the degree of flexion of the hip there may be an additional fracture of the head of the femur or acetabulum.

The more unusual anterior dislocation occurs through forcible external rotation and abduction, again after major violence. The rare central fracture dislocation results from a violent blow to the side, which often produces major damage to the pelvis.

Clinical Features and Diagnosis

A posterior dislocation produces the characteristic appearance of flexion, adduction, internal rotation and

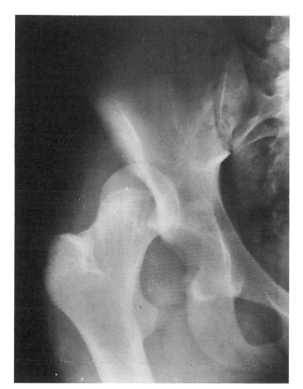

Fig. 5.3 *Anteroposterior x-ray of the hip showing a posterior dislocation.*

shortening of the limb (Fig. 1.9). There is considerable pain and complete loss of function of the limb. Fracture-dislocations produce a similar clinical appearance, but may be very unstable after reduction. The acetabulum is formed from a strong roof with an anterior iliopubic column of bone and posterior ilio-ischial column. A careful radiographic assessment, including anteroposterior, lateral, and oblique films, is necessary to determine stability.

Complications

The most important problem is failure to obtain a satisfactory reduction; incongruity of the articular surfaces will inevitably lead to early osteoarthritis. Nevertheless, provided that the main weight-bearing acetabular dome is intact, surprisingly good function may remain for many years. Injury to the superior gluteal and sciatic nerves is common.

Treatment

Closed reduction is carried out under general anaesthesia with complete muscle relaxation, and considerable force may be necessary. Traction is then maintained for two weeks for dislocations, and up to eight weeks when associated with fractures, followed by a period of protected weight-bearing. If reduction is not concentric, or if gross instability persists, open reduction and internal fixation is carried out.

FRACTURES OF THE NECK OF THE FEMUR

Mechanism

More than 30 000 such fractures occur each year, and the incidence is increasing. They are usually pathological fractures occurring after trivial falls and are largely due to osteoporosis of the ageing skeleton, although up to 60% may be associated with osteomalacia. Fatigue fractures may have occurred before the actual fall, or a fracture may pass through a metastatic deposit.

In younger patients, the neck of the femur may (unusually) be fractured after major violence, and this also happens, rarely, in children. There are two main types of fracture, intracapsular and trochanteric, which are clinically indistinguishable.

Clinical Features and Diagnosis

The patient presents with local pain, restricted movement and inability to bear weight on the leg. When displaced, there is a characteristic shortening and external rotation (Fig. 1.9).

Radiographs confirm the diagnosis and locate the site and displacement (Fig. 5.4). If there is any doubt, the patient should be treated on the basis of the clinical features and confined to bed. Further radiographs, or a radio-isotope bone scan, can be obtained in a few days, when the fracture becomes more obvious.

Treatment

These fractures carry a very poor prognosis; overall

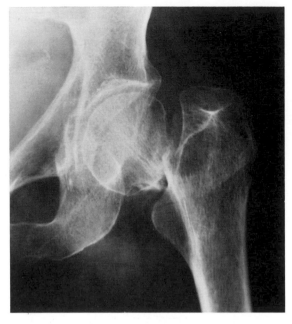

a

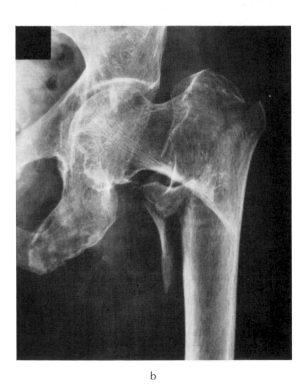

b

Fig. 5.4 *Anteroposterior radiographs of the hip.* (a) *A subcapital fracture.* (b) *A trochanteric fracture.*

mortality is between 30% and 50% within one year. Early mobilisation is the essential principle of treatment; this facilitates nursing care and reduces morbidity from pressure sores, chest and urinary infections, and deep venous thrombosis. Treatment is therefore by operation in the great majority of cases. Better results, with fewer complications, are obtained if the operation is delayed for two or three days so that the patient's general condition can be assessed and any medical problems corrected.

Intracapsular fractures

The blood supply to the femoral head passes mainly in a retrograde fashion, via the retinacular vessels running along the outside of the femoral neck (Fig. 5.5). Ischaemic necrosis of the head is therefore a common problem with these fractures. Displacement is the most reliable guide to vascularity: the more severe the displacement, the worse the prognosis for the head. If the fracture is only minimally displaced, treatment is by closed reduction and internal fixation using pins or screws (Fig. 5.6). If displacement is severe, however, the risk of avascular change is too great and the femoral head should be removed and replaced by a metal prosthesis (Fig. 5.7). The artificial femoral head may, however, wear the acetabulum within five years or so, giving rise to pain and proximal migration. Displaced

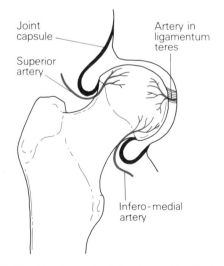

Fig. 5.5 *The blood supply of the femoral head showing its predominantly retrograde direction.*

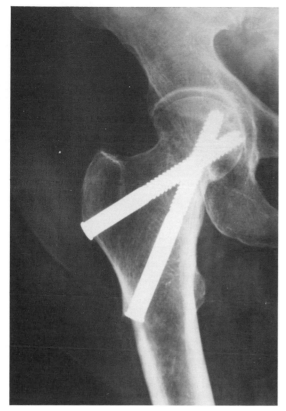

Fig. 5.6 *Anteroposterior x-ray of the hip—a subcapital fracture has been fixed using compression screws.*

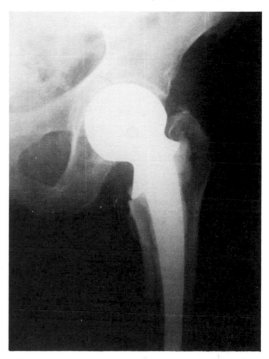

Fig. 5.7 *Anteroposterior x-ray of the hip—this subcapital fracture was too displaced to fix internally. The femoral head has therefore been replaced by the prosthesis of Thompson.*

intracapsular fractures in younger patients should therefore be treated by replacement of both sides of the hip joint, i.e. total hip replacement. Total replacement should also be performed if painful avascular necrosis or non-union follows pinning of minimally displaced fractures.

To the complications of avascular necrosis and non-union can be added dislocation of a prosthetic replacement and deep sepsis, making this injury a very serious problem to an elderly patient.

Trochanteric fractures

While these fractures can be treated very satisfactorily by traction in bed for up to three months, the complications of this conservative treatment outweigh the disadvantages of surgery. Trochanteric fractures are therefore best dealt with by closed reduction and internal fixation using a pin and plate or a one-piece blade plate (Fig. 5.8). In particularly unstable fractures, however, there is a danger of mechanical failure of fixation, when the fracture collapses and malunion takes place in a varus position (Fig. 2.5). This leads to shortening and interference with the abductor mechanism of the hip, causing a limp and difficulty when starting to move.

As with intracapsular fractures, wound infection and venous thrombosis are postoperative threats. Rehabilitation for both types of fractures is generally very slow, and few patients regain normal mobility.

FRACTURES OF THE SHAFT OF THE FEMUR AND THE SUPRACONDYLAR REGION

Fractures of the shaft of the femur are common at any age, and are generally a result of major violence. In the

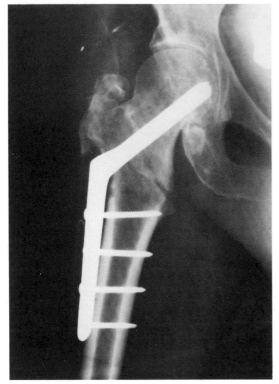

Fig. 5.8 *Anteroposterior x-ray of the hip—a trochanteric fracture has been fixed using a blade plate.*

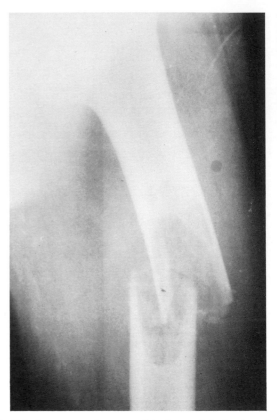

Fig. 5.9 *Anteroposterior x-ray of the femoral shaft—there is a transverse fracture through the upper shaft at the site of a large osteolytic lesion which proved on biopsy to be a secondary malignant deposit.*

elderly, such fractures may be pathological due to secondary deposits or osteoporosis.

Clinical Features and Diagnosis

Since there is obvious pain, swelling, deformity and crepitus, the diagnosis is seldom in doubt. Confirmatory radiographs reveal the fracture type, which to a large extent determines the choice of treatment (Fig. 5.9), though the age and future needs of the patient must also be taken into consideration.

These fractures are often compound, which produces more severe soft-tissue damage. Major arterial injury is unusual, but there may be considerable blood-loss, particularly in an open fracture, and blood transfusion is generally necessary. Injury to the sciatic nerve may also occur.

Interposition of soft tissues between the bone ends may lead to delayed union or non-union. If treated conservatively, maintenance of position may be difficult and can lead to malunion.

Knee stiffness is common after all methods of treatment, especially with fractures of the lower third of the femur. This is minimised by early mobilisation but some restriction of knee-joint movement often remains.

Non-operative treatment

Displaced fractures should be reduced under general anaesthesia and rested on a Thomas's splint. Good alignment can usually be obtained with skeletal traction via a tibial pin. Quadriceps exercises and knee movements are facilitated by using a Pearson knee flexion piece (Fig. 5.10) and, provided length and

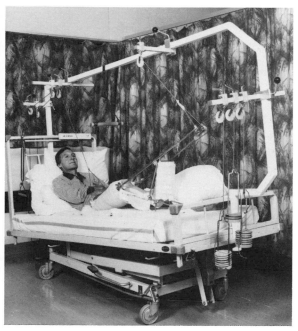

Fig. 5.10 *Conservative treatment for a fractured femoral shaft—the limb is immobilised on a Thomas's splint, traction is applied through a tibial pin counterbalanced by elevation of the end of the bed, and knee movement is facilitated using a Pearson knee flexion piece.*

alignment are maintained, this method can produce very satisfactory results, although the patient is bed-ridden for three months until union takes place.

More recent emphasis on 'functional' treatment, using cast-bracing techniques (Fig. 5.11), allows mobilisation in about six weeks. The brace is applied when there is early callus formation, although the fracture may still be mobile.

The early mobilisation and graded weight-bearing of a cast-brace seem to have a beneficial effect on fracture healing, although it may be six to nine months before full function is achieved, and considerably longer in the elderly.

Operative treatment

Open reduction and internal fixation are indicated when it has not been possible to reduce the fracture or maintain a satisfactory position. If the fracture is part of a multiple injury, it may be helpful to fix the femoral

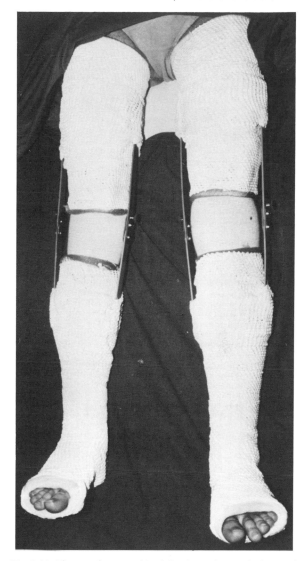

Fig. 5.11 *The cast-brace—skin-tight circumferential plaster of Paris converts the intervening muscles into a fluid which immobilises the femoral fracture: a hinge at the knee allows knee flexion. This young man with bilateral fractures was walking at six weeks.*

fracture to allow easier nursing and management of the other injuries.

Transverse and short oblique fractures of the middle third can be fixed rigidly with an intramedullary nail. This allows immediate weight-bearing, reduces hospitalisation, and facilitates the earliest return to work (Fig. 5.12).

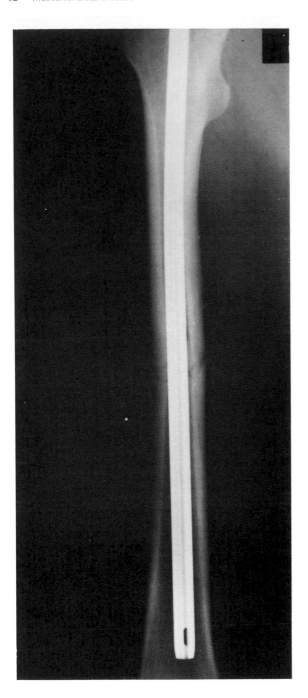

Fig. 5.12 *Anteroposterior x-ray of the femoral shaft—this transverse fracture has been rigidly fixed internally using a Kuntscher nail.*

DISLOCATIONS OF THE KNEE AND PATELLA

Dislocation of the Knee

This is a rare injury involving complete loss of apposition between femur and tibia, and is invariably associated with damage to the popliteal artery. There will also be major ligamentous disruptions and sometimes damage to the popliteal nerves. Reduction is easy but assessment of the associated soft-tissue injuries is more difficult. Repair of any ligamentous injury should be carried out primarily and the knee immobilised in plaster of Paris for at least six weeks.

Dislocation of the Patella

This injury occurs in children and young adults and is particularly common in females. Predisposing factors are a small high patella, genu valgum, and hyperextension deformities. It usually occurs from a fall or blow to the side of the knee. The patella dislocates laterally, and the knee remains flexed until it is reduced. There is an associated tear of the medial capsule and quadriceps expansion.

Reduction is straightforward and may even occur spontaneously with knee extension. After the first injury, it is advisable to immobilise the knee in a plaster cylinder for four to six weeks. Recurrence is common, however, and the condition may require surgical repair. This consists of medial transposition of the insertion of the patellar tendon so that the patella is less inclined to move laterally during knee flexion.

SOFT-TISSUE INJURIES OF THE KNEE

The knee is a complex joint, comprising both tibio-femoral and patellofemoral compartments. Dynamic restraint is provided by the quadriceps muscle, while passive restraint comes from the joint capsule. This capsule is thickened on each side (the collateral ligaments) in order to withstand valgus or varus stresses. In the intercondylar region there are two more ligaments crossing in opposite directions from femur to tibia, the anterior and posterior cruciate ligaments, which resist forward and backward stresses respectively. Between the femoral and tibial articular surfaces lie the two menisci, which have an important load-bearing function. Depending on the mechanism of injury, the ligaments or the menisci may be damaged (Fig. 1.5). A carefully recorded history is therefore essential, because the final common pathway of any of these injuries is a painful swollen knee which is unable to bear weight.

Mechanisms of Injury

These injuries are particularly common in contact sports. Usually only one structure is damaged, but a combination of meniscal and ligament damage may occur in high-velocity injuries. The menisci are most frequently damaged, the medial more often than the lateral. When the weight-bearing and slightly flexed knee receives a blow from the lateral direction, and the femur rotates medially on the tibia, the medial meniscus is damaged. When the similarly-positioned knee receives a blow from the medial direction, and the femur rotates laterally on the tibia, the lateral meniscus is damaged. With the knee extended and weight-bearing, and no rotational component to the injury, a blow from the lateral or medial direction will damage the medial or lateral collateral ligament respectively. A blow to the front of the upper tibia leads to posterior cruciate damage, while hyperextension injuries of the knee produce anterior cruciate damage. With particularly severe violence, the medial collateral ligament, the anterior cruciate ligament and the medial meniscus can all be torn, constituting a triad of soft-tissue injuries.

Clinical Features and Diagnosis

With meniscal or major ligament damage, the patient cannot bear weight and is carried off the field. With incomplete ligament damage, the patient may at first be able to continue the game but goes off later with local discomfort. It is important to establish the timing of the appearance of associated knee swelling. Ligament disruption tears capsular and synovial vessels, giving rise to a haemarthrosis which develops within one hour. The menisci, however, are avascular; when they are damaged, the swelling (a 'sympathetic' effusion) develops slowly over the next 12 to 24 hours.

With meniscal and collateral ligament injuries, the position of discomfort is situated either medially or laterally. The position of maximum local tenderness must then be established (Fig. 1.11).

Meniscal injuries characteristically produce tenderness localised to the joint line, anteromedially for medial meniscal tears and anterolaterally for lateral meniscal tears. Collateral ligament injuries produce tenderness above or below the joint line at the site of attachment of the collateral ligament to bone. Palpation may be difficult in the presence of a tense knee-joint swelling, which may have to be aspirated under local anaesthesia with a wide-bore needle before tenderness can be accurately localised. If the aspirate is straw-coloured synovial fluid, a pure meniscal injury is suggested, but a bloody effusion or pure haemarthrosis strongly suggests ligament damage. Any fat globules present (Fig. 5.13) will indicate bony damage, usually caused by a ligament avulsing a small fragment of bone from one of its insertions.

If there is significant local discomfort, examination should be performed under general anaesthesia. The integrity of the collateral ligaments is tested by stressing the knee in a valgus or varus direction (Fig. 1.18). If the examination is performed without anaesthetic, and gives local pain on stressing but shows no abnormal mobility, then the ligament has only been sprained. With the knee flexed to 90° the integrity of the anterior and posterior cruciate ligaments is now tested.

Late Presentation of Meniscal Damage

In most patients with meniscal injuries, symptoms frequently subside in the short term. The patient returns to training again only to find that, from time to time, the knee locks, cannot be fully extended, and gives way, frequently with some local discomfort. Such symptoms are associated with damage or detachment of the anterior part of the meniscus. If the knee is now examined under general anaesthesia, the integrity of the posterior part of the meniscus can be assessed by McMurray's test (Fig. 1.20), in which the knee is fully flexed and the injury mechanism reproduced (see Fig. 1.5).

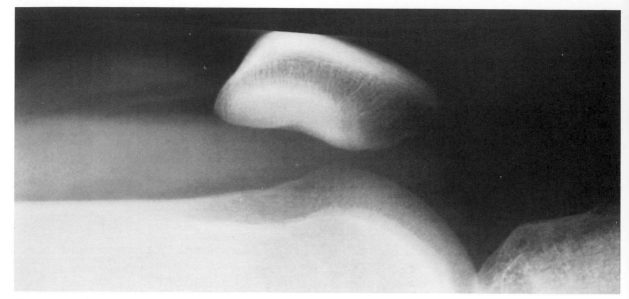

Fig. 5.13 *Lateral x-ray of the knee — the horizontal fluid level with radiolucency indicates the presence of a lipohaem-arthrosis — there must be a fracture.*

In this way, the site of a tear in the incriminated meniscus can be localised. If a patient with a meniscal type injury has a history of locking and giving way, and a positive McMurray's test, then the whole meniscus has been damaged in a bucket-handle fashion.

Arthrography and arthroscopy

These are complementary tests which should be performed to confirm the diagnosis of meniscal damage. Air and radio-opaque dye are injected into the knee joint (double contrast arthrography), when a radiolucent or radio-opaque line through the substance of the meniscus is diagnostic of a tear (Fig. 1.42). A small telescope can be passed into the knee (arthroscopy) and the tear and its site can be visualised; if the detached fragment is small, it can be removed through the arthroscope.

Treatment

Tears of the menisci

The great number of asymptomatic meniscal tears found postmortem indicates that, in most cases,

symptoms will settle without surgical intervention. Meniscal injuries should therefore initially be treated with a compression bandage and a period of no weight-bearing. This is followed by quadriceps exercises, preparatory to a return to normal activities. The majority will settle, and only those with persistent symptoms should undergo operation. Wherever possible, no more than the torn or detached fragment should be excised, leaving a meniscal remnant to act as a shock absorber and thereby minimising the possibility of subsequent degenerative osteoarthritis, which constantly accompanies total meniscectomy.

Tears of the collateral ligaments

Collateral ligament sprains are treated conservatively, with the knee immobilised in a plaster of Paris cylinder for three weeks followed by quadriceps exercises and retraining. Complete tears should be treated by primary repair as early as possible.

Tears of the cruciate ligaments

Again, primary repair as early as possible offers the best hope for restoring stability.

INJURIES OF THE PATELLAR MECHANISM

The four components of the patellar mechanism are the quadriceps muscle, the quadriceps tendon, the patella, and the patellar tendon. Active extension of the knee can be compromised by injury to any of these structures.

Mechanism of Injury

There are two injury mechanisms, indirect and direct. Indirect injury by violent contraction of the quadriceps muscle against resistance may disrupt the patellar mechanism through muscle, tendon or bone. Direct injury to the patella can be sustained in a fall on the knee or (more commonly) in an unrestrained car occupant involved in a road traffic accident, when the patient is thrown forward against the parcel shelf.

Clinical Features and Diagnosis

When the patellar mechanism is interrupted, a gap can be palpated in muscle, tendon or the patella itself. The patient cannot actively extend the knee and flexion is often limited and painful. If the injury occurs through the patella there is a tense haemarthrosis in the knee joint.

Direct injuries cause a more comminuted type of patellar fracture, and again a tense haemarthrosis is present (Fig. 5.14). However, the lateral patellar expansions are not disrupted, displacement is frequently minimal, the patient can actively extend the knee and can often flex the knee quite freely.

Treatment

Injuries to the patellar mechanism must be repaired surgically so that active knee extension can be restored. Disruptions through muscle or tendon are repaired by strong sutures with the knee fully extended, and fractures through the waist of the patella can be wired together. The disrupted expansion on each side must also be sutured. If the avulsion has occurred through the upper or lower pole of the patella, these small

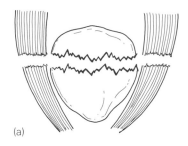

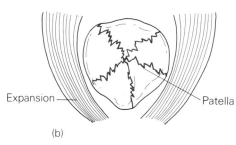

Fig. 5.14 *Patellar fractures. (a) A transverse fracture of the patella—the expansions on each side are also torn. (b) A comminuted fracture of the patella—the expansions are intact.*

fragments of bone can be discarded but the expansions must be firmly repaired. After operation, the knee should be immobilised in the fully extended position for a period of four weeks, followed by quadriceps and knee flexion exercises. These injuries carry a good prognosis, although occasionally re-rupture occurs during the rehabilitation phase.

Direct violence tends to produce comminuted fractures of the patella. These are irreparable; the treatment of choice is patellectomy, lest the patellar fragments give rise to early osteoarthritis of the knee. This does, however, leave the knee significantly weaker in extension.

CONDYLAR FRACTURES OF THE FEMUR AND TIBIA

Mechanism of Injury

These fractures follow either major trauma to the knee, as in road traffic accidents, or trivial falls in elderly osteoporotic patients. Most common is the 'bumper' fracture, usually caused by a valgus or varus strain imposed on a pedestrian by the bumper of a car. Associated ligamentous and meniscal injuries are common.

Clinical Features and Diagnosis

There is a tense haemarthrosis of the knee joint, which is held in semiflexion and cannot bear weight. The knee is grossly unstable to collateral ligament testing (Fig. 1.18). The site of maximal tenderness incriminates the femoral or tibial condylar region as the site of bony injury, and when the haemathrosis is aspirated the presence of fat globules indicates a fracture.

Anteroposterior and lateral radiographs may have to be supplemented by oblique views and tomograms in order to delineate the precise site and direction of the fracture and displacement of the fragments. An important radiological sign on the lateral view is the presence of fat in the joint (Fig. 5.13). This is always diagnostic of a fracture somewhere within the knee joint.

Treatment

Condylar fractures of the femur

If displacement is minimal, alignment of the fragments can be maintained by skeletal traction through a tibial pin. Early knee movement is facilitated with a Thomas's splint and Pearson knee flexion piece, or with a split bed. When the fracture has become clinically stable, a cast-brace allows the earliest resumption of weight-bearing.

In the elderly the above treatment policy should be pursued, even if the fracture is significantly displaced, so that knee-joint movement can be restored as early as possible. However, in the younger patient with significant displacement, open reduction and internal fixation using plates and screws offers the only hope of restoring good knee function.

Condylar fractures of the tibia

If there is no gross displacement of the articular surfaces, the leg should be immobilised in a plaster of Paris cylinder for not more than three weeks, followed

by aggressive quadriceps and knee flexion exercises (Fig. 5.15). In the younger patient with significant depression of the articular surfaces or separation of the fragments, open reduction and internal fixation with plates and screws should be performed, although this

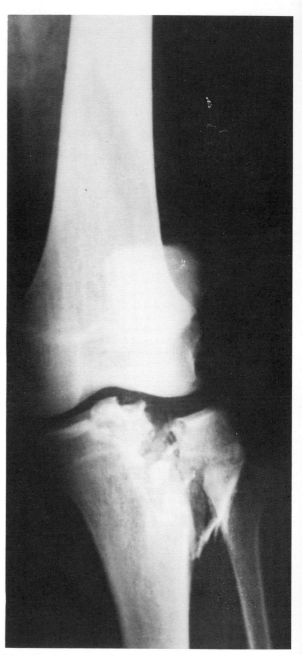

Fig. 5.15 *Anteroposterior x-ray of the knee—there is a fracture of the lateral tibial plateau.*

major reconstruction seldom gives a satisfactory outcome. Operation does, however, afford the opportunity of inspecting the ligaments and menisci so that their repair can be carried out simultaneously.

Degenerative osteoarthritis is an inevitable result of displacement of the articular surfaces, but this may be very slow to appear, often between 15 and 25 years. Meanwhile knee function may be very satisfactory.

FRACTURES OF THE TIBIA AND FIBULA

Mechanism of Injury

Fractures of the tibia and fibula are very common. Low-velocity direct and indirect injuries occur in contact sports. High-velocity direct injuries, causing much more soft-tissue damage often with open wounds, occur in road traffic accidents, where the motorcyclist is particularly vulnerable. Oblique and spiral indirect fractures occur in children through falls with some twisting.

Clinical Features and Diagnosis

Local discomfort, deformity, abnormal movement, crepitus and local bony tenderness make these fractures easy to diagnose. Difficulties in diagnosis do sometimes arise in children; if a child cannot bear weight on the leg, the clinical examination must be particularly careful, and the diagnosis is often obtained radiographically.

The tibia is subcutaneous throughout its length; compound fractures are therefore common. In a motorcyclist, the soft-tissue injury can be extensive enough to put the limb itself at risk. Ischaemia of the deep muscles of the calf may occur as a result of compartmental pressure; this is suggested by excessive pain in the calf muscles, paraesthesia or numbness of the first interdigital cleft, and inability to actively move the toes.

Treatment

The compound wound

Strict principles should be adhered to because of the risk of subsequent sepsis. The wound is first explored and opened to reveal the full extent of the soft tissue damage. All dead and devitalised structures, with the exception of major nerves and blood vessels, are then excised. If the wound can then be closed primarily, like a surgical incision, this should be performed. If there is any tension resisting closure, it is much safer to leave the wound open initially and to close it when local swelling has diminished.

The fracture

If the fracture is undisplaced, it can be immobilised satisfactorily in a long leg plaster. If the facture is displaced it should be reduced under general anaesthesia by traction and manipulation, and if it is stable on reduction it should then be immobilised in a long leg plaster. If the fracture is unstable on reduction, it can be held reduced by means of skeletal traction via a calcaneal pin until it is firm enough to go into a long leg plaster. If the fracture cannot be satisfactorily reduced by closed means, it should be openly reduced and internally fixed using a plate and screws (Fig. 5.16). With significant compounding or soft-tissue damage, the fracture can be held reduced by an external fixation device (Fig. 5.17), which will facilitate attention to the soft tissues.

While these fractures may unite in 10–12 weeks, they often take up to one year. Accordingly, when the fracture is firm enough, a long leg plaster can be exchanged for a cast-brace to facilitate knee and ankle movements.

Non-union and delayed union are common in tibial fractures; the incidence rises from 2% in uncomplicated fractures to about 10% with severe injuries. Deep infection is a particularly serious complication in open or surgically-treated injuries. Treatment is by surgical excision of the septic non-union, followed by bone grafting and prolonged immobilisation, and complete resolution may take 18 months. Most serious deep infections are due to *Staphylococcus aureus* or *Pseudomonas pyocyaneus*. The insertion of 'beads' impregnated with gentamycin has recently achieved good results in a limited number of patients, but amputation is still a common end result of severe infection.

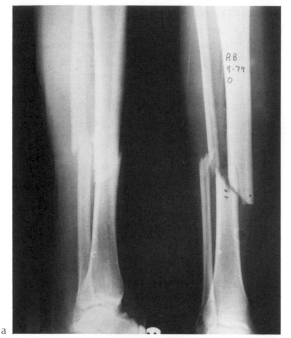

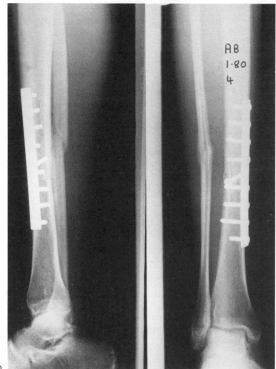

Fig. 5.16 *Anteroposterior and lateral x-rays of a fracture of the tibia and fibula. (a) Initial position of this unstable fracture. (b) Anatomical reduction and rigid immobilisation was obtained using a plate and screws.*

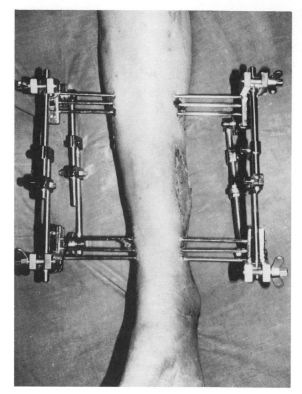

Fig. 5.17 *External fixation of a tibial fracture.*

SOFT-TISSUE INJURIES OF THE ANKLE

The ankle joint is a stable mortice system; the body of the talus fits between the shaped surfaces of the lower tibia and fibula, which are held together by an important ligamentous complex, the inferior tibiofibular group. The hindfoot is stabilised by strong collateral ligaments.

Mechanisms of Injury

The most common injuries occur in the lateral ligamentous complex as a result of inversion strains when the foot twists inwards and the tibia rotates externally on the fixed talus. There are many different combinations, depending on precisely which structures are damaged. Abduction or eversion injuries produce damage to the medial complex. Much rarer is a plantar flexion or dorsiflexion injury, producing damage to the anterior or posterior capsule respectively.

Clinical Features and Diagnosis

Bruising, swelling, inability to bear weight, and restricted movement define the site and severity of the injury. Careful palpation of the bony and ligamentous structures assists diagnosis, although radiographic confirmation is necessary.

Treatment

Traditional treatment of the simple sprain involves protection by strapping or a below-knee walking plaster for 2–3 weeks.

More severe injuries with considerable local swelling, and particularly those with excessive collateral move-

ment, should have anteroposterior and lateral strain radiographs taken to exclude a talar tilt (Fig. 1.19). Complete ruptures may be repaired surgically or treated in a below-knee walking plaster for 4–6 weeks. Inadequate treatment may result in chronic instability, when pain and swelling can persist for many months.

FRACTURES AND DISLOCATIONS OF THE ANKLE

The forces that cause sprains and ligamentous ruptures may, if continued or applied slightly differently, produce fracture-subluxations or dislocations of the ankle. These may be uni-, bi-, or trimalleolar fractures, and many different combinations are possible (Fig. 5.18).

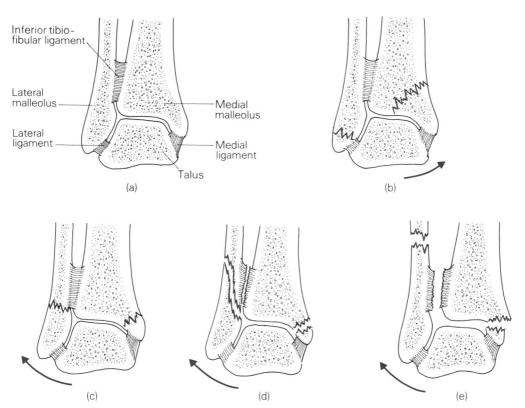

Fig. 5.18 *The ligaments of the ankle region and the types of ankle fracture–dislocation. (a) Front view of the ankle region. (b) A varus stress avulses the lateral malleolus and pushes off the medial malleolus. (c) A valgus stress pushes off the lateral malleolus and pulls off the medial malleolus. (d) A valgus stress with rotation pulls off the medial malleolus, partially disrupts* the interosseus tibio-fibular ligament and causes an oblique fracture of the fibular shaft. (e) A valgus force with extreme rotation avulses the medial malleolus, completely disrupts the inferior tibio-fibular ligament, resulting in a spiral fracture of the fibula much higher.

Mechanism of Injury

A classification based on mechanism of injury is very helpful in carrying out closed treatment, when it is necessary to reverse the deforming process. The most significant and most common fractures are those of the lateral malleolus, often with subluxation. Injuries to the medial malleolus alone are less common. More severe rotational injuries produce damage to both medial and lateral malleoli and, as posterior subluxation of the talus develops, the posterolateral part of the lower end of the tibia (the posterior malleolus) is fractured.

Most ankle injuries are caused when the foot becomes fixed while the weight of the falling body applies a force to the ankle. The degree of subsequent instability depends on how much of the ankle complex is damaged, particularly at the level of the inferior tibiofibular joint.

Clinical Features and Diagnosis

The features resemble those in soft-tissue injuries, but examination reveals maximal tenderness over the fractured bony points. Subluxations and dislocations present with obvious deformity; when this is severe, the overlying skin may be damaged acutely or by later pressure necrosis. The gross deformity of a dislocation may jeopardise the arterial supply to the foot, and any severe deformity must therefore be reduced immediately by heel traction, which relieves skin pressure and restores the circulation.

Treatment

The aim must be to restore perfect joint congruity. There are two main methods of treatment: closed reduction with plaster immobilisation, and open reduction with internal fixation which allows earlier joint movement and quicker rehabilitation. Whatever the treatment, late osteoarthritis is a complication of these injuries, but it is much less common than supposed.

Closed treatment

Unimalleolar or minimally displaced fractures, being relatively stable, can be treated very satisfactorily by a below-knee plaster, often for as little as 4–6 weeks. Bimalleolar fractures and those with significant displacement are best treated by closed methods if there are contra-indications to open operation, such as poor quality skin, a frail elderly osteoporotic patient, and serious contamination or infection of wounds. Provided a satisfactory reduction is obtained, the fractures may be immobilised in plaster for approximately six weeks.

Operative treatment

This is desirable for all fracture-dislocations with significant displacement, in order to restore ankle stability. The most unstable fractures are trimalleolar, but bimalleolar fractures with much lateral displacement are best treated openly (Fig. 5.19).

FRACTURES OF THE FOOT

These are mainly a result of direct violence, either by falls from a height, landing on various parts of the foot, particularly the hind foot, or by crush injury.

FRACTURES OF THE CALCANEUM

Mechanism

These are the most common and most serious injuries to the hind foot caused by a fall from a height onto the heel. They may produce considerable crushing of the cancellous bone of the calcaneum, which leads to great difficulty in satisfactory treatment.

Clinical Features and Diagnosis

There is gross swelling and bruising of the heel and inability to bear weight. Movements of the ankle may be reduced, but subtalar joint movements are extremely painful since the articular surfaces are nearly always involved (Fig. 5.20).

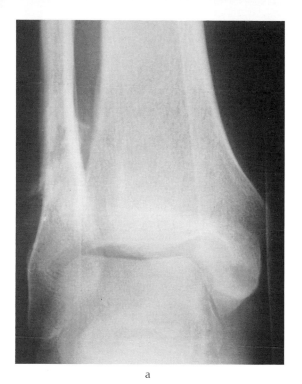

a

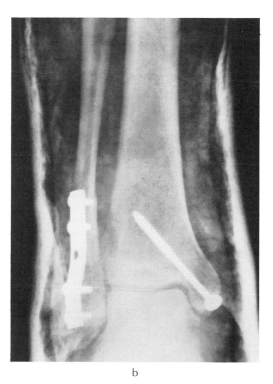

b

Fig. 5.19 *Anteroposterior x-ray of the ankle—this unstable bimalleolar fracture (a) was fixed using screws (b).*

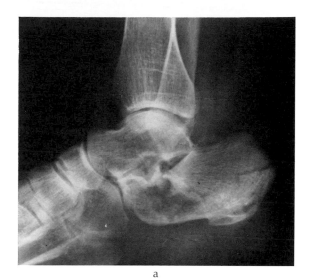

a

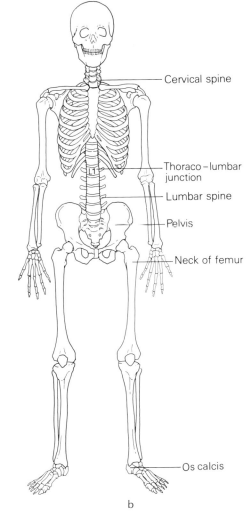

Cervical spine

Thoraco–lumbar junction

Lumbar spine

Pelvis

Neck of femur

Os calcis

b

Fig. 5.20 (a) *Lateral x-ray of the hindfoot showing a comminuted fracture of the calcaneum.* (b) *Other sites of injury when there is a fall onto the feet from a height.*

Treatment

This involves foot elevation with pressure dressings. Ice packs and physiotherapy facilitate early function. When the swelling has reduced and joint movements are returning, the patient may start mobilising in a walking plaster.

Pain often persists, with the development of early osteoarthritis, which sometimes requires arthrodesis of the subtalar joint. People who formerly worked at heights can seldom return to their former occupation.

FRACTURES AND DISLOCATIONS OF THE TALUS

Mechanism

These injuries are uncommon. They occur by forced dorsiflexion of the foot or by severe twisting when the foot is trapped, often in road traffic accidents.

Clinical Features

The most significant injury is a fracture of the neck of the talus (Fig. 5.21). This presents with pain, swelling, deformity and inability to bear weight. Standard radiographs define the fracture satisfactorily, but subluxation and dislocation of the subtalar joint may be difficult to recognise.

Complete dislocations of the talus are serious, and

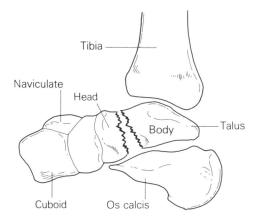

Fig. 5.21 *A displaced fracture of the neck of the talus.*

there may be damage to the neurovascular structures in the sole of the foot.

Treatment

Accurate anatomical reduction is essential for all fractures of the talus, usually implying open reduction and internal fixation. Fracture dislocations often need Kirschner wire fixation before plaster immobilisation, and prolonged prevention of weight-bearing is necessary.

Joint stiffness is common, and avascular necrosis of the body of the talus is a notorious complication giving inevitable arthritic symptoms in the ankle joint.

DISLOCATIONS OF THE TARSOMETATARSAL JOINTS

Injuries to the tarsometatarsal joints are very rare. Treatment consists of elevation followed by immobilisation, but residual joint stiffness is common.

FRACTURES OF THE METATARSALS

These are usually the result of crushing injuries, although stress or march fractures can occur after prolonged physical activity (Fig. 5.22). Crushing causes considerable swelling and bruising, and open injuries are not uncommon.

Radiographs demonstrate crush fractures immediately, but stress fractures are often not diagnosed until callus is present several weeks later.

Treatment is by plaster immobilisation but, with severe displacement, open reduction may be required.

Fractures of the Phalanges

These common injuries are trivial unless they involve the great toe. There is local pain and swelling, and dorsal angulation is common. If malunion occurs there may be subsequent difficulty with footwear.

Simple protective dressings are usually sufficient, but soft-tissue damage requires elevation and plaster immobilisation.

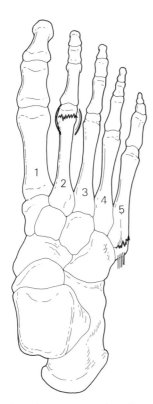

Fig. 5.22 *Front view of metatarsus—there is a stress fracture of the second metatarsal with abundant callus; there is an avulsion fracture of the base of the fifth metatarsal.*

6

Generalised Disorders of
the Skeleton

THE PHYSIOLOGY OF BONE

Bone is metabolically active, and the student should not accept the commonly held view that this tissue is inert. Bone comprises an organic collagen matrix upon which is deposited a mineral phase, composed of calcium and phosphorus and referred to as hydroxyapatite. This tissue is continually formed and removed by specialised cells whose activity is influenced by hormones and by local and mechanical factors. These cells are the osteoblasts, osteocytes and osteoclasts.

Bone Cells

Osteoblasts form the matrix of bone and are also involved in its mineralisation. Osteocytes, derived from osteoblasts, may be found on the surface of bone and also within lacunae in mineralised bone. Osteoclasts, however, are multinucleated cells which resorb bone. Osteoblasts and osteoclasts are derived from different cell lines. Bone resorption is normally followed by formation, but the nature of this link is not known.

Bone is surrounded by an envelope of bone cells, separating bone fluid from the general extracellular fluid and maintaining its specific composition (Fig. 6.1). Mechanical stress stimulates bone formation; many factors increase its resorption, including parathyroid hormone, prostaglandins, osteoclast activating factor, cancer cells and 1,25-dihydroxycholecalciferol (1,25-(OH)$_2$D). In the past, bone cells and haemopoietic cells have been considered separately, but recent work emphasises their close relationship.

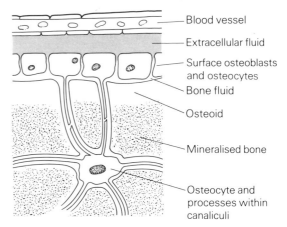

Blood vessel
Extracellular fluid
Surface osteoblasts and osteocytes
Bone fluid
Osteoid
Mineralised bone
Osteocyte and processes within canaliculi

Fig. 6.1 *The relationship between bone and its cells (for clarity the multinucleated osteoclast, which resorbs mineralised bone, is omitted).*

Bone Matrix

The major structural component of bone matrix is collagen (Fig. 6.2). More than 50% of the adult body's collagen is in the skeleton. The collagen molecule is a triple-stranded polymer of three polypeptide or α chains with specific tissue distributions (Table 6.1). Its precursor (procollagen) is formed within the osteoblast and is considerably modified before the collagen fibre is produced; disorders of the skeleton can occur from inherited (osteogenesis imperfecta) or acquired (scurvy) synthetic defects. The fibrils and fibres of collagen, derived from collagen molecules by progressive cross-linking, have great mechanical strength. The arrangement of the collagen molecules leaves areas between them where mineralisation first begins.

Mucopolysaccharides (glycosaminoglycans) are also

COLLAGEN SYNTHESIS   BIOCHEMICAL ABNORMALITIES

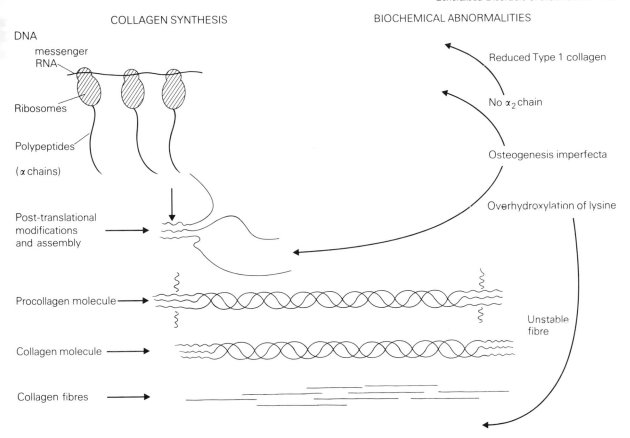

Fig. 6.2 *Steps in the synthesis of the collagen molecule and fibre from constituent polypeptide (α) chains. The position of some of the biochemical abnormalities described in osteogenesis imperfecta is indicated by arrows.*

Table 6.1

The Main Tissue Collagens. Each Collagen Molecule has Three Alpha Chains; the Structure of Type V Collagen is Debated

Type	Tissue distribution	Molecular form
I	Bone, tendon, skin, dentine, sclerae, arteries, uterus	$[\alpha 1(I)]_2\alpha_2$
II	Hyaline cartilage	$[\alpha 1(II)]_3$
III	Skin, arteries, uterus	$[\alpha 1(III)]_3$
IV	Basement membranes	$[\alpha 1(IV)]_3$
V	Basement membranes and other tissues	$\alpha A, \alpha B$

formed by osteoblasts and osteocytes. They are very large branching molecules with a protein core and polysaccharide arms; although of less structural importance than collagen, disorders arising from failure of their breakdown affect the skeleton.

Bone Mineral and Mineralisation

Bone mineral, which contains mainly calcium and phosphorus, is deposited on the collagen matrix, and the matrix is normally almost fully mineralised. How mineralisation occurs is disputed. It probably involves the osteoblasts and structures called calcifying vesicles which are found in mineralising bone and cartilage. Both are associated with alkaline phosphatase which is capable of destroying pyrophosphate, a naturally-occurring inhibitor of mineralisation.

Control of Bone Composition

The factors controlling bone matrix composition are obscure. Bone mineral composition is related to overall calcium metabolism (Fig. 6.3); particularly important are hormones – parathyroid hormone (PTH), 1,25-(OH)$_2$D, and calcitonin – and locally-acting substances such as prostaglandins.

Vitamin D comes mainly from the effect of ultra-violet light on its precursors in the skin (Vitamin D$_3$) as well as from the diet, which may be fortified with vitamin D$_2$. Both D$_2$ and D$_3$ are converted to 25-hydroxycholecalciferol (25-OHD) in the liver, and this is metabolised to 1,25-(OH)$_2$D in the kidney. 1,25-dihydroxycholecalciferol is the most biologically-active metabolite of vitamin D; its production is closely controlled, and it may be regarded as a hormone. Its formation is increased by parathyroid hormone, and by low concentrations of calcium and phosphate. Vitamin D and its metabolites increase the intestinal absorption of calcium and probably have a direct effect on bone. Parathyroid hormone, which is secreted as a precursor and circulates in fragments, increases intestinal calcium absorption, renal calcium reabsorption, and osteoclastic bone resorption; some of its actions are due to its stimulation of 1,25-(OH)$_2$D formation. Calcitonin, a polypeptide derived from the C cells of the thyroid gland, suppresses osteoclastic bone resorption; it appears to increase at times of physiological stress, such as pregnancy.

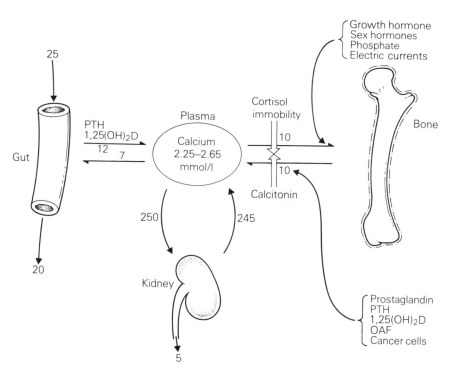

Fig. 6.3 *A diagram of the important pathways of calcium metabolism in the normal adult and the factors which influence them. Amounts in millimoles per day. To convert to milligrams multiply by 40. (PTH, parathyroid hormone; OAF, osteoclast-activating factor.)*

OSTEOPOROSIS

Mechanisms

In osteoporosis, the most prevalent generalised bone disorder, the mass of bone is reduced without any change in its composition (Fig. 6.4). An alternative term is osteopenia. Osteoporosis is clinically important only when it is sufficiently severe to lead to structural collapse. In the young adult, the rates of bone formation and resorption are linked and equal, but from about the age of 30 bone mass begins to fall as the formation rate falls below the resorptive rate.

Bone trabeculae become thin, and some disappear; in the long bones, periosteal new bone formation is lower than endosteal bone resorption. At age 70, for instance, the femoral cortex is much thinner than at age 30, although its external diameter is slightly larger (Fig. 6.5). In young adult women, bone mass is smaller

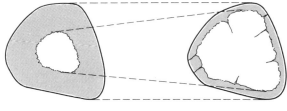

Age   30 years   70 years

Fig. 6.5 *The appearance of a cross-section of the femoral shaft at the age of 30 and 70 years. At 70 most trabeculae are lost and the cortex has been narrowed by a disproportionate increase in the internal diameter.*

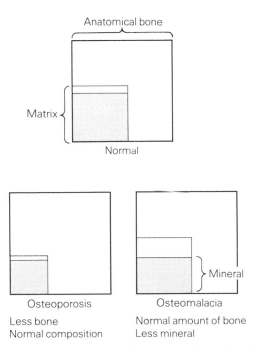

Fig. 6.4 *A diagram to compare the amount of bone tissue in its anatomical space (for example, vertebral body or femur) in normal, osteoporotic and osteomalacic bone. In osteoporosis there is a reduction in bone tissue but the composition is normal; in osteomalacia the amount is normal, but there is a lack of mineral.*

than in men; after the menopause it declines more rapidly. Osteoporotic fractures particularly affect the vertebrae, femoral necks, and forearm bones, and are far more common in elderly women than men. Decreasing mobility contributes to age-related bone loss, since the formation of bone depends on the stress through it. Thus the main factors leading to osteoporosis are age, immobility, and the menopause.

Some individuals lose bone more rapidly than is normal, which leads to accelerated osteoporosis. It can be superimposed on age-related bone loss, or occur in the young where the cause may be obvious (e.g. immobility, Cushing's syndrome, hypopituitarism, Turner's syndrome) or unknown (idiopathic osteoporosis). Several causes for osteoporosis may occur in a single patient.

Clinical Features and Diagnosis

Osteoporosis leads to fracture, deformity and pain. The main deformity is loss of height due to vertebral compression. Back pain initially occurs only with fracture, but later occurs without it.

X-rays show loss of trabeculae, a thinning of the cortex and often wedge-shaped vertebral collapse (Fig. 6.6). Biochemical measurements are often normal, except for hypercalciuria in the immobilised young patient.

In diagnosis it is important to exclude multiple myeloma, metastatic deposits in bone, and other 'metabolic' bone disorders (in which the biochemistry is abnormal) such as osteomalacia or parathyroid bone

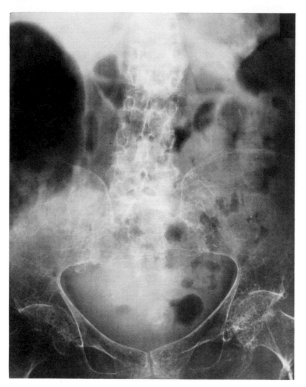

Fig. 6.6 *An anteroposterior x-ray of the spine and pelvis of a patient with osteoporosis—there is widespread vertebral collapse and marked loss of density.*

disease. Where possible, the main cause for the osteoporosis should be identified.

Osteoporosis most frequently produces its effects in postmenopausal women. In this age group, femoral neck fracture is common and most individuals are osteoporotic (Fig. 5.4). The relation between fracture rate and osteoporosis is not close and other factors are important; for instance, elderly people fall more often than the young. The economic and medical effects of femoral neck fractures are important; in the USA the annual cost of the primary treatment alone is estimated at more than one billion US dollars.

Treatment

The rapid loss of bone after the menopause, related to the decline of female hormones, leads to an imbalance between bone resorption and formation. This suggests that osteoporosis, and hence fracture rate, could be reduced by giving oestrogens to women at the menopause. Young women who have had both ovaries removed at the time of a hysterectomy lose bone more rapidly than those who have had hysterectomy alone; this bone loss may be prevented or even reversed by giving oestrogen but, when the oestrogens are discontinued, loss of bone is very rapid. How far these observations can be applied to 'normal' postmenopausal bone loss is not clear. Giving oestrogens to postmenopausal women appears to increase the incidence of uterine cancer and vascular thrombosis. The cancer risk may be reduced by giving progestogens as well as oestrogens, or by prior hysterectomy.

Physical exercise and continuing mobility are important in building up and maintaining bone mass. To prevent further bone loss in the osteoporotic female, calcium and oestrogens are most commonly given. The pain of vertebral collapse requires analgesics and often some form of spinal support.

OSTEOMALACIA AND RICKETS

Mechanisms

Lack of vitamin D, or a disturbance of its metabolism, produces defective mineralisation of bone with osteomalacia in adults and rickets in children; hypophosphataemia can produce similar effects.

Since matrix formation is normal, there is an excess of unmineralised bone collagen (osteoid) which is thicker and covers more bone surfaces than normal. In rickets, the removal of the poorly-mineralised calcified cartilage is defective and the formation of new bone is disorderly. Excessive osteoid (hyperosteoidosis) may also occur if bone turnover is sufficiently rapid to outstrip normal mineralisation, as in Paget's disease or thyrotoxic bone disease.

The causes of osteomalacia relative to the pathway of vitamin D metabolism are shown in Fig. 6.7. In the UK, vitamin D deficiency in the elderly and in Asian immigrants is the most common cause; insufficient exposure to sunlight is all-important. Coeliac disease, partial gastrectomy, intestinal resection and bypass, and liver disease all contribute to malabsorption; disorders of the kidney, both tubular and glomerular,

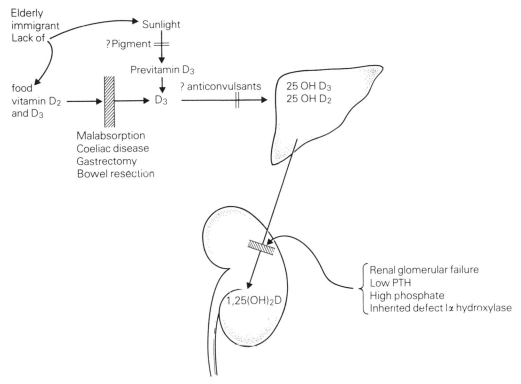

Fig. 6.7 *The main causes of osteomalacia related to the known metabolism of vitamin D. In some subjects, particularly Asian immigrants, the relative contribution of lack of sunlight and of dietary deficiency of vitamin D is still debated.*

can also cause osteomalacia. These two renal groups must be distinguished; the commonest renal tubular disease leading to rickets is inherited (X-linked) hypophosphataemia; in contrast, renal glomerular failure produces a complex sequence of events, where defective mineralisation and excessive bone resorption predominate (Fig. 6.8).

Clinical Features and Diagnosis

Bone pain, deformity, and proximal myopathy are the clinical features. The bones may be universally tender. The deformities of rickets depend partly on the age of the child; they include enlarged epiphyses and costochondral junctions, bossing of the skull, knock knees and bow legs. Osteomalacia may produce loss of height and a triradiate pelvis. Proximal muscle weakness (whose cause is obscure) leads to a waddling gait,

difficulty in climbing stairs and in getting out of low chairs. Other features of the underlying disease, e.g. anaemia or steatorrhoea, or of hypocalcaemia, e.g. overt or latent tetany, may be seen.

Most frequently, the plasma calcium and phosphate are low and the alkaline phosphatase is increased

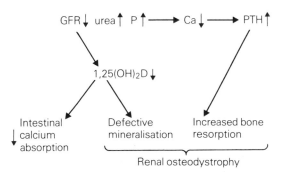

Fig. 6.8 *To show how renal glomerular failure may lead to renal osteodystrophy. (GFR, glomerular filtration rate.)*

(derived from osteoblasts) but variations do occur. The urinary calcium is usually very low.

Radiographs of rickets show a widened growth plate, with a widened, ragged and cupped metaphysis (Fig. 6.9); in osteomalacia, the diagnostic feature is a Looser zone or pseudofracture, which is a linear area of defective mineralisation. Such zones are common in the pelvis, the long bones, the ribs, and the scapulae.

Examination of undecalcified bone obtained at biopsy shows extensive osteoid and often a variable

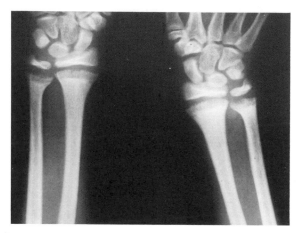

Fig. 6.9 *Anteroposterior x-ray of the wrists of a patient with rickets—there is epiphyseal and metaphyseal widening.*

degree of osteoclastic bone resorption due to secondary hyperparathyroidism.

The diagnosis of rickets presents no difficulty. Osteomalacia is often missed because it is not considered; pain may suggest arthritis and myopathy suggests polymyalgia rheumatica. Histology is diagnostic, and a therapeutic trial with vitamin D provides final confirmation.

Treatment

The treatment of osteomalacia depends on its cause. All patients require vitamin D, and those with simple vitamin D deficiency respond to daily microgram doses. Patients with renal glomerular osteodystrophy are best treated with 1α-hydroxylated vitamin D metabolites.

PAGET'S DISEASE OF BONE

Mechanisms

In Paget's disease, both formation and resorption of bone are excessive and disorderly, although they remain linked. The abnormal bone is vascular, enlarged, deformed and mechanically weak. Histology shows numerous osteoblasts and multinucleated osteoclasts, excessive fibrosis and an irregular mosaic pattern. The cause is unknown, but the abnormal osteoclasts appear to contain virus-like particles. Paget's disease is more frequent in the elderly; it is present in up to 4% of persons over 40, and is more frequent in men than in women. The pelvis, spine and skull are commonly affected. The striking geographical variations are not understood: it is most frequent in Northern industrial England and in Lancashire; and very rare in Scandinavia and Japan.

Clinical Features and Diagnosis

The clinical features are bone deformity, pain, fracture, nerve compression, heart failure and sarcoma. Deformities include a bowed and enlarged tibia, bowing of other long bones, or a large overhanging skull vault. Pain is a common symptom, often related to nearby degenerative arthritis. Multiple microfractures (fissure fractures) occur on the convexity of affected bones (Fig. 6.10), and complete fractures through Pagetic bone may heal slowly. Nerve compression contributes to deafness, paraplegia, and cranial nerve palsies. Heart failure is common in patients with Paget's disease; it may follow from the increased cardiac output (high-output heart failure), or be coincidental. Bone sarcoma is the most serious complication; it occurs in probably less than 1% of those with symptoms, and the upper humerus is a typical site.

The considerable increase in plasma alkaline phosphatase and urine hydroxyproline (derived mainly from bone collagen) reflects the accelerated bone turnover.

Radiographs show many appearances. Excessive resorption, with an obvious resorbing front, is a common early feature (Fig. 6.11, p. 112); later the affected bone is larger, the trabeculae are coarse, and the cortex is often thick.

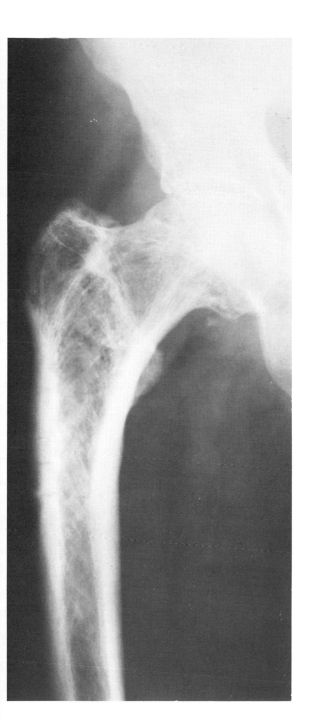

Fig. 6.10 *Anteroposterior x-ray of the upper femur—fissure fractures on the convexity of bones are typical of Paget's disease.*

Diagnosis is based on biochemistry and radiology. It is important to exclude other conditions with a raised alkaline phosphatase, e.g. osteomalacia and osteitis fibrosa, and osteoblastic secondary deposits (particularly from the prostate). Isotope bone scan, which shows localised areas of very high uptake, and bone biopsy may both be necessary.

Treatment

Probably less than 5% of those with Paget's disease have symptoms. Pain often responds to simple analgesics. The young, and those with complications or pain unresponsive to analgesics, should be considered for treatment with drugs known to reduce bone turnover; these are diphosphonates, calcitonin, or mithramycin. All these have specific effects on bone cells, particularly osteoclasts.

PARATHYROID BONE DISEASE

Overactivity of the parathyroid glands stimulates osteoclastic bone resorption, and may eventually produce cyst-like lesions containing fibrous tissue in the bones; hence the term osteitis fibrosa cystica. In primary hyperparathyroidism, which is most often due to an autonomous parathyroid adenoma, clinical bone disease occurs in less than 20% of patients (although histological changes may be present in most). Where the parathyroid overactivity is due to prolonged hypocalcaemia, as in osteomalacia, bone resorption is universal.

Primary hyperparathyroidism is most often detected by multichannel biochemical screening and by investigation of nonskeletal features such as renal stones, peptic ulceration, renal failure, pancreatitis, or the effects of hypercalcaemia (thirst, nocturia, constipation, anorexia, depression). It is distinguished from other causes of hypercalcaemia, particularly malignant disease, by the clinical and biochemical evidence, the circulating concentration of immunoreactive parathyroid hormone, and the response of the hypercalcaemia to corticosteroids.

Where osteitis fibrosa occurs, the bones are painful and tender to percussion. X-rays may show localised

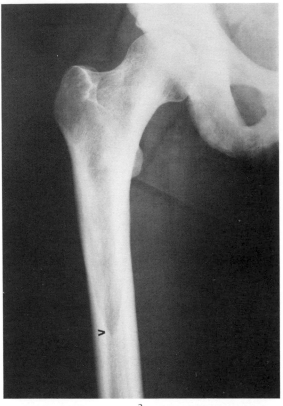

a

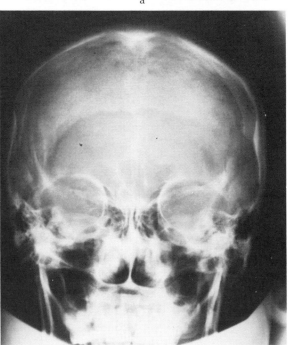

b

cysts in the long bones or expanded lesions in the ribs. The most characteristic finding is subperiosteal resorption of the phalanges of the hand. The biochemistry is diagnostic; plasma calcium is high, phosphate low, and alkaline phosphatase increased.

Patients with primary hyperparathyroidism who have clinical bone disease tend to have larger parathyroid adenomas and a higher plasma calcium than those without. Treatment is by neck exploration and removal of the adenoma. 1α-hydroxylated vitamin D metabolites, which act quickly, can be used to prevent severe postoperative hypocalcaemia.

OSTEOGENESIS IMPERFECTA: THE BRITTLE BONE SYNDROME

This group of disorders, which arise from primary inherited defects in collagen synthesis, have the common feature of bone fragility.

The commonest form (Type 1, Table 6.2) is mild and dominantly inherited; although multiple fractures occur, deformity is uncommon. Blue sclerae, deafness, hypermobility and cardiac valve lesions are associated. Less common sporadic cases are more severe, often

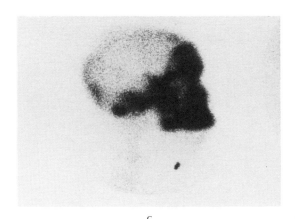

c

Fig. 6.11 (a) *Antero-posterior x-ray of the upper femur showing a well-marked resorbing front due to Paget's disease in the mid-shaft of the femur (arrowed). The cortex of the proximal femur is widened and abnormal due to the disorganised formation of new bone. The skull x-ray (b) and bone scan (c) of a woman of 48 with pain around the upper central teeth. The x-ray (b) shows a front of resorption; the isotope scan (c) shows that the affected area has a very high uptake.*

Table 6.2

*Recognisable Types of Osteogenesis Imperfecta
(The Brittle Bone Syndrome)*

Type	Clinical features	Inheritance
1	Commonest form Mild bone disease Blue sclerae Extraskeletal changes	Dominant
2	Lethal severe, many fractures at birth	Some recessive
3	Fractures at birth. Progressive deformity and scoliosis	Some recessive
4	Fragile bones, normal solerae, often abnormal teeth	Dominant

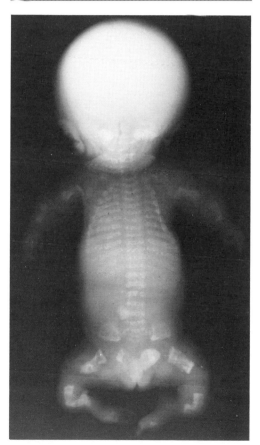

Fig. 6.12 *The appearance of the skeleton in lethal osteogenesis imperfecta (Type 2). The vault of the skull is uncalcified, there are multiple rib fractures and the bones of the limbs are short, deformed and structureless.*

showing fractures at birth. Some of these patients survive, with considerable deformity but few extra-skeletal features. Others (Type 2) are lethal (Fig. 6.12). Abnormal dentine (composed of collagen) is most often found in association with severe bone disease.

The commonest biochemical abnormality appears to be defective synthesis of sufficient type I collagen, particularly the $\alpha 1(I)$ chain. This greatly affects the skeleton, since bone contains type I collagen only.

The bone pathology reflects the severity of the disease. In the mild (type 1) disorder there is merely a reduction in the amount of bone (i.e. a form of inherited osteoporosis); in severe osteogenesis imperfecta, fibrous bone is excessive and the arrangement of the abnormal collagen bundles is entirely haphazard.

Treatment is unsatisfactory. Fractures, which heal easily, are dealt with conservatively. The main difficulty is in severely affected, deformed and dwarfed children who are unable to walk. The bones may be straightened by the insertion of intramedullary rods, but multiple operations are necessary and walking is rarely possible. Power-driven wheelchairs provide an acceptable alternative. No medical treatment is of proven use.

THE MUCOPOLYSACCHARIDOSES

These disorders arise from a lack of the specific enzymes which break down large mucopolysaccharide (MPS) molecules, and MPS therefore accumulates in the tissues. Some, e.g. MPS I H, affect many tissues and lead to mental backwardness and early death (the Hurler syndrome), whilst others, e.g. MPS IV, particularly affect the skeleton (the Morquio syndrome).

The physical features of the recessively-inherited Hurler syndrome include dwarfism, coarse facial appearance (hence its previous name 'gargoylism'), short neck, and a lumbar gibbus. The eyes are prominent, with corneal clouding, there is variable deafness, a large abdomen with hepatosplenomegaly, and broad stiff trident hands. X-rays show an abnormal-ly-shaped skull, a slipper-like sella turcica, beaking of the thoracolumbar vertebrae, and bullet-shaped phalanges. After mental and physical deterioration, death often occurs in late childhood. Patients with MPS IV, on the other hand, have normal intelligence but striking skeletal deformity and dwarfism (Fig. 6.13).

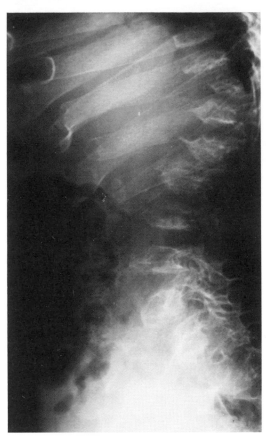

Fig. 6.13 *Lateral x-ray of the spine of a patient with Morquio's syndrome—there is characteristic vertebral flattening (platyspondyly).*

THE SKELETAL DYSPLASIAS

In some disorders, skeletal changes are only one aspect of a generalised disease; in others, the skeleton alone (bone and cartilage) appears to be affected. This second category includes many conditions grouped together as the skeletal dysplasias. Present knowledge of the skeletal dysplasias is purely descriptive.

The commonest of these is achondroplasia. In this condition, which is either dominantly inherited or occurs as a new mutation, there is selective failure of the epiphyseal growth cartilage. Bulbous masses of cartilage appear at the end of the long bones. Periosteal and membrane bone formation and the repair of bone are normal. There is a striking disproportion, obvious at birth and within the first year of life, between the normal trunk and the very short limbs. This shortness is greater proximally, the limbs look broad, with deep creases, and the hands are trident-like (Fig. 6.14). The vault of the skull appears large in comparison with the

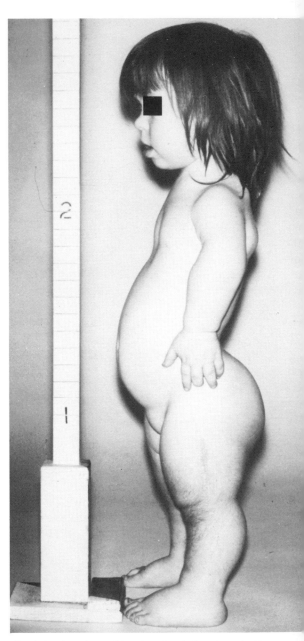

Fig. 6.14 *A patient with achondroplasia—there is disproportion with a normal trunk and short limbs with trident-like hands. (Courtesy of Mr M. A. Nelson, FRCS.)*

small face and flat nasal bridge. The spine shows an increased lumbar lordosis and progressive narrowing of the interpedicular distance in the lower vertebrae (the reverse of normal). Children with achondroplasia are of normal intelligence. The main complications, which arise from skeletal disproportion, include early osteoarthritis, obstetric difficulties, hydrocephalus and paraplegia.

FIBROUS DYSPLASIA

In fibrous dysplasia, areas of bone are replaced by fibrous tissue. This may occur in one bone (Fig. 10.7), such as a rib or femur, or in several bones, and most commonly presents as a fracture. Monostotic fibrous dysplasia is the most frequent variety but more interest attaches to the polyostotic form because of its association with unilateral pigmentation (on the same side as the bone lesions), sexual precocity in girls, and (rarely) overactivity of other endocrine organs such as the thyroid, adrenal cortex, and pituitary. The reason for these associations remains obscure.

The skeletal lesions may lead to gross deformity of the upper femur and femoral neck (producing the 'shepherd's crook' deformity), asymmetry of the skull and long bones, and spinal cord compression. Hypophosphataemic osteomalacia is a rare association. Unilateral bone lesions, pigmentation, and (rarely) osteomalacia also occur in osseous neurofibromatosis, which shows clear evidence of dominant inheritance; the changes in the bones may be bizarre, with asymmetrical overgrowth or undergrowth (Fig. 6.15) and characteristically there is a sharp kyphoscoliosis.

ENDOCRINE DISORDERS OF BONE

In addition to parathyroid hormone, calcitonin, and 1,25-$(OH)_2$D, the skeleton is affected by many other hormones, by both physiological stress and pathological changes. Thyrotoxicosis, Cushing's syndrome and hypopituitarism all cause osteoporosis; hypothyroidism delays skeletal maturation; and hyperpituitarism increases bone formation.

The thyroid hormones increase collagen turnover,

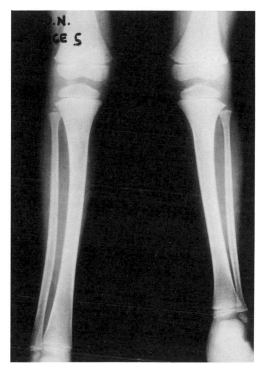

Fig. 6.15 *Anteroposterior x-ray of the legs of a patient with neurofibromatosis—there is unilateral gigantism.*

including that of bone, with disproportionate increase in bone resorption. Thyrotoxicosis increases urinary hydroxyproline excretion, and the levels of plasma alkaline phosphatase and often plasma calcium (and phosphate). Mineralisation lags behind matrix formation, so that there is an increase in osteoid; there is also excessive cellular activity and fibrosis. In adult hypothyroidism, the hydroxyproline excretion is low but the skeleton is not clinically abnormal; in infancy and childhood, hypothyroidism causes a striking delay in bone age, and the epiphysis of the femoral head is markedly fragmented. In Cushing's syndrome (either spontaneous or due to corticosteroid treatment) the accelerated bone loss leads rapidly to osteoporosis and structural collapse.

Hypopituitarism in the child leads both to infantilism and to osteoporosis. Overactivity of the pituitary will cause excessive bone formation. Hypogonadism (whether primary or secondary to pituitary disease) also leads to osteoporosis, which responds to hormone replacement.

OTHER GENERALISED DISORDERS OF BONE

There are many other conditions associated with a generalised bone disorder, most of which are rare. However, the effects of neoplasia and parenteral nutrition on bone are commonly encountered.

Neoplastic Deposits in Bone

Infiltration of bone with malignant disease (Figs 10.8 and 10.11), such as the reticuloses, myeloma, and metastases from tumours elsewhere, has complex effects which are not entirely mechanical. In neoplastic disease, bone is resorbed in many different ways, including the direct effect of the tumour, the local production of prostaglandins, and the stimulation of osteoclastic activity.

Bone Disease and Parenteral Nutrition

In subjects receiving prolonged parenteral nutrition, periarticular pain and impaired mineralisation of bone can occur. These patients are invariably ill, often have malabsorption, may have specific deficiencies such as those of copper and zinc, and are often immobile.

7

Local Lesions and Deformities

CERVICAL SPINE

Torticollis

This is tightness of the sternomastoid muscle, whose action tilts the head towards the shoulder on the *same* side while rotating the chin to the *opposite* side. The condition, popularly known as 'wryneck', may be divided into primary and secondary types; the primary type, which may be subdivided into postural and structural varieties, is confined to infants.

Postural torticollis in infancy

This common condition presents soon after birth. The child holds its head in the characteristic attitude. Passive movements of the neck are unrestricted and palpation of the sternomastoid reveals no abnormality. Spontaneous resolution can be expected within a few months, but the importance of the condition lies in its occasional association with more serious congenital defects, e.g. congenital dislocation of the hip.

Infantile structural torticollis (sternomastoid tumour)

In this condition a true contracture develops in the sternomastoid muscle. In over half of cases there is a history of difficult delivery of the head, with breech or face presentations.

The initial feature is the appearance of a firm swelling, about the size of a pea, at the junction of the middle and lower thirds of the muscle. Deformity is seldom pronounced at this stage, and may be absent altogether. Over the next few months, the tumour disap-

pears while the sternomastoid contracts to develop a cord-like appearance and the head assumes the characteristic attitide (Fig. 7.1). Rotation of the head towards the affected side and lateral movement away from the affected side are restricted. Facial asymmetry and plagiocephaly (asymmetry and twisting of the head) soon develop.

Although spontaneous resolution may occur, stretching exercises, performed first by the physiotherapist and later by the mother, should be instituted. In a few instances, the muscle is resistant to stretching and an open tenotomy must be performed.

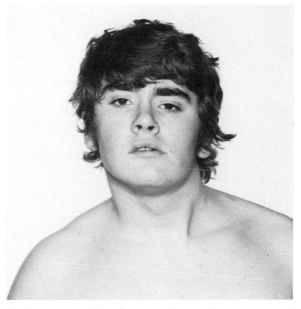

Fig. 7.1 *Untreated infantile structural torticollis (sternomastoid tumour)—contracture has shortened the sternomastoid and tilted the head towards the same side but rotating it to the opposite side. There is marked facial asymmetry.*

Secondary torticollis

This may arise as a result of muscle spasm produced by infective foci in the neck and pharynx, particularly tuberculosis. It may also be seen, in an acute form, secondary to fractures of the upper end of the cervical spine.

Spasmodic torticollis is a postural deformity which affects adults. The deformity characteristically disappears when the patient lies down. Many patients exhibit behavioural psychiatric disturbances, and orthopaedic surgery has nothing to offer.

Klippel–Feil Syndrome

This non-familial condition is a result of abnormal fusion between cervical vertebrae which, in severe cases, may be total. The neck is short; the head appears to grow directly from between the shoulders; and the trapezius muscle may give the impression of webbing. Neck movements are restricted, especially lateral rotation, and the posterior hairline is unusually low. The radiological changes are unmistakable (Fig. 7.2).

The problems are mainly cosmetic and the condition is not amenable to treatment.

Sprengel's Shoulder

In normal development, the scapula arises in the cervical region and then descends to its definitive

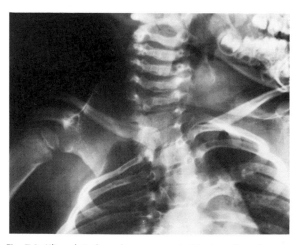

Fig. 7.2 *Klippel–Feil syndrome—cervical fusion gives rise to a short neck and there is often an elevated scapula.*

position. Arrest of this process leads to a congenitally high scapula with obvious asymmetry. The condition may be bilateral; it is then easily confused with the Klippel–Feil syndrome, with which it may coexist.

The scapula itself is abnormally small and is often fixed to the spinal column by either a bony or firm fibrous band. Normal rotation of this bone is not possible and abduction of the shoulder therefore is limited. Treatment is not beneficial.

Cervical Disc Lesions

Between each pair of vertebrae there is a disc, consisting of a liquid nucleus pulposus surrounded by a fibrous annulus adherent to the anterior and posterior longitudinal ligaments, which are rich in sensory nerve endings. When nuclear material bulges the annulus, the term protrusion is appropriate. When nuclear material has forced its way through the annulus, it is termed a prolapse (Fig. 7.3). During the process of disc degeneration which leads to protrusion or prolapse, the nuclear material becomes fleshy and resembles crab meat.

Disc lesions may present as an acute episode or, more frequently, as a gradual development, and are often unrelated to previous trauma. There is stiffness and an aching pain in the neck, often referred to the occipital region. These symptoms reflect stimulation of the nerve endings in both the annulus and posterior longitudinal ligament under pressure. On examination, there is reduced movement of the neck, with discomfort particularly on flexion and rotation, and often considerable spasm of the paravertebral musculature.

If the protrusion is big enough or if there is a frank prolapse of nuclear material, the local nerve root may be compressed to give a radicular pain down the distribution of the root, sensory symptoms in its dermatome, weakness of muscles supplied, and reflex suppression (Fig. 1.3). Flattening of the normal cervical lordosis, shown on lateral radiographs, indicates significant muscle spasm (Fig. 1.24). Cervical myelography may demonstrate distortion of a nerve root by a disc prolapse, and confirms the anatomical level.

The great majority of cases respond to conservative treatment. Painful muscle spasm is relieved by the local rest and warmth of a cervical collar. Discomfort localised to one intervertebral level is often relieved by

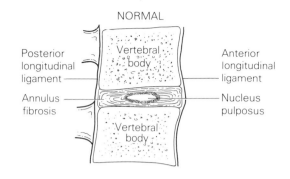

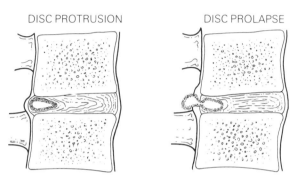

Fig. 7.3 *In a disc protrusion, nuclear material bulges the annulus and posterior longitudinal ligament: In a disc prolapse, nuclear material has herniated through to lie against a nerve root.*

local manipulative treatment with the added anti-inflammatory effect of local ultrasound. If symptoms persist, with evidence of nerve-root pressure at one level confirmed by myelography, anterior inter-body fusion following nerve root decompression is the treatment of choice.

Cervical Spondylosis

This usually involves an older age group. There are degenerative changes in the cervical spine, often at multiple levels. Long-standing disc degeneration leads to narrowing of the disc spaces and marginal new bone formation, which may encroach on local nerve roots or even the spinal cord. Characteristically the patient presents with pain in the cervical spine radiating to the shoulder and often to the occipital region. There is limitation of movement, often with neurological signs in the upper limb appropriate to the root involved. Radiographs demonstrate disc space narrowing, with marginal bony spurs. Conservative treatment is again favoured, but progressive neurological signs are an indication for surgery. Nerve-root pressure is relieved by removal of the offending bony spur with enlargement of the nerve root foramen, and spinal cord pressure responds to decompressive laminectomy.

THORACOLUMBAR SPINE

Scoliosis

Although the term is used for all forms of lateral deviation of the spine, deformity is often more complicated than this and is frequently accompanied by rotation of the vertebral bodies. In the dorsal region, rotation is very obvious because of its effect on the ribs and this is largely responsible for the hump-back deformity which is such a prominent feature of the condition (Fig. 1.27). In the lumbar region, where there are no ribs, the cosmetic aspects are much less striking.

The condition may be classified in a variety of ways, but a fundamental distinction exists between structural and non-structural curves.

Idiopathic structural scoliosis

This is the most important type of structural curve. It is much commoner in girls and, curiously, is almost always convex to the right in the dorsal region. It usually begins in late childhood or early adolescence but is frequently not recognised for several years. Mild curves are present in 5% of teenagers. The natural history is a slow progression of the deformity during growth, with an ugly rib hump. Serious degress of deformity can lead to cardiopulmonary embarrassment, with significant diminution of expectancy and quality of life.

The diagnosis from other forms of scoliosis is mainly by exclusion. Even mild degrees of the deformity can be seen if the patient is asked to bend forward, when the rib hump becomes much more evident. The radiological changes are characteristic, with structural changes including lateral wedging of the vertebral bodies and evidence of rotation (Fig. 7.4).

Treatment is difficult and often disappointing. For

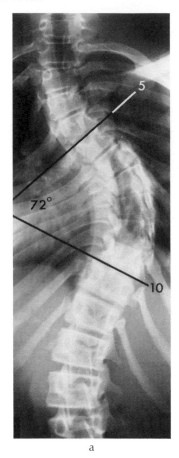
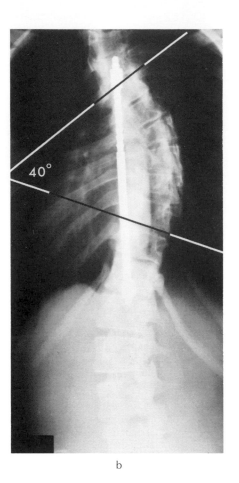

a   b

Fig. 7.4 (a) *Anteroposterior radiograph of a patient with idiopathic scoliosis demonstrating the lateral curvature of the spine with rotation responsible for rib asymmetry. (b) Anteroposterior radiograph of the same patient after operative correction using a metal distraction rod.*

this reason, early diagnosis is essential and, because the majority of these patients are often shy schoolgirls, some form of positive screening of children at the appropriate age is essential. If the condition is picked up early and monitored regularly, and progression then occurs, bracing will be required using the Milwaukee brace (Fig. 1.1). This apparently barbaric device extends from the pelvis below and supports a padded ring below the patient's chin and occiput. The muscular efforts involved in keeping the chin clear of the upper ring provide a dynamic corrective force which helps to prevent curve progression. Deterioration tends to cease at maturity.

If the curve is already severe when diagnosed, bracing will be ineffective and surgery is necessary both to reduce the deformity and to arrest progression by spinal fusion. Although correction can be achieved by external methods using plaster casts, modern techniques usually rely on some form of internal instrumentation.

It might be expected that such corrective treatment would also improve cardiopulmonary function, but this is by no means certain. Unfortunately, the cosmetic improvement is often disappointing because vertebral rotation is difficult to eliminate and the rib hump frequently persists.

Infantile idiopathic scoliosis

This presents in the first year of life, and may be accompanied by plagiocephaly. Cot-positioning in the prone position protects against curve development. The curve is structural, as evidenced by the fact that it will not correct completely when the child is suspended by its head. Fortunately, the great majority of these curves undergo spontaneous resolution, but 10% progress to extremely unpleasant structural curves which are, for unexplained reasons, usually convex to the left. Treatment is difficult; in the early stages it involves casting or bracing, often employing gravitational forces to aid correction.

Secondary structural scoliosis

This usually arises secondary to a paralytic condition such as poliomyelitis or spina bifida, although in the latter condition congenital malformations of the vertebrae also play an important part. There is also an association with neurofibromatosis. The treatment of these curves is on the same lines as (adolescent) idiopathic scoliosis. Where paralysis is extensive, however, the use of a brace is inappropriate and recourse is more often made to surgery, which has to be performed both anteriorly and posteriorly (Fig. 7.5).

Congenital structural scoliosis

This is the result of congenital malformation of the vertebrae, often in the form of single or multiple hemivertebrae. There may also be abnormal areas of fusion between individual vertebrae (Fig. 7.6). The deformity is usually only slowly progressive, so that the condition often does not become evident until well into childhood. Once demonstrated, however, progression is inexorable; it is uninfluenced by bracing, and surgical treatment is required for curves that are sufficiently severe to warrant correction. Fortunately, in many instances the deformity is not great, rotation tends not to be a marked feature, and the cosmetic problem is correspondingly smaller.

Non-structural scoliosis

This derives from such conditions as leg-length inequality and pelvic tilting due to contractures at the hip

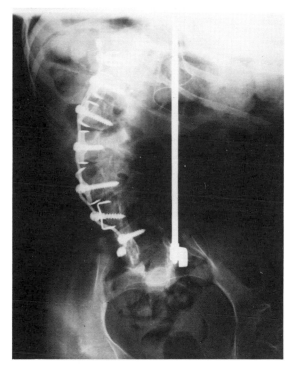

Fig. 7.5 *Anteroposterior x-ray of a scoliosis in association with spina bifida—such curves can only be corrected by anterior and posterior instrumentation and fusion.*

joint. The curve disappears when the patient bends forwards or when he sits with his buttocks on a level surface.

The primary condition is treated. A special case of postural scoliosis is the so-called sciatic scoliosis most commonly seen in association with a prolapsed intervertebral disc. This is the result of muscle spasm due to nerve-root irritation.

Kyphosis

This is the name given to a curvature of the spine in the sagittal plane, the convexity being posterior. A mild kyphosis is normal in the dorsal spine but is abnormal in other areas of the spine. It may exist in two forms, localised and generalised.

Localised kyphosis can occur in any portion of the spine. The segment involved is usually short but the

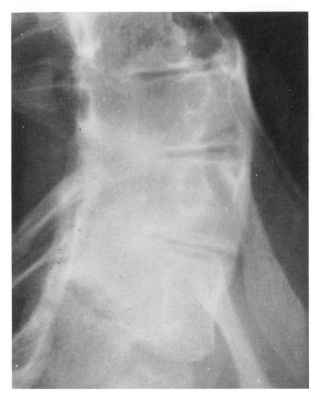

Fig. 7.6 *Anteroposterior radiograph of a scoliosis showing a congenital unilateral fusion at the apex.*

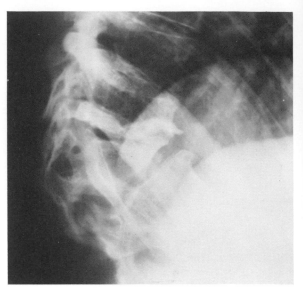

Fig. 7.7 *Lateral radiograph of the spine demonstrating a localised kyphosis due to tuberculous infection.*

angular deformation is considerable. The result is a prominent knuckle of spine, described as a gibbus or kyphus. It is usually a result of destruction of the vertebral bodies, most commonly by tuberculous or other infection (Fig. 7.7). The condition can also be caused by severe damage to one or more vertebral bodies as a result of injury.

Generalised kyphosis arises from generalised vertebral disease. In adolescence, the condition is usually due to a form of osteochondritis which affects the vertebral endplates (Scheuermann's disease) producing a characteristic rigid round-back deformity with its apex in the lower thoracic region (Fig. 1.26). The deformity increases with growth, and rapidly-progressive cases should be treated with a Milwaukee brace.

Ankylosing spondylitis is the usual cause for such curves appearing in young adults, while osteoporosis is a common cause in the elderly (Fig. 6.6).

Lordosis

This is the opposite of kyphosis and is a normal feature of the lumbar and cervical spine. It is seldom a fixed deformity and is usually secondary to some other condition. Excessive muscle spasm in the erector spinae often exaggerates the normal lordosis and this is particularly noticeable in spondylolisthesis (see below). It often arises secondary to conditions in the hip, particularly fixed flexion deformities, and in young children it is a prominent feature of bilateral congenital dislocation of the hips. Treatment is aimed at the underlying condition.

Spondylolisthesis

This literally means the slipping forward of one vertebra upon another, but the term is usually reserved for conditions in the lower lumbar spine (Fig. 7.8). Two main forms of the condition exist, spondylolytic and degenerative. In the former there is a defect in the pars interarticularis of the 4th or, more commonly, the 5th lumbar vertebra. This defect, spondylolysis, is thought to be acquired as the result of a stress fracture which has failed to unite, while the anterior part of the

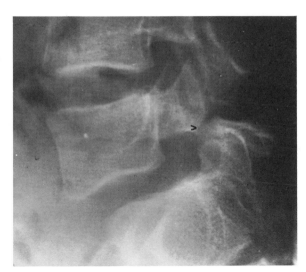

Fig. 7.8 *Lateral radiograph of the lumbosacral region showing a spondylolytic spondylolisthesis. There is a defect in the pars interarticularis.*

vertebra has moved forward, carrying the upper portion of the spinal column with it. The condition may be symptomless and only noted incidentally on x-ray. It may present, particularly in adolescence, with backache, muscle spasm and an increase of the normal lumbar lordosis. Sometimes the deformity is actually palpable or even causes a visible additional local skin crease.

Occasionally a nerve root may become entrapped and the condition can present as sciatica. Treatment depends upon symptoms; sciatica is treated on the same conservative lines as a protruded intervertebral disc, but persistent backache due to instability may require spinal fusion and, in some rare instances, progression of the slip may also be an indication for fusion. A degenerative variety of the condition occurs later in life and is due to instability of the facet joints through osteoarthritis. This is almost invariably at the L4–5 level, leading to a moderate degree of forward slip of L4.

Lumbar Disc Lesions

Clinical features and diagnosis

Males are affected twice as frequently as females, usually in the 20–50-year age group. When the disc protrusion is small, there is typically acute low back pain (lumbago) with sudden stiffening of the spine, usually in flexion. There is frequently a history of indirect trauma, e.g. lifting heavy loads. Pain may be referred to the buttocks and thighs and is of a dull nature. On examination there is paravertebral muscle spasm, often pulling the spine into a non-structural scoliosis. Movements of the lumbar spine are reduced, particularly flexion. There are usually no neurological symptoms or signs. Nuclear material is bulging the richly-innervated annulus and posterior longitudinal ligament, but is not sufficient to compromise the local nerve root (Fig. 7.3).

When nuclear material prolapses through the annulus, usually posterolaterally, it compresses the local nerve root. In this situation the low back pain is less severe, but is compounded by radicular symptoms of lancinating pain shooting down the leg, often to the foot, with objective neurological evidence of nerve-root pressure in the form of either ankle reflex suppression with S1 nerve root pressure, or reduced power in extensor hallucis longus with L5 nerve-root pressure (Fig. 1.22). These signs correspond with disc prolapses at the L5–S1 and L4–5 levels respectively, which represent the great majority of cases. Occasionally the disc prolapse occurs at the L3–4 level, in which case the L4 nerve root is compressed with diminution of the knee jerk and the power of the quadriceps. Straight leg raising is reduced because this manoeuvre stretches the lumbosacral nerve roots over the prolapse (Fig. 1.28). If the prolapse is more central, there may be bilateral neurological signs and loss of bladder control. With disc prolapses higher in the lumbar spine, the femoral nerve stretch test is positive.

Conservative management

The great majority of lumbar disc protrusions settle uneventfully with two weeks strict bed rest helped by sedative and anti-inflammatory drugs. No patient should be referred for specialist advice until this regime has been tried. Nor should the spine be x-rayed at this stage; it has been estimated that plain radiography is only of value in one in 6 250 cases, and such rare cases, who may have a tumour or ankylosing spondylitis, will remain symptomatic after the period of bed rest. It is customary then to prescribe 'physiotherapy', and a variety of corsets, none of which is of any proven value.

One of the only really useful measures is attendance at a 'back school' run by physiotherapists, where the object is to teach patients about the structure and function of their back so that they will be less inclined to abuse it in the future.

For those who fail to benefit from the bed-rest regime, and particularly those with disc prolapses and objective neurological signs, further investigations are necessary. Plain radiography is rarely helpful; though it occasionally shows disc space narrowing in the younger patient or widespread degenerative changes in the older, its real value is in excluding more sinister pathology, particularly ankylosing spondylitis in the younger patient. Accordingly, the sacroiliac joints, which are always visible on the anteroposterior view of the lumbar spine, should be scrutinised for erosive disease or irregularity although these joints appear obliquely from the front.

The final common pathway for radicular symptoms is mechanical irritation of the nerve root over the prolapsed disc, with local inflammation and oedema. Therefore a further period of rest with the spine immobilised in either a plaster jacket or a high corset firm enough to increase intra-abdominal pressure may relieve symptoms.

Operative management

For those with a persistent radiculitis and neurological signs, surgical removal of the displaced nucleus is indicated. This can easily be performed through an approach between the contiguous laminae by removal of the ligamentum flavum, thus obviating the need to remove significant portions of bone, which might lead to local instability. The compressed nerve root is identified, dissected clear and retracted, and the underlying nuclear material excised. Anatomical variations in the exit of nerve roots from the spinal canal are frequently found, so preoperative myelography is most helpful (Fig. 1.42). A sample of cerebrospinal fluid is also removed during myelography and its protein content determined. A high level of protein in association with an atypical myelographic appearance indicates the presence of the more unusual intradural tumour.

The central disc prolapse with impending loss of bladder control constitutes one of the direst emergencies in surgical practice. The patient should be operated upon immediately, without any of the foregoing investigations, since delay may render the neurological situation irreversible.

Adolescent disc lesions

The older child and the adolescent also sustain intervertebral disc protrusions. The clinical picture is, however, much less clear, and the lesion often occurs high in the lumbar spine or even in the thoracic region. Protrusions are the rule and prolapses the exception so that local symptoms of pain, muscle spasm, scoliosis and limited movement are common but objective neurological signs rare.

Diagnosis is not easy and, combined with the difficulty of treatment, is responsible for the protracted clinical course which characterises this condition. Plain x-rays are only helpful in excluding other pathology, notably infective discitis. Treatment is conservative and may involve the use of a plaster jacket for several months before symptoms settle. When persistent neurological signs are present, myelography cannot often help because the protrusions are usually not significant enough to distort the dye column. Surgical intervention is also unrewarding as the nuclear material is often liquid rather than the tougher crabmeat of the adult.

When plain films demonstrate disc-space narrowing with irregularity and erosion of the endplates of contiguous vertebrae (Fig. 7.9), this indicates infective discitis, which presents in the same manner as a disc protrusion. There is no systemic upset, no history of ill-health, sedimentation rate is seldom raised, and bacteriological investigations including blood titres and culture of disc material obtained at biopsy are unhelpful in the great majority of cases. The condition may indeed not be of infective origin at all and this is reinforced by the fact that the clinical course is self-limiting and eventually settles spontaneously whether or not antibiotics are empirically prescribed.

Lumbar Spondylosis

Low back pain in the older patient is likely to be due to degeneration of the intervertebral discs rather than nuclear displacement. In such patients the normal process of ageing has been accelerated and is frequently observed at multiple levels. Loss of disc-space

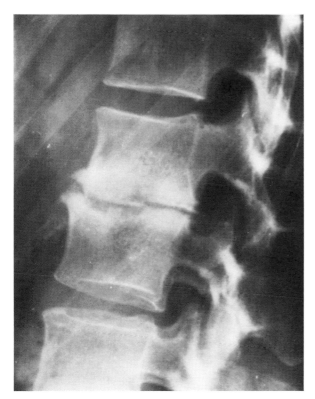

Fig. 7.9 *Lateral x-ray of the spine—disc space narrowing with irregularity and erosion of the endplates of contiguous vertebrae is characteristic of discitis.*

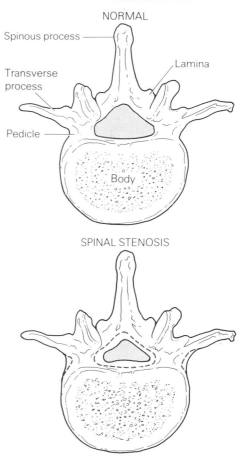

Fig. 7.10 *In spinal stenosis the dimensions of the spinal cord are compromised by new bone formation occurring in association with degenerative disease.*

height is associated with instability and degenerative change in both the intervertebral syndesmoses (spondylosis) and the posterior facet joints (osteoarthritis).

Clinical features and diagnosis

Low back pain is a dull pain, frequently continuous, often exacerbated by movement and relieved by rest, and associated with referred pain in the buttocks and thighs. New bone formation occurring posteriorly at intervertebral level may narrow the dimensions of the spinal canal, causing spinal stenosis (Fig. 7.10). The patient may then describe symptoms of spinal claudication, with muscular aches and cramps in the thighs and calves occurring at a certain walking distance, relieved by rest, and in the presence of normal peripheral vasculature.

Plain radiography demonstrates posterior facet joint osteoarthritis with joint space narrowing, irregularity

and sclerosis, and intervertebral spondylosis with sclerosis and marginal syndesmophytes (Fig. 7.11). It is, however, seldom useful for localising symptoms to a particular level. In patients with spinal stenosis, myelography may show symmetrical waisting at multiple intervertebral levels.

Treatment

The majority of patients achieve some symptomatic improvement on adopting a less vigorous lifestyle combined with anti-inflammatory analgesics. Particularly irritable backs may be helped by a supportive lumbar corset or manipulative therapy. Intractable spinal stenosis can be relieved by widening the spinal

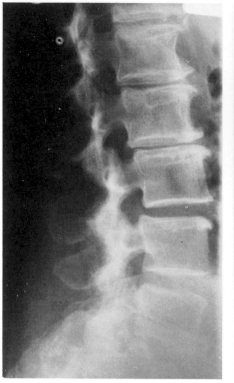
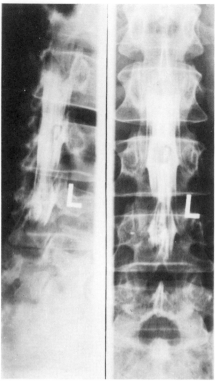

a

b

Fig. 7.11 (a) *Lumbar spondylosis with marginal syndesmophyte formation.* (b) *Myelogram of a patient with spinal stenosis showing intervertebral waisting with a block at L4–5.*

canal by means of decompressive laminectomy, although the results are frequently short-lived.

ELBOW

Cubitus Valgus

This term refers to an increase in the carrying angle of the elbow. Bilateral cubitus valgus is a feature of certain generalised skeletal disorders; when it is unilateral, the usual cause is a childhood fracture involving the lateral humeral condyle with a corresponding growth disturbance (Fig. 4.7). Functional incapacity is usually not great; the main significance of the condition is its association with the development, many years later, of an attrition neuritis of the ulnar nerve (tardy ulnar nerve

palsy), which should then be decompressed by anterior transposition of the nerve.

Cubitus Varus

This is a reversal of the carrying angle giving an unsightly deformity sometimes known as 'gunstock elbow'. It usually occurs after malunion of a supracondylar fracture sustained in childhood (Fig. 4.6). Interference with function is minimal, but correction by osteotomy of the lower end of the humerus may be undertaken if the appearance is unacceptable.

Osteochondritis Dissecans

The articular surface of the capitulum is usually affected. Necrosis of the subchondral segment of bone occurs over a fairly wide area and the overlying cartilage may become detached. It is believed to be an avascular necrosis of bone and is usually found in the second decade of life, in boys more than girls. The loose body may be symptomless but, if it locks in the joint, may lead to pain and loss of movement. The loose body may be visible on x-ray. Treatment in the early stages consists of resting the elbow but if symptoms persist the loose body should be removed.

WRIST AND HAND

Madelung's Deformity and Radial Club Hand

There is marked radial deviation of the whole hand and undue prominence of the lower end of the ulna (Fig. 7.12). Essentially this is a consequence of a disparity of

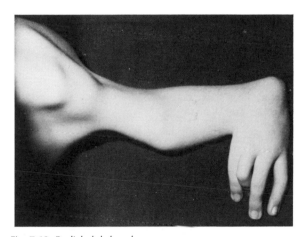

Fig. 7.12 *Radial club hand.*

length between radius and ulna, either due to congenital shortening or absence of the radius, or due to injury or disease of the lower end of the radius. In the former case there may be associated abnormalities in the thumb and radial side of the hand. Function is usually surprisingly well preserved but reconstructive surgery is sometimes necessary.

Kienboeck's Disease

Spontaneous avascular necrosis of the lunate bone occurs in this condition, which can cause pain and discomfort in the wrist joint. There is tenderness over the lunate with a reduction of wrist movement. Radiographs demonstrate a sclerotic collapsed lunate bone.

Treatment consists of resting the wrist but if symptoms persist the lunate should be excised.

Congenital Digital Anomalies

Syndactyly

The fusion of digits is often multiple, and may involve both hands and feet. Surgical separation in the upper limb is indicated to improve hand function and is normally carried out at about the age of four.

Polydactyly

Additional digits are very common in both upper and lower limbs. In some cases the attachment is by a small skin pedicle, and can be amputated soon after birth. If the digit is well formed, surgery should be delayed until the age of four or five, when function can be more fully assessed.

Congenital absence of digits

These may be single or multiple; the reduction may be total, or significant parts of the digit may remain. Reconstruction should be delayed until the age of four or five, when the function of the hand can be properly assessed.

HIP

Disorders of the developing and growing hip joint tend to occur within particular age ranges (Table 7.1). Age is therefore a useful aetiological guide when a child presents with a hip problem. The vast majority of congenital hip dislocations are diagnosed within a few days of birth by routine hospital screening. Occasionally they are missed and present later, most commonly as a result of the first school medical examination at the age of five. Perthes' disease typically presents between 4 and 9 years; slipping of the upper femoral epiphysis occurs between 9 years and maturity, when the epiphyses close.

Table 7.1

Hip Disorders in Children

Age	Condition
0–5	Congenital dislocation
2–10	Irritable hip and infective arthritis
4–9	Perthes' disease
9–maturity	Slipping upper femoral epiphysis

The irritable hip syndrome and infective arthritis can occur at any time during growth, usually within 10 years of birth.

Congenital Dislocation

Mechanisms

The aetiology is probably multifactorial. At birth, the acetabulum is a relatively shallow cavity and dislocation readily occurs for a variety of reasons. There is a familial tendency, and abnormal intra-uterine positions also contribute; the dislocation is ten times more frequent in breech deliveries. Excessive joint laxity and anteversion of both femoral neck and acetabulum, are also important factors.

Clinical features and diagnosis

Girls are affected six times more frequently than boys and, although some cases are bilateral, most are unilateral, with the left side much more commonly affected for unknown reasons. The diagnosis should be made at birth, using the tests of Ortolani and Barlow (Fig. 1.17). If it is overlooked at birth, it is more easily detected radiographically after the age of six months (Fig. 7.13). Clinical suspicion should be aroused by limited abduction of the hip, asymmetrical skin creases, or any other form of asymmetry, such as plagiocephaly or torticollis.

Treatment (Table 7.2)

When diagnosed at birth, treatment consists of splinting the hip in the reduced position of moderate flexion and abduction until stability is achieved (usually 6–8

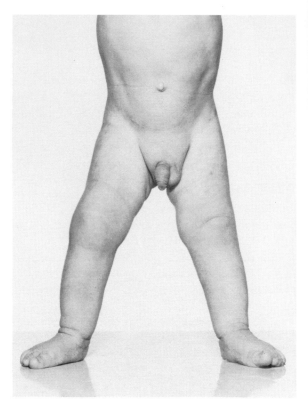

a

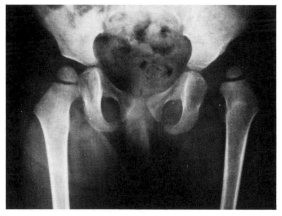

b

Fig. 7.13 (a) *The clinical appearance of congenital dislocation of the left hip with asymmetric skin creases. (b) Anteroposterior radiograph of an infant's hips. The left hip is dislocated. The ossific nucleus of the capital epiphysis does not lie inside the horizontal line drawn through the triradiate cartilages (Hilgenreiner's line), and a vertical line passing through the lateral edge of the acetabulum (Perkins's line).*

Table 7.2
Treatment of Congenital Hip Dislocation

Age	
0–1 month	Abduction splint
1–9 months	Pavlik harness
9–18 months	Frame/open reduction and femoral osteotomy
18 months–7 years	Pelvic osteotomy
7 years–maturity	No treatment
Adulthood	Total hip replacement

weeks). These splints are made of waterproof material and should not be removed until the end of treatment. A check x-ray is necessary in the splint to ensure that the hip is in the reduced position. If the diagnosis is made at the three-month child assessment clinic by the family doctor or health visitor then a Pavlik harness should be applied. This is a gentle means of encouraging gradual reduction of the hip by increasing abduction. A great majority will stabilise with this treatment, and the prognosis is good as the primary problem has been corrected before the secondary problems of hip dysplasia can arise. If the diagnosis is made at the time of the commencement of walking then the prognosis diminishes appreciably. On no account should such a hip be manipulated back into position, as there is a serious risk of jeopardising the tenuous blood supply to both the femoral head and the upper femoral epiphysis, with the disastrous complications of avascular necrosis and progressive growth asymmetry.

Reduction must therefore be a gradual process on some form of abduction frame, and for a complete dislocation a full three weeks should be allowed for this process to reduce the risks of avascular necrosis, although a shorter time is permissible for a subluxation. If an x-ray then shows that the head will not seat concentrically into the acetabulum, then an open reduction operation is necessary to divide the capsule and to remove whatever soft tissue is preventing full relocation. The hip is then plastered until the capsule contracts around the reduced position. To save time the femur can be osteotomised below the trochanters to bring the leg to the neutral position, while leaving the head properly located.

Even later diagnosis implies that secondary dysplasia on the pelvic side has occurred and attention should then be directed to the acetabular side of the joint.

Division of the pelvis above the acetabulum allows the upper part of the hip joint to be moved so that the femoral head is better covered. If the diagnosis is made at the unusually late time of seven years of age or older no treatment should be offered lest more harm (avascular necrosis, stiffening, pain) is done. Many of these cases, even after seemingly satisfactory initial treatment, develop early secondary osteoarthritis and a total hip replacement in early adulthood is frequently required.

Perthes' Disease

This is a condition which affects the head of the femur in growing children between 4 and 10 years. Boys are more commonly affected than girls, and the condition is usually unilateral. The basic pathological change appears to be an obstruction to the blood supply of the femoral head resulting in avascular necrosis of part of its centre of ossification (Fig. 7.14).

The child presents with a painful limp, which is more marked when tired and increases as the disease progresses. Pain is often referred to the ipsilateral knee and it is essential to examine the hip of a child complaining of knee pain. There is limitation of hip movement, notably abduction and internal rotation.

The presentation may be so acute as to simulate septic arthritis, particularly in the younger child. The

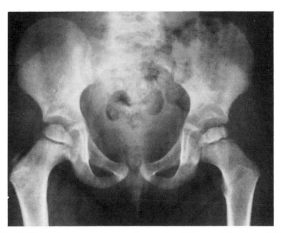

Fig. 7.14 *Anteroposterior radiograph of the pelvis of a child with Perthes' disease of the left hip. There is sclerosis and fragmentation of the ossific nucleus of the femoral capital epiphysis.*

erythrocyte sedimentation rate and white cell count should be ascertained and, in particularly severe cases, joint aspiration may be necessary to exclude infection. Radiographs, however, show the typical features of irregularity, sclerosis and collapse of the femoral head. There is also often irregularity of the epiphyseal plate, particularly on the metaphyseal side.

In the first instance, treatment is by bed rest with skin traction until local symptoms have settled. Thereafter the most important factor determining the outcome is whether or not the hip joint is subluxated laterally. Without subluxation, no treatment is necessary; revascularisation and reconstitution of the shape of the femoral head will occur uneventfully. If there is evidence of subluxation, however, the hip joint should be properly located and this can be conveniently performed by way of a varus derotation subtrochanteric osteotomy. Persistent subluxation is associated with persistent local deformity and early osteoarthritis is inevitable.

Irritable Hip

Children frequently present with a painful hip and a limp to which no definite cause can be attributed. Pain presents in the groin or thigh and may radiate into the knee. The only positive findings are pain and limitation of movement, particularly of rotation. Infection, inflammatory disorders and Perthes' disease must be excluded. Treatment consists of bed rest for a few days until the pain resolves.

Medial Femoral Torsion (Persistent Fetal Alignment)

This occurs mainly in girls, presenting as an intoeing gait (pigeon toes), and is usually seen from 6 to 7 years onwards. When the child stands with her feet together, the patellae can be seen to point medially and examination of hip rotation in extension shows that, while the total range is normal (about 90°), there is a preponderance of medial rotation, which frequently approaches 90° while external rotation may be confined to only a few degrees. When the child is young, she tends to stand with her knees rotated medially, hence the intoeing gait. Correction nearly always

occurs spontaneously with growth, and treatment is not indicated.

Coxa Vara

Here the angulation between the neck and shaft of the femur is increased, the trochanter is raised and Trendelenburg's sign is positive. There is true shortening of the leg and abduction is obviously reduced. The cause is often indicated by the age of the patient.

Congenital coxa vara

This is due to abnormal development of the upper epiphysis of the femur and is usually bilateral. The child develops a characteristic waddling gait and the condition is difficult to separate clinically from congenital dislocation. The radiological appearances are, however, characteristic. Treatment is by valgus osteotomy, which may have to be repeated several times during growth.

Adolescent coxa vara

This is the result of slipping of the upper femoral epiphysis (Fig. 7.15). Although there is an acute form of this condition, which is effectively a fracture-separation of the upper femoral epiphysis, the majority of cases are insidious. Characteristically it affects children who are overweight in the early stages of puberty, often presenting with a limp rather than pain. The physical

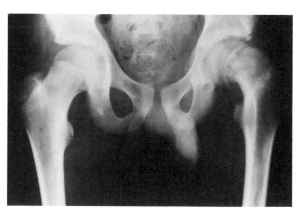

Fig. 7.15 *Anteroposterior radiograph of the hip of an adolescent with slipping upper femoral epiphysis. The slip is much more noticeable on the left side.*

signs are also characteristic, with shortening and loss of abduction. The leg lies in external rotation, but flexion of the hip causes a position of extreme lateral rotation which is diagnostic.

Treatment depends on the extent of the slip. If this is moderate, the position can usually be held by internal fixation with metal pins until the epiphysis closes. If the slip is more severe, reconstructive surgery including an osteotomy of either the femoral neck or the upper shaft will be required. Unfortunately these procedures, especially the former, carry a serious risk of avascular necrosis.

KNEE

Genu Varum (Bow Leg)

This is extremely common in children at the toddler stage. The deformity is typically mild and symmetrical. Spontaneous resolution of the condition can confidently be anticipated – indeed it is sometimes referred to as 'physiological bow leg'. Before making this diagnosis, however, rickets and Blount's disease should be excluded.

With rickets, the deformity is often quite marked and appears to involve the lower third of the tibia as well as the region of the knee. The usual stigmata of the rib rosary and frontal bossing are frequently present, but in doubtful cases an x-ray of the wrist is advisable (Fig. 6.9). Blount's disease is a rare condition in which congenital hypoplasia of the medial half of the upper tibial epiphysis results in a varus deformity.

In adults, bow leg most commonly arises from osteoarthritis, but osteomalacia and other bone-softening diseases such as Paget's disease should also be borne in mind.

Genu Valgum (Knock Knee)

Like bow leg, this condition is most commonly seen as a physiological variant. Children affected are, however, a little older, often 6–7 years old when the condition is first noticed. Again, spontaneous correction is the rule, but there are exceptions who will require an operative procedure to reduce growth on the medial side of the

epiphyses around the knee, usually by the insertion of a metal staple. Rarely, osteotomy may be indicated. Such children are nearly always overweight. This should be noted when the condition is first diagnosed.

Excessive shoe wear sometimes occurs on the inner side, in which case an inner heel 'raise' may improve gait and will certainly lead to longer shoe life. It will, however, have no effect whatever on the deformity itself. Again, rickets should be excluded.

In adults, osteoarthritis, osteomalacia, and Paget's disease are all common causes.

Chondromalacia Patellae

As the name implies, there is softening of the articular cartilage on the under-surface of the patella, usually on the medial side. The condition characteristically affects adolescents and young adults, and females predominate. The clinical feature is a dull retropatellar pain, particularly when the knee is flexed and the patello-femoral joint is therefore loaded. Thus, sitting for long periods or going down stairs brings on the discomfort. The cartilage softening is associated with irregularity, and the patient may be conscious of a grating sensation under the kneecap which imparts crepitus to the examining hand. Intermittent effusion, quadriceps wasting, and giving way are also common. X-rays are not helpful. The condition can be regarded as either primary or secondary.

The primary condition, although troublesome to the patient and difficult to treat, is self-limiting; it lasts up to a year with no tendency towards subsequent osteoarthritis. Anti-inflammatory drugs, quadriceps exercises, and splintage in plaster are the mainstays of treatment. Surgery is not indicated.

The condition may be secondary to an abnormality in the tracking of the patella through the intercondylar region of the femur. Thus individuals with genu valgum, genu recurvatum (natural hyperextension of the knee, Fig. 1.12), or generalised ligamentous laxity, are prone to develop symptoms of chondromalacia secondary to the mechanical problem. Similarly, adolescents or young adults with a tendency to subluxate or even dislocate the patella laterally present with symptoms of chondromalacia.

It would seem logical to create a more normal patellar tracking mechanism surgically by moving the insertion of the patellar tendon downwards and medially, thus minimising the likelihood of the patella moving laterally during knee flexion. This is indeed performed in recurrent dislocation of the patella for mechanical reasons, but any alteration of patellar alignment must lead to asymmetrical loading of the patellofemoral joint, with the increased risk of developing osteoarthritis. Surgery should therefore be withheld unless the patient continues to have severe symptoms.

Osteochondritis of the Knee

Mechanical derangement of the immature knee does not occur through a mensical tear. In youth a fragment of articular cartilage with attached subchondral bone loosens and may eventually shear, usually from the lateral aspect of the medial femoral condyle. The aetiology of this condition is not clear but it appears to be associated with an impairment of blood supply, either occurring spontaneously or as the result of an osteochondral fracture. The patient is typically an immature male of athletic ability presenting with local discomfort, effusion, quadriceps wasting and a history of locking or giving way. In the process of separation, the lesion is visible radiographically; radio-opaque dye introduced at arthrography may track between the fragment and its base (Fig. 7.16). When detached, the loose body is usually not visible, but the residual crater provides the diagnosis. If the fragment is not separated, it can be pinned back into position. A loose body requires removal.

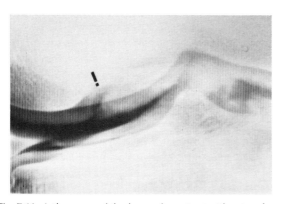

Fig. 7.16 *Arthrogram of the knee of a patient with osteochondritis dissecans showing dye tracking beneath the fragment, indicating impending total detachment.*

Occasionally, mechanical derangement of the immature knee is due to a congenitally misshapen meniscus which, instead of being semilunar, is discoid in shape. The condition is nearly always symptomatically self-limiting; whenever possible, the cartilage should not be removed because removal will certainly lead to early osteoarthritis.

FOOT

Club Foot (Talipes)

This congenital abnormality can be considered in two ways; the first takes into account the anatomy of the deformity, while the second makes the important distinction between postural and structural forms (Fig. 7.17).

Calcaneovalgus deformity

This exists only in a postural form and is therefore a benign condition. The appearance of the foot at birth is, however, very striking. There is extreme dorsiflexion so that the dorsum of the foot may lie against the shin and the forefoot is twisted into valgus. The postural nature of the condition is shown by the fact that, with gentle manipulation, the deformity can be corrected. It probably arises because the foot has occupied a cramped ~~space~~ in utero during the latter weeks of pregnancy. Spontaneous resolution invariably occurs.

Equinovarus deformity

Most cases are structural, the condition is serious, and urgent action is called for. The foot is plantarflexed and inverted, as the name suggests, but when an attempt is made to restore the neutral position it is evident that the condition is fixed by soft-tissue contractures.

The condition is commoner in boys, and is usually bilateral. The involvement is almost never symmetrical, however, and symmetry suggests muscle imbalance from some underlying neurological cause such as spina bifida. There is marked wasting of the calf, which may present a 'pipestem' appearance, and another unfavourable prognostic factor is that the os calcis is small and difficult to feel.

early surgical release of the contracted structures on the posteromedial aspect of the foot. If this condition is neglected, very severe and disabling deformity results.

There is a rare postural form of the condition in which calf wasting is absent, the heel is well developed, and the foot can be brought to neutral or near neutral. Obviously the distinction between this and a mild form of the structural condition is difficult to make and it is safer to use some form of corrective splintage.

Pes Planus

A flat foot is referred to as a valgus foot because of the eversion of the heel. It implies that the arch has collapsed by falling over sideways as a result of the eversion movement. Flat foot may be a result of muscle imbalance, which allows the peronei to pull the foot into the valgus position. However, in the majority of instances no underlying cause can be detected.

The postural nature of the deformity is illustrated when the patient attempts to stand on tiptoe, when the arch is restored. Minor problems do arise; excessive shoe wear is common, which, in a small child, may be helped by an inner heel 'raise'. Later in life, secondary degenerative changes may supervene, giving rise to a rigid flat foot. Very rarely, the pain may be so severe as to require joint arthrodesis.

Pes Cavus

This deformity, which usually presents in late childhood and adolescence, may involve abnormalities of forefoot, midfoot and hindfoot (Fig. 7.18). In the former there is clawing of the toes. In the midfoot, the longitudinal arch is markedly raised, and in the hindfoot there is varus of the heel.

Even in the most severely affected cases the deformity is seldom crippling. Many are associated with neurological conditions; peroneal muscular atrophy is the commonest, closely followed by spina bifida. It also occurs in rarer conditions, such as Friedreich's ataxia. Treatment is directed towards whichever of the deformities is the most prominent; an attempt to straighten the toes is usually the most rewarding.

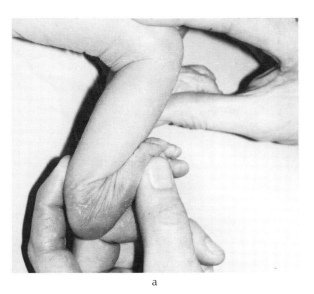

a

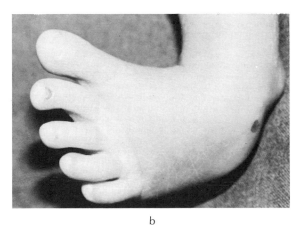

b

Fig. 7.17 (a) *Calcaneovalgus deformity—an unimportant and self-limiting condition.* (b) *Equinovarus deformity—an important and progressive condition.*

The aetiology is unknown and, although the condition behaves like a paralytic deformity, neurological disease can only be identified in a very small number of cases. Treatment should be begun on the day of birth, since even a delay of a few days may compromise the end result. Essentially this consists of gentle manipulation and either serial plasters or some form of retentive strapping. In some cases a satisfactory correction can be obtained in a matter of weeks but splintage then has to be retained for the next 12 months. Many other cases prove resistant to such treatment and will require

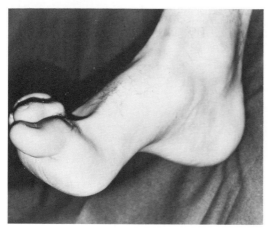

Fig. 7.18 *Pes cavus—the longitudinal arch is elevated, the metatarsal heads press downwards into the sole and the toes are compensatorily clawed.*

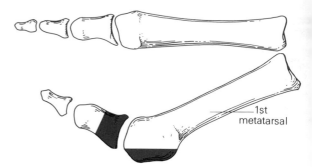

Fig. 7.19 *Hallux valgus. The first metatarsal is in varus and the toe in valgus. In Keller's operation the shaded areas are resected.*

Claw Toes

Both interphalangeal joints are held flexed and calluses often form over them. These may occur in association with pes cavus, but the cause is usually unknown. When the joints are mobile, the flexor tendons may be transferred to the extensors to act as intrinsics. When the metatarsophalangeal joints are completely dislocated, excision of the proximal phalanx is the only solution.

Hammer Toes

The proximal interphalangeal joint is flexed, but the distal joint is hyperextended. If the toe causes problems with shoe fitting, it may be straightened by an arthrodesis of the terminal joint.

Hallux Valgus

This is the commonest toe deformity and afflicts mainly females in later life although it can occur in the adolescent or young adult (Fig. 7.19). The first ray is too long and the big toe buckles at the metatarso-phalangeal joint, so that the metatarsal head projects medially and the toe laterally. It only occurs in shod races and the shoe rubs against the metatarsal head producing an exostosis and a painful overlying adventitious bursa, a bunion. The bunion may become inflamed and infected.

In the older patient the symptomatic condition is best dealt with by Keller's procedure, removal of the exostosis and the proximal half of the proximal phalanx with tightening of the medial capsule. In the younger patient a lateral displacement osteotomy of the metatarsal neck is preferred.

Osteochondritis of the Foot

Sever's disease (osteochondritis of the heel), Kohler's disease (osteochondritis of the navicular) and Freiberg's disease (osteochondritis of the metatarsal heads) are characterised by radiographic sclerosis and fragmentation of these bones in childhood or adolescence. The conditions are self-limiting, seldom lasting for more than two years, and local pain is the mode of presentation. If pain is severe or protracted then the foot should be rested in a plaster cast.

These self-limiting conditions seldom give rise to severe symptoms but plaster immobilisation is occasionally necessary.

8

Soft Tissue Lesions

Soft tissue lesions of the musculoskeletal system are common. Although many eventually settle spontaneously, some may cause considerable morbidity which can be reduced by early recognition and treatment. Some, e.g. bicipital tendonitis and trigger finger, are often occupational, being caused by repetitive movements. Others, e.g. hamstring strains and shin splints, are mainly sporting injuries. With increased leisure time, interest in athletics and jogging has increased, and with it the number of sports-related injuries.

SHOULDER AND UPPER ARM

Frozen Shoulder

This is a common condition of unknown aetiology. Symptoms are often precipitated by using the shoulder with the arm elevated, causing pain, which may last for months but which eventually subsides and is followed by a progressive loss of movement. This stage represents the true frozen shoulder, and may last for many months.

In the early stage, pain is helped by short-wave diathermy and gentle exercise. The late stage with grossly restricted movement can be dramatically improved by a careful manipulation under anaesthetic to break down the adhesions, followed by an immediate course of intensive physiotherapy.

Painful Arc Syndrome

This is another variety of painful shoulder, but the pattern is different. At rest, with the arm hanging by the side, and at full abduction, the shoulder is comfortable. However, pain is felt over the top of the shoulder when the arm is abducted between 60° and 120° (Fig. 8.1). On continuing elevation, the pain diminishes. This arc of movement is painful because, when the bulk of the greater tuberosity of the humerus slides under the acromion, there is increased tension in the restricted

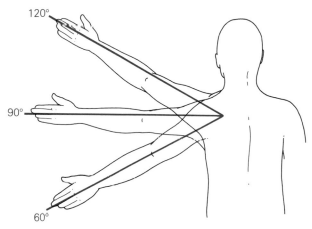

Fig. 8.1 *Painful arc syndrome. The patient complains of pain when abducting the shoulder between 60° and 120°. Beyond these limits movement of the shoulder is comfortable.*

subacromial space. Causes include an incomplete tear of the supraspinatus tendon, degenerative supraspinatus tendonitis, calcification within the supraspinatus tendon, and subacromial bursitis.

If the symptoms do not settle with simple measures such as short-wave diathermy, an injection of steroid and local anaesthetic may be necessary. Calcific deposits may require surgical removal.

Tenosynovitis of the Biceps Tendon

The tendon of the long head of biceps runs in the intertubercular groove, where it may be subject to repeated strain causing tenosynovitis. The major clinical sign is tenderness to palpation along the bicipital groove in front of the humerus. Flexing the shoulder against resistance provokes pain.

Mild cases usually respond to rest and short-wave diathermy or ultrasound. More severe cases are helped by a steroid injection together with local anaesthetic into the synovial sheath. Care should be taken not to inject the steroid into the tendon itself as this may result in weakening or even rupture.

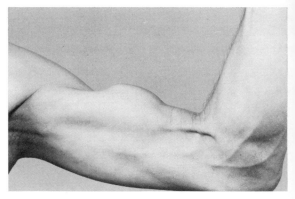

Fig. 8.2 *Rupture of the long head of biceps. The biceps muscle presents as a soft tissue mass in the front of the lower arm when the elbow is flexed.*

Rupture of the Long Tendon of Biceps

The tendon of the long head of biceps can rupture, allowing the muscle belly to bunch up in the lower part of the arm (Fig. 8.2). This occasionally follows injection but the great majority of cases occur spontaneously, probably as a result of constant friction where the tendon enters the bicipital groove.

Once the acute pain of the rupture has settled, the functional disability is slight and treatment is not indicated.

ELBOW AND FOREARM

Lateral and Medial Epicondylitis of the Elbow (Tennis Elbow and Golfer's Elbow)

Lateral epicondylitis (tennis elbow) is an inflammation of the common extensor origin at the site of attachment to the lateral epicondyle of the humerus. It is due to overuse or strain of the forearm extensor muscles. Pain is felt on the outside of the elbow and extends down the forearm. Tenderness is localised to the front of the lateral epicondyle. Extending the wrist and fingers against resistance often aggravates the discomfort. Movements are full.

Injections of local anaesthetic with a steroid are frequently effective. Short-wave diathermy or ultrasound may help and, in very resistant cases, surgical detachment of the common extensor tendon from the lateral epicondyle is indicated.

Medial epicondylitis (or golfer's elbow) is a similar condition but not as common. Treatment is along the same lines as for tennis elbow.

Olecranon Bursitis

There is usually a superficial bursa between skin and the attachment of the triceps tendon to the olecranon. It is liable to become inflamed, often following trauma or in association with gout, and may fill with clear fluid. If this is painless it can be left alone, as aspiration is frequently unsuccessful. Persistent or painful bursitis should be treated by careful excision. Septic bursitis always requires surgical drainage.

Volkmann's Ischaemic Contracture

Fibrous contracture of the extrinsic and intrinsic muscles of the forearm and hand is the late result of ischaemia. In children, the commonest cause is a displaced supracondylar fracture of the humerus (Fig. 4.6), whereas in the adult it is a crush injury to the forearm with the development of a 'compartment syndrome'. The deep muscles of the flexor compartment have the most precarious blood supply and are constrained by surrounding fascia.

The early sign is flexor spasm. The classical symptoms

and signs — severe and unrelenting pain following trauma, loss of the radial pulse, paraesthesia, weakness, and pallor — are late, and usually indicate that irreversible damage has already occurred. Early fasciotomy of the muscle compartments of the forearm is required to relieve compression of the main vessels and muscle capillary beds. The earlier this is carried out, the less the damage. If the lesion is due to damage to the brachial artery, urgent repair is indicated.

The late case presents with flexion contractures of the wrist and fingers. The wrist can be partly extended if the fingers are flexed maximally, and the fingers can be partly extended when the wrist is fully flexed (Fig. 8.3).

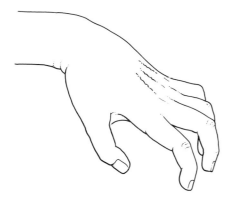

Fig. 8.3 *Volkmann's ischaemic contracture. In the fully established case, fibrosis of the forearm muscles is associated with a flexion contracture of the wrist and fingers. If the wrist is maximally flexed, then extension can take place at the metacarpophalangeal and interphalangeal joints.*

Treatment of the established contracture depends upon its degree. Mild contractures may be treated by dynamic splinting to maintain finger extension. More severe contractures require tendon lengthening or muscle slide procedures to move the origin of the flexor mass distally.

WRIST AND HAND

Ganglia

Ganglia are firm but fluctuant cysts filled with a colourless gelatinous fluid; they transilluminate bril-

liantly if large enough. The commonest sites are on the back or front of the wrist (Fig. 8.4). They also occur on the flexor tendon sheath at the level of the metacarpal head. Here the ganglion is tense and tender, and may simulate trigger finger.

Ganglia arise by degeneration in the fibrous lining of

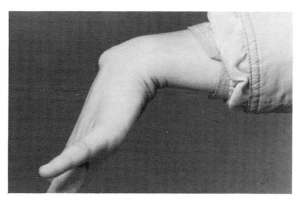

Fig. 8.4 *Ganglion. The commonest site is on the dorsum of the wrist, the lesion presenting as a firm but fluctuant swelling.*

joints and tendons and remain fixed to these underlying structures.

They may disappear spontaneously, but tend to recur. They can sometimes be burst by digital pressure. Careful surgical excision of the entire ganglion is the procedure of choice.

De Quervain's Tendovaginitis Stenosans

This is a contracture of the fibrous sheath of the extensor pollicis brevis and abductor pollicis longus tendons over the radial styloid, with local synovitis, resulting in pain on the radial side of the wrist with extension and abduction of the thumb. Repetitive frictional trauma is the most likely cause. The condition may resolve spontaneously; three weeks' immobilisation in a plaster cast may resolve it; but operative treatment with longitudinal incision of the sheath of the two tendons, is most effective.

Dupuytren's Contracture

Dupuytren's contracture is caused by a proliferative fibrosis of the subcutaneous palmar aponeurosis (Fig.

8.5). The lesions may be nodules tethered to the skin, or bands running longitudinally from the palm to the digits, causing flexion contractures. It occurs more commonly in men, is associated with epilepsy, alcoholism and diabetes, and is frequently bilateral. The incidence increases with age and there may be a positive family history. The ring finger is most often affected. There may be an associated contracture of

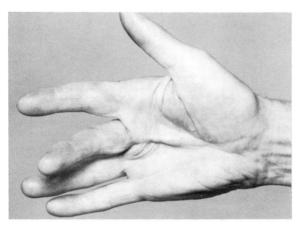

Fig. 8.5 *Dupuytren's contracture. Thickening of the palmar aponeurosis with contracture of the middle finger.*

the plantar aponeurosis and more rarely a contracture of the fibrous tissue of the penis.

In the absence of contracture, no treatment is required. Selective fasciectomy, with excision of the contracted bands, is the treatment of choice. In severe cases with fixed contractures of the interphalangeal joints of the little finger, amputation may be necessary.

Trigger Finger and Thumb

Triggering of the digits is caused by the development of a nodule in the flexor tendon just proximal to the mouth of the fibrous sheath at the level of the metacarpal head, which is a region of constant friction. Triggering also occurs in rheumatoid patients whose sheaths are filled with diseased synovium. On attempting to extend the fully flexed finger, the nodule in the tendon is impeded as it moves into the fibrous tunnel, resulting in a jerk. In severe cases the affected finger may be locked in the flexed position and the patient has

to passively extend it. On clinical examination a tender nodule can be felt in the flexor tendon overlying the metacarpal head. The same pathology is responsible for flexion contractures of the thumb in infants.

Mild cases settle spontaneously. If it is severe, the best form of treatment is surgical division of the mouth of the proximal fibrous tunnel to allow free sliding of the swollen tendon.

HIP AND THIGH

Trochanteric Bursitis

Inflammation of the trochanteric bursa may be irritative, caused by friction between the fascia lata and the greater trochanter of the femur. Injection of steroid and local anaesthetic is of value.

Occasionally the bursa may be the site of pyogenic or tuberculous infection. If pus is present, incision of the bursa is necessary to allow free drainage and culture to identify the organism. Tuberculous trochanteric bursitis has a more insidious presentation. If an acid-fast bacillus can be identified, excision should be undertaken with appropriate antituberculous chemotherapy.

KNEE AND LEG

Prepatellar and Infrapatellar Bursitis

Prepatellar bursitis (housemaid's knee) may follow a direct blow to the front of the knee, but it is more frequently a result of constant irritation such as prolonged kneeling. The bursa is subcutaneous and covers the lower half of the patella (Fig. 8.6), and when irritated it fills with fluid which may become infected.

Infrapatellar bursitis (clergyman's knee) is a similar condition that follows frictional pressure below the patella. The resulting bursa lies superficial to the patellar tendon.

Small bursae with no symptoms require no treatment. Larger, painful or tender bursae may warrant excision, ensuring that the deep space is carefully closed at surgery. An infected bursa requires incision, drainage, and appropriate antibiotics.

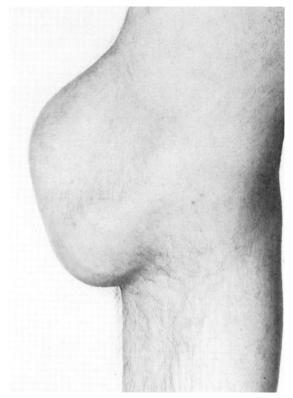

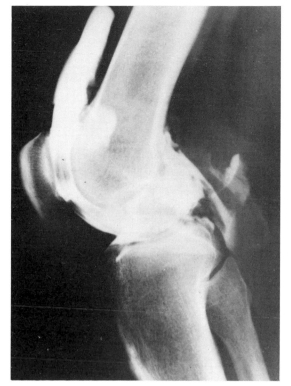

Fig. 8.6 *Prepatellar and infrapatellar bursitis in the same patient. Prepatellar bursitis occurs in front of the patella, and infrapatellar bursitis occurs in front of the patellar tendon.*

Fig. 8.7 *Lateral arthrogram of the knee showing a popliteal cyst posteriorly from which dye is escaping, thus indicating rupture.*

Popliteal Cyst

When a swelling in the popliteal space is located centrally, it is called a popliteal cyst. It is more easily palpable when the knee is extended. When the knee is flexed, the cyst becomes lax. It is formed as a 'blow-out' of fluid from the knee through the posterior capsule. It frequently communicates with the knee joint, but cannot be emptied by pressure because flow is unidirectional from knee to cyst. It may be secondary to osteoarthritis or rheumatoid disease.

Occasionally, a popliteal cyst may rupture into the calf, producing symptoms similar to a deep vein thrombosis. The diagnosis is confirmed by arthrography, when the dye is seen to pass from the knee to the calf (Fig. 8.7).

Treatment is directed at the underlying condition in the knee but, if the cyst is extensive and symptomatic, excision is indicated.

Semimembranosus Bursa

This is the commonest swelling behind the knee in children. The bursa lies between the medial head of the gastrocnemius and the semimembranosus tendon. The swelling is tense when the knee joint is extended, and does not communicate with the knee joint.

The bursa tends to disappear spontaneously. Excision is usually avoided unless the cyst becomes large and uncomfortable.

ANKLE AND FOOT

Ganglion

Ganglia can be found around the foot and ankle and usually present as a painful lump on the dorsum of the foot. Excision is indicated if they produce symptoms due to pressure from footwear.

Conditions of the Tendo Achillis

Rupture

Complete rupture of the tendo Achillis is symptomatically typical. The patient feels sudden pain at the heel or calf, describing it as if he has been kicked, and is then unable to bear weight. Soon after injury there may be a palpable gap in the tendon. The patient may be able to actively plantarflex but cannot raise the heel from the ground whilst standing only on the affected leg. The gap rapidly fills with haematoma and is obliterated. Treatment is by surgical repair of the torn tendon; this carries a lower incidence of rerupture than conservative treatment in plaster.

Tendonitis

Achilles tendonitis is due to inflammation of the tendo Achillis paratenon by excessive friction. The patient is usually an active young adult, complaining of local pain aggravated by exercise. The tendon is tender, and a localised thickening may also be felt. Treatment is by rest in a below-knee walking plaster for four weeks. Steroid injections must never be given into the tendo Achillis because of the danger of rupture, but injections into the paratenon may help.

Bursitis

Repeated friction between the back of the heel and the shoe produces chronic inflammation and thickening of a bursa behind the insertion of the tendo Achillis. This occurs most frequently in young women, and symptoms are aggravated by walking. There is an obvious swelling at the back of the heel and the overlying skin is thickened and inflamed. Mild cases can be controlled by protecting the heel with dressings; if the bursitis persists, however, the bursa should be excised.

Tibialis Posterior Tenosynovitis

The tendon of the tibialis posterior muscle runs in a sheath behind and below the medial malleolus. Repeated friction may produce a tenosynovitis, which presents as pain brought on by activity. The area is tender and a localised thickening may be palpable. Rest in a below-knee walking plaster for four weeks is usually effective, but sheath division is occasionally necessary.

Painful Heel Pad

The patient complains of pain under the heel on standing or walking, probably due to a simple contusion. Tenderness is localised over the heel pad.

A steroid injection may speed recovery, and a sponge-rubber insole also relieves symptoms.

Plantar Fasciitis

This is thought to be due to an inflammation or strain at the site of the attachment of the plantar aponeurosis to the calcaneum. It presents as pain beneath the anterior part of the heel on standing or walking, often extending into the sole. Usually there is marked local tenderness.

Conservative measures, e.g. excavating the heel of the shoe and filling it with sorbo rubber, usually suffice. Local injection of steroid is occasionally required.

Anterior Metatarsalgia

This is due to flattening of the transverse arch producing an anterior flat foot. The patient presents with pain under the forefoot. The foot may be splayed, with callosities beneath some or all of the metatarsal heads, which are prominent in the sole of the foot. There is usually associated clawing of the toes, with local callosity formation (Fig. 8.8). The condition is commonly associated with rheumatoid disease of the metatarsophalangeal joints.

In young patients, intrinsic foot exercises may help. In older patients, a fitted insole to redistribute pressure under the foot often suffices. If symptoms are severe and fail to respond to conservative treatment, surgery may be indicated either in the form of resection of the metatarsal heads or osteotomy of the metatarsal necks with dorsal displacement.

Morton's Metatarsalgia

The patient, often a middle-aged woman, complains of pain in the forefoot radiating into adjacent toes. This is due to a neuroma of the common digital nerve to the cleft between the 3rd and 4th toes, rarely the 2nd and 3rd toes. Tenderness is usually localised to the affected nerve, and aggravated by transverse compression of the metatarsal heads. The treatment is by surgical resection of the neuroma.

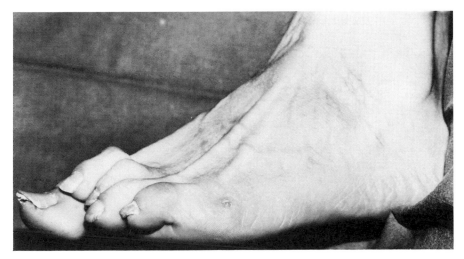

Fig. 8.8 *Flattening of the transverse arch makes the metatarsal heads prominent in the sole. The toes are compensatorily clawed.*

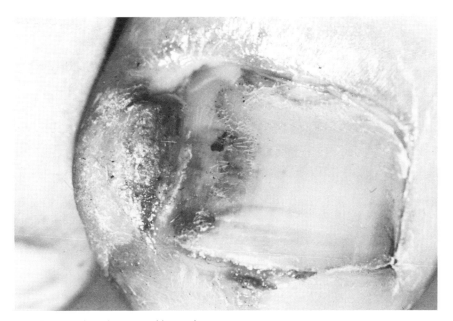

Fig. 8.9 *Ingrowing toenail—note the infection and heaped up granulation tissue, particularly at the front of the nail.*

Nail Deformities

Ingrowing toenail

Ingrowing toenail usually affects the big toe (Fig. 8.9). In this condition the side of the nail embeds itself into the local soft tissues. It occurs as a result of incorrect cutting of the toenail. When cutting the nail, its sides should be left long enough to project beyond the terminal pulp.

The patient complains of local pain and the affected corner of the nail is tender. There is exuberant granulation tissue and superadded infection. In severe cases, with obvious suppuration and exuberant granulation tissue, avulsion of the nail is required, with careful supervision of the growth of the new nail to ensure that the lesion does not recur. In recurrent cases, permanent ablation of the nail by excision of the nail bed is necessary.

Onychogryphosis

The deformed nail, usually of the big toe, is enormously thickened and curved. This usually affects elderly patients and may cause problems with footwear. Careful trimming by a chiropodist may help, but in many cases radical excision of the nail and nail bed is required.

9

Infections of Bone and Joint

OSTEOMYELITIS

This is an infection of bone caused by pathogenic organisms which reach the bone either from a wound or via the bloodstream from an infection elsewhere.

Acute Pyogenic Osteomyelitis

There is usually bacteraemic spread from an infected skin lesion. It is much commoner in children than adults and about 50% give a history of trauma.

Bacteriology

The commonest organisms causing acute osteomyelitis in Britain today are *Staph. aureus*, 90%; *Strep. pyogenes* or *pneumoniae*, 4%; *Haemophilus influenzae*, 4%; *E. coli*, *Proteus*, *K. aerogenes*, *Neisseria meningitidis* and *Salmonella* comprise the remaining 2%.

Pathology

The spongy vascular metaphyseal region collects the organism because of the end artery system near the epiphyseal growth plate. Rapid bacterial multiplication occurs, the trabeculae liquefy, and pus is formed (Fig. 9.1). In untreated cases, this medullary abscess grows and penetrates the cortex to lift up the periosteum on the outer surface. Pus then spreads extracortically and liquefaction continues within the bone. A piece of cortex then becomes isolated from its blood supply and dies, forming a sequestrum. The elevated periosteum lays down new bone on its cortical surface and attempts to surround the dead bone with new bone,

the involucrum. Pus can then damage the epiphyseal growth plate, enter the adjacent joint, spread elsewhere by septicaemic spread, or penetrate the skin to form sinuses. Thrombosis of vessels aids destruction of bone and hinders antibiotic penetration.

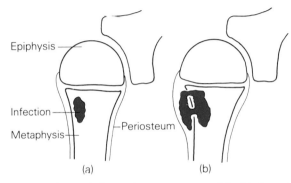

Fig. 9.1 *The pathology of acute osteomyelitis. (a) Bacteria multiply in the metaphysis while x-rays remain normal. (b) Pus then breaks through the cortex and elevates the local periosteum. This stimulates the periosteum to lay down new bone, which is often the first radiographic sign of bone infection.*

Clinical presentation

The disease starts when pathogens localise in a long-bone metaphysis. The commonest sites are the knee, the upper end of the humerus, and the lower end of the radius, but any bone can be involved. Osteomyelitis of the spine usually presents as a severely painful and extremely stiff spine. When it occurs in the pelvic bones, the disease can present as a pyrexia of unknown origin (PUO). There is local pain, loss of function, heat, swelling and redness of the overlying skin. Tenderness is acute and is localised to the metaphysis. Pyrexia, toxicity, and raised ESR and WBC are common. Blood culture may isolate the organism. It is important to know that radiographs do not show any change for 7–14 days, when osteoporosis and, later, cortical erosion with subperiosteal new bone formation occur.

Treatment

The essential steps are rest and antibiotic therapy. Immediate operation in the acute phase is not advised as the site can often not be determined accurately enough, and bone destruction is not lessened. The patient should be admitted to hospital and the affected part should be splinted in the position of rest. Blood culture takes 36 hours to show a positive growth and at least another 18 hours for antibiotic sensitivity testing. There is not always a bacteraemia, however, and cultures from blood are often negative. Therefore antibiotic therapy should be started immediately and should ensure effective early serum concentrations. Because *Staph. aureus* is the commonest pathogen, cloxacillin is given for 48 hours intramuscularly in a dose of 100 mg/kg/day and then changed to a combination of fusidic acid and erythromycin orally in doses of 30 mg/kg/day each for three weeks. If the blood culture develops *H. influenzae*, the regime is changed to ampicillin 100–150 mg/kg/day, again for three weeks.

In one-third of all cases the blood culture will not grow the infecting organism. There are many antibiotics available to which the most common infecting organism, *Staph. aureus*, is sensitive. The combination of fusidic acid and erythromycin is favoured because they have a synergistic effect and the former penetrates into both pus and infected bone with a lower incidence of toxic effects.

The role of surgery

Operation is only indicated when a fluctuant abscess forms, which occurs in about 50% of cases. The earlier that effective antibiotics are commenced, the less likelihood there is for operation. If an abscess forms, however, it must be opened; the cortex is drilled, the entire cavity and subperiosteal zone is irrigated with saline impregnated with cloxacillin, the wound is closed, and the splintage reapplied.

Clinical course

Early antibiotic treatment results in clinical improvement within 48 hours. Pain and skin tension diminish, the temperature settles, and there is improvement in the range of local joint movement. If this response is not forthcoming, and the infecting organism has not been isolated, then surgery is indicated in order to obtain local material for bacteriological culture. To persist with an inappropriate antibiotic against an unknown organism may lead to epiphyseal growth plate damage, local septic arthritis, septicaemic spread, and the development of chronic infection with sinus and sequestrum formation (Fig. 1.38).

Chronic Pyogenic Osteomyelitis

Chronic bone infection implies the presence of sequestra and gross distortion of the bone due to multiple abscesses throughout the medullary tissues. This results from inadequate treatment of the acute infection. The organism is usually *Staph. aureus*, although there may be secondary infection from the sinuses. Chronic sinus formation leads to amyloidosis and the possibility of carcinomatous change in the sinus lining. Typically the condition lasts indefinitely, with intermittent episodes of purulent discharge followed by apparent healing.

Treatment

Treatment consists of a radical operation to remove all dead and infected tissue, laying open by guttering the affected medullary cavity. Surgical treatment is supported by a prolonged course of the appropriate antibiotic and therefore all material removed at operation should be sent for bacteriological culture in order to determine any change of organism or sensitivity. Erythromycin or gentamycin may be required if organism resistance develops. Unfortunately, chronic osteomyelitis is difficult to eradicate, even by aggressive surgical treatment, and repeated operations may be necessary. Not infrequently the end result is amputation, particularly if amyloidosis or malignant change develops. Such a sequence of disasters can only be prevented by adequate treatment of the initial acute phase.

Brodie's abscess

This is a chronic pyogenic abscess in the metaphysis of a long bone, showing radiographically as a small central cavity surrounded by dense cortical bone (Fig. 9.2). The lesion is usually caused by staphylococcal infection, but it develops insidiously without an acute phase. There is a local chronic aching pain over many years, with intermittent local swelling and loss of function.

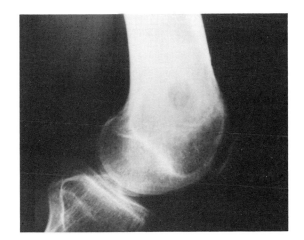

Fig. 9.2 *Lateral radiograph of the lower femur showing the central lucency without periosteal reaction of a Brodie's abscess.*

Treatment is surgical, comprising the complete evacuation of the contents of the cavity followed by irrigation with saline impregnated with cloxacillin.

SEPTIC ARTHRITIS

Pyogenic infections of joints follow the local spread of an intracapsular osteomyelitis, via the bloodstream from a focus elsewhere, or from a penetrating wound. In the first two instances the organisms are likely to be the same as for acute osteomyelitis, but wounds often produce an infection by more than one organism. *Pseudomonas* or *Clostridium* can therefore be encountered, and wounds penetrating joints should be repeatedly cultured.

Pathology

The organism causes an infected synovial effusion with local swelling, redness, warmth, intense pain and markedly limited joint movement. The presence of pus inside a joint erodes the articular cartilage and can thereby destroy the joint surfaces. Unless the infection is promptly treated, proliferation of granulation tissue occurs within the cavity, obliterating the joint space. Ultimately this leads to joint stiffening – a fibrous ankylosis. If the articular cartilage is completely destroyed, the fibrous tissue may ossify – bony ankylosis.

Clinical Features

In infants, the spread of infection is extremely rapid. The affected joint is hot, tender and rigid. Radiographs always show extensive involvement of bone at the time of presentation. There is pyrexia, malaise, and failure to gain weight. Multiple joint infections are common at this age. The hip joint in infants is particularly prone to dislocate in the presence of pyogenic infection (Smith's arthritis, Fig. 9.3).

In older children, the presentation may follow acute osteomyelitis locally, when the clinical features also include local metaphyseal infection. If the infection is the result of haematogenous spread to the synovium, the presentation is of a hot effusion without any preceding bony change.

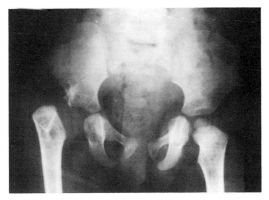

Fig. 9.3 *Anteroposterior x-ray of the pelvis of an infant with a septicaemia and dislocated hip—Smith's arthritis.*

Treatment

The diagnosis can be confirmed by joint aspiration, which provides material for bacteriological culture and reduces local discomfort. In the earliest cases it may be possible to thoroughly irrigate the joint via the aspiration needle, through which cloxacillin can also be introduced for suspected staphylococcal infection. However, in order to clean out an infected joint radically, open arthrotomy is necessary. Systemic antibiotic treatment is also administered.

Bed rest with the articulation splinted in its position of rest is also necessary. All aspirations and dressings should be performed in a strictly aseptic manner in view of the dangers of secondary infection. If the infection has given rise to considerable joint damage, then the joint should be rested in a splint or a caliper until all possibilities of re-infection have passed, when arthrodesis in a position of function is performed.

TUBERCULOSIS

Tubercle bacilli infect joints either by primary synovial infection or spread from an adjacent bone focus. The infection is secondary to a tuberculous lesion in the lung or abdominal glands.

Clinical Features and Diagnosis

Any joint at any age can be involved. Usually the infection is seen in children from lowly social circumstances. There is slow development of pain, stiffness, and swelling of a joint. Muscle wasting is marked. The history is usually months in duration and regional lymph node enlargement is common. The swollen joint is cool, painful and severely restricted in movement. The patient is ill, with loss of weight and pallor. All joints affected by tuberculosis tend to flex and adduct. This is common in the hips, giving rise to apparent shortening.

Investigations

The sedimentation rate is important in gauging the severity of infection. Radiographs should be taken of the chest and of the affected joint. Biopsy is essential to prove the diagnosis. Synovium should be sent to both pathology and bacteriology departments, to give the best possible chance of arriving at a correct diagnosis and appropriate antibiotic therapy. Excision of a lymph node was popular, but a direct attack on the joint is desirable because excision of diseased tissue – a necessary part of healing – can be carried out at the same time. Radiographs always show severe osteoporosis, and often ill-defined cavities.

Treatment

Prolonged rest in a healthy environment is a necessary general treatment. The affected joint is rested in a position such that, when healing occurs, the joint will be as functional as possible. The patient should be treated in the recumbent position on a plaster bed for spinal infection, recumbent on an abduction frame for hip infection, and recumbent on a Thomas's splint for knee infection. All abscesses should be drained by aspiration under the strictest aseptic conditions; secondary pyogenic infection greatly worsens the outcome. After resolution of the infection, arthrodesis is often necessary to produce a useful stable joint in a functional position. Progress is monitored by the patient's weight, appetite, ESR, and the degree of calcification seen radiographically.

Adequate antituberculous chemotherapy is essential.

Tuberculosis of the spine

Infection starts in the vascular endplate of a vertebral body, usually in the lower thoracic or upper lumbar region (Fig. 7.7). Spread occurs quickly through the disc so that the contiguous margins of two vertebral bodies and the intervening disc are involved. As the bone becomes structurally weak, a kyphosis develops, resulting eventually in an angular gibbus. Necrotic material and pus become extruded and lie on the sides of the bony column, giving rise to a paravertebral abscess (Fig. 9.4). Pus then tracks up and down the spine and may enter the sheath of the psoas muscles to present below the inguinal ligament as a psoas abscess in the groin. In addition, necrotic material may extend posteriorly, aided by the kyphosis, to press on the front of the spinal

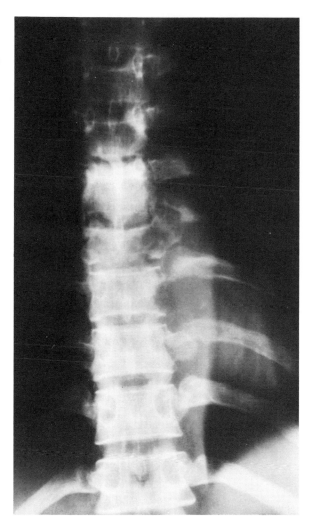

Fig. 9.4 *Anteroposterior x-ray of thoracic spine of a Vietnamese boatperson with a lower thoracic level paraplegia. There is a large paravertebral abscess in association with tuberculosis of the spine.*

cord – Pott's paraplegia. On healing, calcification follows bone destruction.

Pain, stiffness and local spasm usually precede the kyphosis. There is pallor and malaise and a raised ESR and radiographs demonstrate the collapse of two adjacent vertebrae. An unsteady gait, spasticity, or bowel and bladder dysfunction indicate spinal cord pressure from a paravertebral abscess.

Early cases with no abscess formation can be treated by a spinal support and antituberculous chemotherapy. Paravertebral abscesses must be drained, and

this should be performed urgently if there are signs of impending paraplegia. The spinal cord is compressed from the front and therefore the decompression procedure should be performed through an anterior approach. At the same time, necrotic or infected bone can be removed and replaced by a healthy autogenous graft. Rest in a plaster bed leads to graft incorporation and resultant spinal stability. Again, antituberculous chemotherapy is required.

Tuberculosis of bone

Any bone can be affected by bacteraemic spread, but most-commonly affected, besides the vertebrae, are the long bones such as femur and tibia, and the small bones of the hands and feet (Fig. 9.5). The condition may be accompanied by tuberculous arthritis, especially when long bones are involved. Radiographs demonstrate local osteoporosis, but if the infection is diaphyseal there may be cortical thickening. The cavities produced by tuberculous infection, due to caseous destruction of tissue, are ill-defined and poorly-visualised in contrast with a Brodie's abscess.

Treatment is by rest and antituberculous chemotherapy. Abscess formation requires surgical drainage.

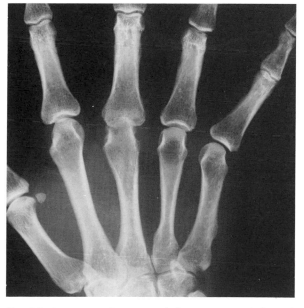

Fig. 9.5 *Anteroposterior x-ray of the metacarpophalangeal joints showing destruction of the middle finger metacarpophalangeal joint due to tuberculous arthritis.*

10

Tumours of the Musculoskeletal System

Primary malignant tumours of bone are so rare that a general practitioner has only a 3% chance of seeing one in his lifetime. Metastatic tumours in bone, on the other hand, may be found in 75% of disseminated malignancies. Unless a tumour presents with obvious swelling, the diagnosis is unlikely to come to mind. Most serious tumours present with pain of gradual onset, either felt in the region of the tumour or referred, and so must be considered in the differential diagnosis of obscure limb pain. Each cell type occurring in normal bones, cartilage, periosteum and marrow is liable to give rise to tumours, which may be benign or malignant. Tumours may thus be classified by the cell of origin (Table 10.1).

Diagnosis

Diagnosis always requires a clinical and radiological examination. The age of the patient is important, because certain tumours occur more frequently in definable age groups (Fig. 10.1). The most important local physical signs are tenderness, swelling, and joint stiffness. The regional lymph glands, though rarely enlarged, must be examined. Deformity may occur with fractures and there may be neurological signs caused by pressure on the cord or on the peripheral nerves.

Radiographs of good quality, taken in at least two planes, are essential. Where tumours are found in one side of the body, films of the opposite side are taken for comparison. Tomography is valuable to show the detail of deep-seated or dense lesions. If the diagnosis remains uncertain, a biopsy specimen may be taken from the tumour for histological study. Generally this is

Table 10.1

The Classification of Primary Tumours of Bone

Origin	Benign	Malignant
Bone	Osteoma Sub-ungal exostosis Osteoid osteoma	Osteosarcoma
Cartilage	Chondroma Chondromyxoid fibroma Chondroblastoma	Chondrosarcoma
Fibrous tissue	Benign fibroma	Fibrosarcoma
Marrow	Histiocytosis 'X' Eosinophilic granuloma	Myeloma Ewing's sarcoma Malignant lymphoma
Vascular	Haemangioma	Angiosarcoma
Uncertain origin	Solitary and aneurysmal cysts Adamantinoma Giant cell tumour	Malignant cell tumour

conclusive and therefore the most important examination in diagnosis.

Haematological and biochemical tests are made according to the suspected nature of the tumour. Malignant tumours require further investigation, to determine the extent of local spread, to seek metastases, or to find the primary lesion if the bone tumour is secondary. Bone scanning picks up bony metastases at an earlier stage than radiography.

148

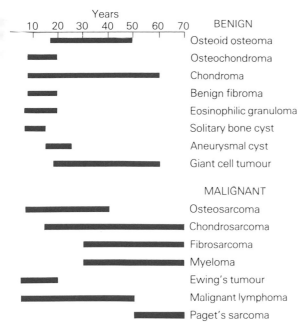

Fig. 10.1 *Diagram to show the usual age of presentation of primary tumours of bone.*

Treatment

Surgery, radiotherapy and chemotherapy are the three main curative or palliative methods of treating bone tumours. Before operation, computerised tomography and angiography may be required to determine the exact margin of the tumour, its relationship to major vessels and nerves, and its vascularity.

TUMOURS OF OSTEOBLASTIC ORIGIN

Osteoma

Single outgrowths of dense bone occur under the nail beds of fingers or toes (subungual exostoses), usually in children. These cause painful, tender, hard rounded swellings under the nail. Treatment is removal of the exostosis taking care to avoid damage to the nail bed.

Ivory dense osteomata occur on the membranous bones of the skull as painless round swellings. Unless they are within the nasal cavities, these are simply cosmetic defects and do not need to be removed.

Osteoid Osteoma

This is a benign tumour forming osteoid and bone. It is a rare, isolated lesion which occurs in young adults, causing chronic pain severe enough to disturb sleep. It may occur in any bone, but is commonest in long bones of the legs, characteristically showing on radiographs as an area of translucency surrounded by an area of dense sclerosis due to bone reaction (Fig. 10.2). Benign osteoblastoma is a similar but larger lesion.

Treatment is by surgical excision.

Osteosarcoma

Clinical features and diagnosis

Also called osteogenic sarcoma, this is a primary malignant tumour derived from primitive bone-forming cells. It consists of spindle-shaped sarcoma cells, with variable amounts of osteoid and cartilage. Osteosarcoma is one of the commonest lethal primary tumours of bone; compared with secondary malignant tumours, though, it is rare. Only about 150 cases are reported annually in Britain. Most patients are between 10 and 15 years old; the incidence then falls until, after the age of fifty, there is a second peak caused by osteosarcoma complicating Paget's disease of bone.

No bone is immune but the larger bones, notably the pelvis, femur, tibia and humerus, are most commonly affected. Tumours of long bones usually arise in the metaphyseal region, and cause gradually increasing local pain and swelling which becomes tender. The radiological features are variable; it is rare for all the typical changes to be found in one patient. A mixture of osteolysis and patchy sclerosis develops in the medulla. The cortex becomes expanded, eroded, and later broken through. The periosteum overlying the tumour may become calcified and, at the margin of the tumour mass, a calcified triangle (Codman's triangle) may be seen. Occasionally, calcified striae radiate out (sunray spiculation) from this bone into the extra-osseous tumour (Fig. 10.3). In 50% of cases the serum alkaline phosphatase is raised.

Osteosarcomata spread in all directions by invasion and destruction, except in metaphyseal tumours, which are restrained by the epiphyseal plate. Involvement of regional lymph glands is rare, but metastasis by

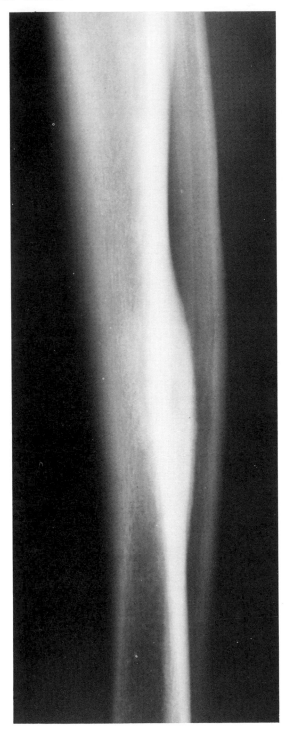

Fig. 10.2 *Anteroposterior x-ray of the tibia showing an osteoid osteoma. There is a uniformly dense zone with a small central lucency.*

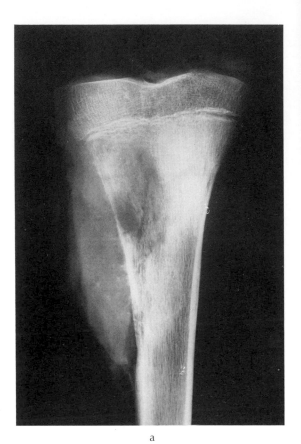

a

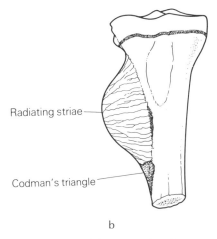

Radiating striae

Codman's triangle

b

Fig. 10.3 *Osteosarcoma of the upper tibia. (a) Anteroposterior radiograph of the upper tibia after amputation, showing an ill-defined area of bone destruction with radiating ossification outside bone. (b) Diagram of the same lesion.*

the bloodstream occurs more often than not. The lung is the most common site of secondary deposits, but they may occur in any part of the body. More than 50% of cases develop visible pulmonary metastases within a year of diagnosis and, of these, many must have had invisible micrometastases at the time of diagnosis.

Treatment

A biopsy specimen must be taken from the tumour for histological examination before treatment is started. Limb tumours are treated by amputation if there are no visible lung metastases. Ineradicable tumours with lung metastases are treated by high-energy irradiation. Removal of isolated pulmonary metastases is occasionally successful.

Surgery and radiotherapy are supplemented by chemotherapy. Methotrexate and doxorubicin, given in combination, are the two main drugs used. Methotrexate administration is immediately followed by folinic acid rescue, and treatment is given at monthly intervals for about a year. Because of the many side-effects, including lethal cardiac toxicity, careful monitoring is essential. Adjuvant chemotherapy has possibly increased the five-year survival rate to about 20%.

Osteosarcoma in Paget's disease

Osteosarcoma as a complication of bone disease was described by Paget himself; it is most common between the ages of 60 and 80 years. Unlike primary osteosarcoma, it is more common in the spine than long bones, and paraplegia is a frequent complication. It may also occur in the skull, which is commonly affected by Paget's disease.

Paget's sarcoma may be multifocal in origin and is liable to metastasise to other bones. Radiographically it has the appearance of osteosarcoma superimposed on Paget's disease. Its behaviour is similar to primary osteosarcoma but it is even more lethal. This is reflected in the more pleomorphic histological features. The average survival is from 1–2 years. Pathological fracture is a common basis of presentation. Amputation is rarely advisable; palliative radiotherapy is the treatment of choice for most patients.

TUMOURS OF CARTILAGINOUS ORIGIN

Osteochondroma

This tumour consists of bone capped with cartilage and may be single or multiple. Osteochondroma is the most common tumour of bone; it occurs more often in males than females, and is hereditary in about 75% of patients. It occurs only in bones formed from cartilage and originates in the metaphysis of long bones (especially femur, humerus and tibia), with growth gradually moving away from the epiphysis. The number of lesions in one patient can vary from one to hundreds.

A painless swelling which has come to attention through a minor injury is the usual mode of presentation. Tumours of the upper end of the radius or fibula may cause local paralysis of slow onset by pressure on the adjacent nerves. Large tumours near joints occasionally restrict movement.

Tumours grow into various shapes and to different sizes (Fig. 10.4), tending to become arrested when the

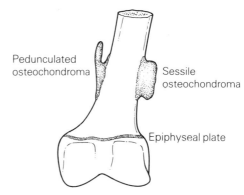

Fig. 10.4 *Osteochondromata of the femur. These are found close to the epiphyseal plate and are of two varieties—pedunculated or sessile.*

epiphyseal plate closes. A few of those which continue to grow and arise from long bones develop chondrosarcoma.

Only osteochondromata causing significant symptoms or impairing of function, and ones which are suspected of becoming malignant, need to be excised. To avoid recurrence, all the cartilaginous tissue must be removed.

Chondroma

This benign cartilaginous tumour of bone is less common than osteochondroma. It may be single or multiple. The commonest sites are the phalanges and metacarpals of the hands, followed by the large limb bones and pelvis (Fig. 10.5). Growth usually begins within the medullary cavity. Tumours in the hand

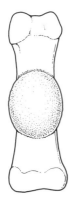 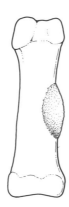

Central enchondroma   Periosteal enchondroma

Fig. 10.5 *Chondroma of the phalanx. There are two varieties—central (enchondroma) and periosteal (ecchondroma).*

usually present because of pathological fractures. Elsewhere, local discomfort or swelling are the usual complaints.

Fractures unite with splintage. Small chondromata occasionally heal spontaneously, but most need to be curetted out and bone-grafted. Chondromata of large bones are liable to malignant change.

Ollier's disease

Multiple chondromata of bone were first described by Ollier. Tumours preponderate on one or other side of the skeleton and many phalanges and metacarpals become affected, causing ugly deformities. Chondrosarcoma develops in 25% of patients.

Chondroblastoma and Chondromyxoid Fibroma

These are rare, solitary benign tumours that occur in adolescence, and should be removed.

Chondrosarcoma

This is a malignant cartilaginous tumour arising in bone or from a pre-existing cartilaginous abnormality. Unlike osteosarcoma, it has no peaks of frequency. The commonest sites are pelvis, ribs, femur, humerus, spine and scapula. Because chondrosarcoma is slow-growing, it usually presents with a painless swelling.

Radiographs show central tumours as expanded osteolytic zones with thinning and erosion of the cortex (Fig. 10.6). Extraosseous tumours develop irregular masses of calcified tissue. Unlike the osteosarcoma, there is no change in the periosteum.

An untreated chondrosarcoma may grow to a great size and, especially in the pelvis, may cause great distress to the patient. Metastasis via the bloodstream causes secondary deposits in the lungs, though this occurs less frequently and often later than with osteosarcoma.

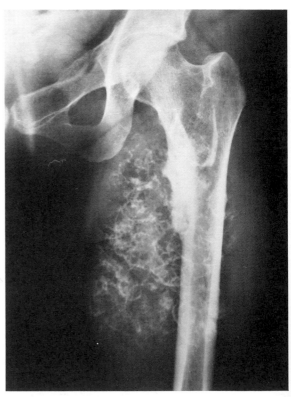

Fig. 10.6 *Anteroposterior radiograph of the left upper femur showing a chondrosarcoma. There is a large irregularly calcified extra-osseous tumour with erosion of the medial femoral cortex.*

The only effective treatment is by amputation of limb tumours, with prosthetic replacement where possible. Radiotherapy is used as a palliative for painful tumours which cannot be extirpated. Chemotherapy is of no value. Overall, the five-year survival is 60%.

TUMOURS OF FIBROUS ORIGIN

Fibrous Dysplasia

This is a fibro-osseous defect of bone of unknown origin. It may be a developmental defect rather than a true tumour. There are two types of fibrous dysplasia: monostotic, where one bone is diseased; and polyostotic, where many bones are involved. The rarer polyostotic form may be associated with patches of brown skin pigmentation, precocious sexual development in females, and premature growth and maturation of the bone (Albright's syndrome). The long bones of the lower limb, the ribs, and the skull are most commonly affected, but no bone is immune.

The condition is usually discovered in childhood after a pathological fracture. Such fractures heal but often occur in turn at various levels and may lead to permanent severe deformity. Lesions of skull and ribs cause visible swellings.

On radiographs, lesions appear as round or oval defects and the cortex becomes thin and expanded, but not eroded (Fig. 10.7).

No treatment is required except for fractures, which usually heal without difficulty.

Fibrosarcoma of Bone

This primary malignant fibroblastic bone tumour is rare; it occurs mostly between the 3rd and 6th decades and is liable to arise as a late complication of inflammation or other bone pathology. Most tumours occur in the lower limb bones, causing local pain and swelling or, occasionally, pathological fracture.

Radiographically this is an ill-defined osteolytic lesion caused by destruction.

The appearances vary from a fasciculated spindle cell tumour to a much more pleomorphic tumour with little fibrous differentiation. Treatment is then by either

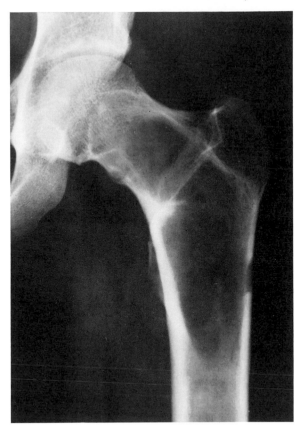

Fig. 10.7 *Anteroposterior x-ray of the left upper femur showing an area of fibrous dysplasia. There is a large well-defined cavity in the neck and shaft with an incomplete fracture of the calcar femorale.*

extirpation or irradiation, but not chemotherapy. The five-year survival is about 30%.

TUMOURS ARISING FROM CELLS OF THE MARROW

Histiocytosis 'X'

Histiocytosis 'X' includes three conditions – eosinophilic granuloma, Hand–Schüller–Christian and Letterer–Siwe syndromes – with the same histological appearance.

The most common is the eosinophilic granuloma, usually single, which occurs in children and may be found in any bone. It presents with pain of short duration and local tenderness. On radiographs it appears as a sharply-defined central lucency, with a thin expanded cortex under one or more layers of calcification. Lesions of vertebral bodies cause collapse and appear dense; at one time these were called Calve's epiphysitis.

Eosinophilic granulomata heal spontaneously in a few months; apart from diagnostic biopsy, they need no treatment.

Myeloma

This is a malignant tumour of the skeleton formed of plasma-like cells.

Clinical features and diagnosis

After carcinoma this is the commonest malignant tumour of bone, affecting middle aged and elderly patients. It is rare under the age of thirty years. It is usually multifocal. The commonest sites are the vertebrae, ribs, skull and pelvis.

The disease has many modes of presentation, depending on the site and extent of the lesions. Tumours of limb bones and ribs cause pain due to pathological fractures. There may be pain in the spine, with gradual increase in curvature, and widespread decalcification which is often mistaken on radiographs for senile osteoporosis. Individual vertebral bodies may collapse, causing paraplegia or tetraplegia. The first symptoms may be due to the systemic effects of the disease: loss of weight, fever, abnormal bleeding and anaemia.

On radiographic examination, the characteristic change in affected bones is the appearance of sharply punched-out holes, of which there may be many in the skull. The vertebral bodies and pelvis become demineralised and individual bodies may collapse and become wedge-shaped (Fig. 10.8). The diagnosis is established by the clinical, radiological, haematological and biochemical investigations, together with marrow puncture and, in isolated lesions, biopsy.

Treatment

Treatment is required for the disease itself, for its systemic effects, for disease of the kidneys, and for lesions of bones and their complications.

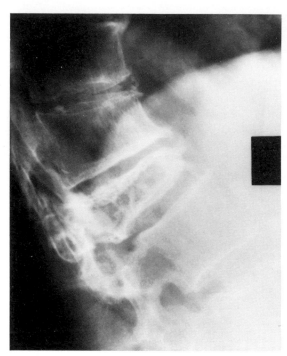

Fig. 10.8 *Lateral x-ray of the thoracolumbar junction showing vertebral collapse due to myeloma.*

In the treatment of the skeletal element of the disease, radiotherapy is used to relieve pain and promote healing. Fractures which do not heal with immobilisation require internal fixation. The prognosis for myeloma is poor; survival is 1–2 years.

Ewing's Sarcoma and Malignant Lymphoma

These are two rare malignant tumours of bone in which the cells tend to be round in appearance. Ewing's sarcoma usually occurs in children and malignant lymphoma in young adults. They may arise in any bone but are more liable to affect the larger bones.

CYSTS OF BONE

Solitary Cyst

The benign unicameral (single chamber) cyst arises in the metaphyseal region of growing bones, usually presenting between the ages of 5 and 10 years, and occurring most commonly in the upper end of the humerus with the upper end of the femur as the second most common site. Pain caused by fracture through the cyst is nearly always the cause of presentation. The lesion appears radiographically as a sharply-defined central, osteolytic lesion, often abutting on the epiphysis with fusiform enlargement and thinning of the cortex (Fig. 10.9). Cysts last for years, but they eventually heal. Repeated fractures may require surgical treatment: the cyst, with most or all of its osseous wall, is resected subperiostally and the cavity filled with bone chips.

Aneurysmal Cyst

This type of cyst is a benign expansile lesion of bone with irregular blood filled cystic spaces and occurs in the 2nd and 3rd decades of life. It affects any bone, but is usually found in the long lower limb bones or vertebral column, presenting with pain or (rarely) slow onset paraplegia. Though benign, it is a rapidly-growing lesion which causes pathological fractures. It appears radiographically as an eccentric expanded cavity. Treatment is a combination of surgery, curettage and grafting, and irradiation.

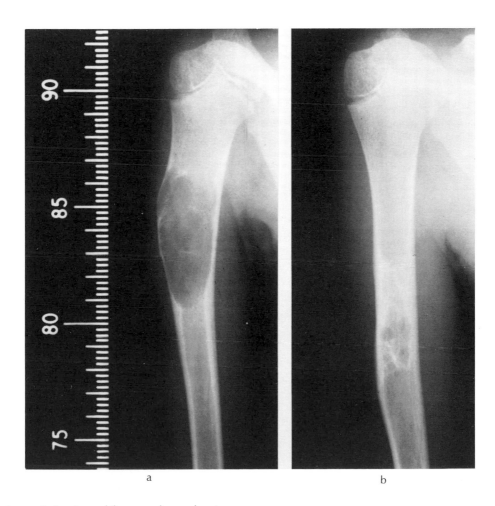

a   b

Fig. 10.9 *Anteroposterior views of the upper femur showing a solitary cyst of the humerus. (a) At presentation. (b) After resection and bone graft—note that the lesion has moved distally with growth.*

Chordoma

This is a rare and highly malignant primary tumour arising from the notochord, most commonly occurring in the sacrum and coccyx but also found in relation to the spheno-occipital part of the base of the skull. Treatment is by a combination of surgery and irradiation. The prognosis is poor.

Giant Cell Tumour

Giant cell tumour, or osteoclastoma, is a neoplasm composed of a vascularised network of spindle shaped and ovoid cells interspersed with multinucleated osteoclast cells. It usually develops in the third decade, and is most common in the large limb bones, especially the lower end of the femur and the upper end of the tibia, followed by the vertebral column, but may appear in any bone. It appears radiographically as a fairly sharply-defined central, cusped and trabeculated lesion; later it expands and erodes the cortex, which may fracture. It involves both epiphysis and metaphysis abutting on the joint (Fig. 10.10).

Diagnosis requires a biopsy and estimation of the blood serum calcium, phosphorus, and alkaline phosphatase to exclude a parathyroid tumour (of which it may be a complication). The histological examination permits grading into a benign or malignant lesion. The prognosis for the benign lesion is, however, uncertain; 30% of tumours recur after surgical treatment other than total removal either by block excision or amputation. Malignant forms metastasise early to the lungs, and are hard to eradicate.

Surgical treatment aims at total removal, and may require prosthetic replacement or amputation. Radiotherapy is reserved for recurrent or inaccessible lesions. Occasionally, a fibrosarcoma or osteosarcoma may develop at the site, several decades later.

CARCINOMA METASTASISING TO THE SKELETON

This is the most common malignant tumour of bone, arising either by metastasis or by direct invasion. An

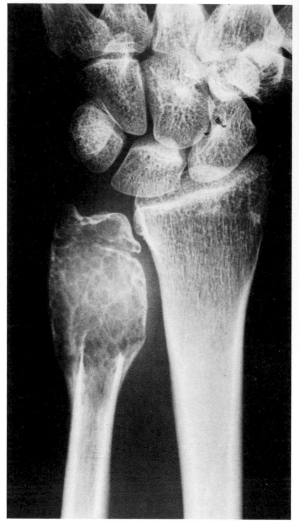

Fig. 10.10 *Anteroposterior x-ray of the right wrist showing a giant cell tumour of the ulnar neck. There is an expanded osteolytic tumour which has eroded the cortex across the epiphyseal plate.*

analysis of 1000 autopsies of patients with carcinoma found that over 25% had bone lesions. No bone is immune, but the vertebral column, pelvis, femur and skull are most commonly affected. The main primary sites of origin, in order of frequency, are the breast, lungs and bronchi, prostate and thyroid. Metastases from tumours of the alimentary tract distal to the stomach are unusual. In children, neuroblastoma is the commonest origin of bony metastases.

Pain is the usual presenting symptom. Eroded bones

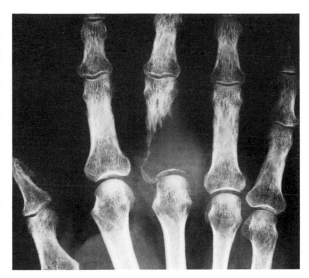

Fig. 10.11 *Anteroposterior view of part of the right hand, showing a metastatic carcinoma of the proximal phalanx of the middle finger. There is destruction of most of the phalanx by tumour, which has eroded through the cortex into the soft tissues without expanding bone whose margins are ill-defined.*

may fracture, and vertebral tumours cause paraplegia. The most common radiographic change is a zone of lucency with an ill-defined margin (Fig. 10.11), but radio-isotope scanning shows metastases earlier than radiographs. Sclerotic secondaries also occur; they are common in the spine, particularly from carcinoma of the prostate gland.

Efforts to trace the primary lesion are not always successful; it may be difficult to find even at autopsy. When the primary lesion is in an endocrine gland, secondaries are more likely to respond to treatment.

Pathological fractures are common and usually respond to immobilisation and irradiation.

TUMOURS OF THE SOFT TISSUES

Desmoid Tumour

Desmoid tumours are lesions of fibroblastic origin which arise from the connective tissues, usually in the rectus abdominis muscle in the abdominal wall of multiparous women, but they may occur elsewhere on the trunk or limbs (musculo-aponeurotic fibromata).

They are locally invasive non-metastasising tumours which can be difficult to remove and are liable to recur. In females, who are more often affected than males, they may regress in the menopause.

Haemangioma

Cavernous or capillary haemangiomata may occur anywhere in the connective tissues, producing soft collapsible swellings if superficial. They are painful only when thrombosing, after which calcification may become visible on radiographs. Lesions may be single or multiple, small or large. Removal is rarely necessary, and only feasible for localised lesions. Massive and widespread haemangiomata may cause serious impairment of function in a limb.

Glomus Tumour

This rare, tiny, benign tumour, derived from the neuromuscular structures that control blood-flow and temperature in the corium and subcutaneous tissue, occurs typically in the fingertips, where it may involve the periosteum and underlying bone. Severe and persistent pain, aggravated by pressure or change of temperature, and sharply-localised tenderness over the lesion, are constant findings. Removal is curative.

Benign Synovioma and Pigmented Villo-nodular Synovitis

The benign synovioma occurs in tendons, tendon sheaths, bursae and joints. It is seen as a grey or yellow, often ovoid, tumour and is treated by surgery, which must be thorough to avoid recurrence.

Pigmented villo-nodular synovitis is classified with benign synovioma; both have a similar histological appearance and may have a common derivation. They also have a similar distribution and a predilection for joints. A mat of brown or red villous and nodular material spreads over the synovium. This gradually destroys articular cartilage, causing secondary osteoarthritis. Sudden bleeding into the joints causes pain, swelling and stiffness, the three symptoms with which it usually presents. Treatment is by surgical removal of the lesion. Whether or not these conditions are truly neoplastic is disputed; many of their features are suggestive of a reactive lesion.

Fibrosarcoma

Malignant tumours of connective tissues are more common than primary malignant tumours of bone. About one-half are fibrosarcomata, which are six times as common as osteosarcomata of bone.

Fibrosarcomata of connective tissues and of bone are similar in behaviour and histological appearance. They occur throughout adult life, presenting with a hard fixed swelling, which is often painful and tender, most commonly on the trunk, buttocks and thighs (Fig. 10.12). If untreated, they may grow to a great size. Metastasis occurs via the blood stream, and pulmonary secondaries are common.

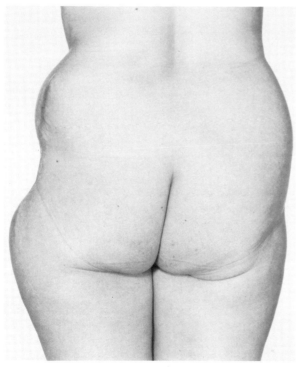

Fig. 10.12 *Fibrosarcoma of the left pelvis and upper thigh. The growth is restrained by the bony pelvis but bulges above and below.*

Early and complete removal of the tumour is the treatment of choice. This requires either amputation or total excision of the tumour, with the whole of any muscles which it may involve. Radiotherapy is used only for ineradicable tumours and for the relief of pain. The five-year survival is 25–30%.

Liposarcoma and Rhabdomyosarcoma

These are rare sarcomata which originate from fat and skeletal muscle respectively.

Neurilemmoma

This is the commonest tumour of the peripheral nerves, and has a characteristic histological appearance. There may be one or more tumours, tending to involve large rather than small nerves, and presenting with pain or local swelling. It is thought to originate in Schwann cells, and forms a smooth oval swelling within the nerve, from which it must be 'shelled out', leaving the surrounding nerve fibres undamaged.

Neurofibroma

A nodular or plexiform tumour of a nerve may complicate neurofibromatosis. Because the tumour, which originates from surrounding cells, merges into the normal surrounding nerve tissue, it cannot be removed without nerve tissue damage and surgical removal is avoided if possible. The neurofibroma is liable to occur in the spinal canal, from which it may extend outwards through an intervertebral foramen, producing a dumb-bell swelling. Severe pain and gradual paresis make surgery essential.

Neurofibrosarcoma

Neurofibrosarcoma may occur as a primary lesion or complicate neurofibromatosis. It is a highly lethal tumour for which there is no effective treatment.

11

Disorders of Nerve and Muscle

CEREBRAL PALSY

This is a fixed non-progressive brain lesion, or lesions, occurring before, during or after birth with interference of the developing central nervous system. Normal brain tissue is replaced by fibrous tissue, with the site providing the differing manifestations. There may be lack of motor control, with or without mental retardation, convulsions, and impediment of speech, sight and hearing.

Prenatal Cerebral Palsy

This is caused by a developmental malformation occurring during the early months of pregnancy; rubella and x-irradiation are the commonest precipitating factors. Rubella gives rise to a spastic paraplegia with athetosis and congenital cataracts. The most frequent neuroradiological effect is diplegia and ataxia, often with epilepsy.

Perinatal Cerebral Palsy

Hypoxic

In the last trimester of pregnancy, ante-partum haemorrhage and pre-eclamptic toxaemia can cause fetal hypoxia by disturbing placental nutrition. Maternal cardiopulmonary insufficiency is also a cause. During labour itself the umbilical cord can be prolapsed or twisted, reducing the oxygen supply to the fetus. Neonatal apnoea is also an important factor, with prematurity, hypoxia during pregnancy, or delivery

with atelectasis as related factors. Hyaline membrane formation, pulmonary oedema, or aspiration of gastro-intestinal contents are all established hazards.

Traumatic birth

Prolonged labour, delivery by forceps, or a breech extraction may directly traumatise the child. Subdural haemorrhage or tears of the dural ligaments are the most obvious manifestation.

Toxic injury

This can be caused by rhesus incompatibility producing an excess of bilirubin. Additional causes are maternal uraemia, diabetes, and infections such as pyelitis.

Postnatal Cerebral Palsy

In postnatal life intracranial trauma, abscess formation, thrombosis and embolism produce unilateral or asymmetrical lesions. Meningitis and encephalitis produce symmetrical lesions. In general, brain damage is due to anoxia producing extrapyramidal syndromes, while damage caused by primary trauma and haemorrhage give pyramidal syndromes.

Clinical Features

Spasticity

This implies increased tension when a muscle is passively lengthened due to exaggeration of the muscle-stretch reflex. It is typical of lesions of the cerebrum and descending pyramidal pathways. This is distinguished from rigidity by the typical 'clasp knife' waxing and waning of the resistance. Deep tendon reflexes are exaggerated and the pathological reflex of Babinski is present with clonus.

Spastic paralysis has a predilection for certain muscle groups. In the upper extremity the shoulder is held adducted, flexed and internally rotated while the elbows, wrists and fingers are flexed with the thumb adducted into the palm (Fig. 11.1). When the lower limb

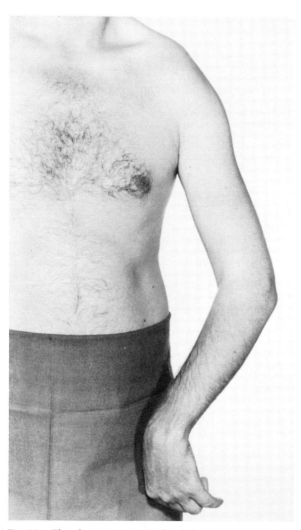

Fig. 11.1 *The characteristic attitude of the upper extremity in spastic paralysis—the shoulder is held adducted, flexed and internally rotated. Flexion of the wrist markedly impairs hand function.*

is affected, the hip is adducted, flexed and internally rotated while both knee and ankle are flexed.

Other features

These include athetosis, ataxia, asynergy and dysynergy, dysdiadochokinesis or adiadochokinesis, dysmetria, hypotonia, and rigidity. Athetosis is characterised by the persistence of involuntary writhing or squirming movements which are irregular, coarse and continuous but disappear during sleep. Pathological changes are mainly in the basal ganglia. Ataxia is caused by lesions in the cerebellum, producing loss of coordination and control with loss of posture and balance with the eyes open or closed. Midline lesions give a wide-based gait. Asynergy and dysynergy refer to loss or disturbance of the coordination of muscle groups which normally act synchronously. Thus phonation can be slurred or there may be a jerky or explosive speech type. Hyperreflexia is common when the action of the synergistic muscle restraining power is lost. Dysdiadochokinesia and adiadochokinesia refer to alternate movements, e.g. pronation and supination, carried out slowly, irregularly and clumsily. Dysmetria implies loss of the ability to judge distance, space and speed. Hypotonic muscles tire easily and have intention tremors. Rigidity is due to diffuse brain damage. There is a steady and equal increase in agonist and antagonist muscle groups, producing a continued resistance described as 'waxy' or 'lead pipe'. Irregular resistance is described as 'cog wheel'.

Incidence and prevalence

Cerebral palsy affects two or three per thousand children. Spasticity is a feature in 50–60% of cases while 20–25% are athetoid. Rigidity occurs in 5–7% of cases, and ataxia in less than 2%.

Spastic Hemiplegia

There is a right to left ratio of 6:4, with the right side producing the greater disability because the majority of individuals are right-handed. Initially there is a flaccid paralysis with absence of movement on the affected side; this is then followed by automatic movements, while spasticity may take weeks or months to develop.

The characteristic spastic hemiplegic posture is adopted, with a subsequent tendency for contractural deformities to occur in that position (Fig. 11.2).

The condition is seldom diagnosed at birth, but a history of the mother observing the baby to be clearly right- or left-handed under the age of one year should arouse suspicion. There is a clenched fist with lack of use of the hemiplegic arm, and an equinus posture of the foot which may not be noticed until the child starts to stand. Motor development, particularly walking, is delayed. The grasp reflex persists on the affected side after having disappeared on the contralateral side, and the plantar reflex response remains extensor in the hemiplegic foot as it becomes flexor on the normal side.

Epilepsy is frequent; it correlates unfavourably with the intellectual status in general prognosis. The majority of cases have some sensory disturbance.

All hemiplegics are able to walk independently; all have one normal hand and therefore can participate in some type of occupation. Behavioural abnormalities, mental retardation and epilepsy are the principal obstacles to competitive performance in adult life.

Spastic Quadriplegia

Again there is usually a delay of some six months before the classical picture becomes apparent. There are three stages:

Hypotonic stage

This lasts for six weeks to six months or more, and the longer this stage the worse is the prognosis. The striking clinical feature is minimal movement and, unless epilepsy is present, the child may be thought to be normal.

Dystonic stage

This has an onset from 2 to 12 months; there is sudden muscular rigidity, more severe in the lower extremities, with sudden extension of the neck and head. Rigidity is markedly increased in all limbs when the child is held in the vertical position.

Rigid spastic stage

The posture is similar to that of the hemiplegic but the attitude is bilateral and usually the legs are more affected than the arms. In these children mental impairment is usually considerable and it is rare to find normal intelligence. Contractural deformities produce a poor base for balance, and one-third never achieve standing balance adequate for independent walking.

Extrapyramidal Cerebral Palsy

This is the second largest group presenting with marked retardation of motor development, and is usually seen between the ages of 6–12 months. Delay in head balance or sitting balance are common presenting

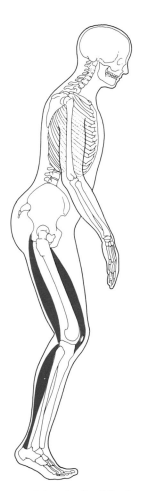

Fig. 11.2 *The characteristic attitude of the lower extremity in spastic paralysis—there is flexion of pelvis, hip, knee and ankle.*

features. At this stage there is a hypotonic expression-less face with a drooling open mouth. Deep tendon reflexes are normal but the tonic neck reflex persists, often up to 18 months, to be followed by varying degrees of involuntary movement. In the security of the mother's lap, tension and involuntary movements disappear. On the examination couch, however, tension athetosis becomes marked. Contractural deformities usually develop, and uncontrolled movements hinder effective walking, sitting or head control throughout life. Interestingly, these are the most intelligent group in the whole range of cerebral palsies.

Mixed lesions are not uncommon and the diagnosis of tetraplegia in the first year of life may be followed by extrapyramidal signs. Others start as pure athetoids and subsequently develop spasticity.

Minimal Brain Dysfunction

This is characterised by learning and behavioural disorders, with short attention spans, impulsiveness, and impaired control of motor functions. There is a tendency for improvement to occur with ageing, however, which supports the theory of delayed brain maturation. The parents may present to an orthopaedic surgeon with a 'clumsy' child.

General Principles of Treatment

A multidisciplinary care programme is needed to cover the changing requirements that occur with development, growth and maturation of the central nervous system. Diagnosis, prognosis and parent counselling are the essential factors in patient management, but surgery has a definite role in the management of cerebral palsy depending on the particular neurological pattern. Initially, an attempt should be made to find out why the child cannot perform certain tasks and what the present and future implications of that failure of performance would be.

In the spastic type of cerebral palsy, preventive measures are the most useful. These may involve exercises and soft-tissue operations, which are seldom indicated in non-spastic types. The athetoid child's active muscle coordination is disturbed, and tendon releases, transfers and neurectomies are very likely to

be followed by recurrence of the original deformity or even the opposite one. In cerebral palsy with extrapyramidal involvement, therefore, surgery is mainly indicated when unfavourable skeletal deformities are fixed in an inappropriate position. Operations should thus be limited to bony procedures, such as joint fusion, after assessment by the use of splints or orthoses over a period of time. The tolerance of plaster fixation in athetoid patients may be enhanced by the use of tranquillising and relaxant drugs.

Conservative treatment

As with any contractural situation, passive manual stretching regularly by day and the use of corrective splints at night are most useful. Deformities can be improved by the use of progressive corrective plasters in association with dynamic orthoses.

Surgical treatment

Accurate patient assessment is essential. Surgery should not be performed under the age of five, when the patient usually has the minimum level of intelligence for cooperation. It is particularly important to assess the child's span of attention preoperatively so that trainability after surgery can be envisaged. Parents should be made aware that, while their child's motor handicap can be substantially improved by surgery, it will never become a normal child or adult. Before any soft-tissue surgical procedure is carried out, an accurate analysis of the deforming muscles or muscle groups must be established (Fig. 11.3). The degree of fixation of ligament and capsule is also important in assessing whether a joint contracture is fixed or passively correctable.

FRIEDREICH'S ATAXIA

This is a hereditary spinocerebellar ataxia with degenerative changes in the dorsal and ventral spinocerebellar tracts, the corticospinal tracts, and the posterior columns. In the cerebellum there is atrophy of Purkinje cells and the dentate nuclei, and there may be changes in the brain stem.

The aetiology is unknown and males and females are

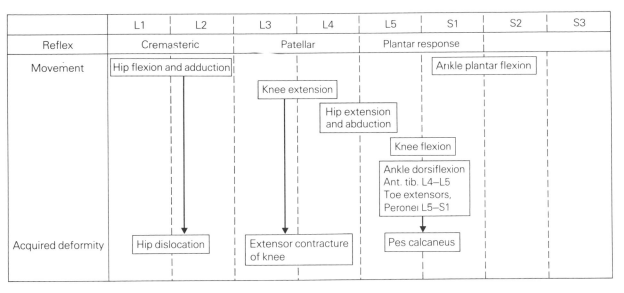

	L1	L2	L3	L4	L5	S1	S2	S3
Reflex	Cremasteric		Patellar		Plantar response			
Movement	Hip flexion and adduction		Knee extension	Hip extension and abduction	Knee flexion / Ankle dorsiflexion Ant. tib. L4–L5 Toe extensors, Peronei L5–S1	Ankle plantar flexion		
Acquired deformity		Hip dislocation	Extensor contracture of knee		Pes calcaneus			

Fig. 11.3 *Diagram to show how deformities of the lower extremities are produced by paralysis at different neurological levels. (After Mr W. J. W. Sharrard.)*

equally affected. A hereditary factor is, however, incriminated: an autosomal recessive gene can often be traced through a number of generations, although the condition may occur in a mild and incomplete form in some members of the family.

There is an insidious onset, usually between the ages of 7–10, with an unsteadiness of gait, a tendency to stagger and fall, and difficulty on sudden turning. While lower limb symptoms progress, the upper limb ataxia develops. The diagnosis is most frequently made by the orthopaedic surgeon, who is presented with a secondary musculoskeletal deformity such as pes cavus with clawing of the toes and a progressive scoliosis (Fig. 11.4).

Unfortunately, treatment has little to offer and the prognosis is a steady progression to complete disability. An early onset is a poor prognostic sign. The control of foot deformities should be conservative, using special insoles or shoes to distribute load maximally.

SPINA BIFIDA

This is a developmental defect in the spinal column, involving failure of fusion of the vertebral arches with or without protrusion or dysplasia of the spinal cord and

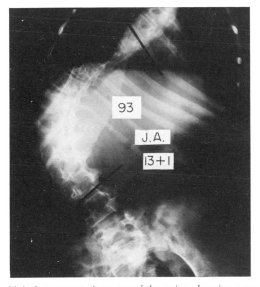

Fig. 11.4 *Anteroposterior x-ray of the spine showing a severe scoliosis in association with Friedreich's ataxia.*

its membranes. There are three types: in spina bifida occulta there is no sac present; in meningocele and myelomeningocele there is both a sac and dysplasia of the spinal cord (Fig. 11.5), although in meningocele cord function can be normal.

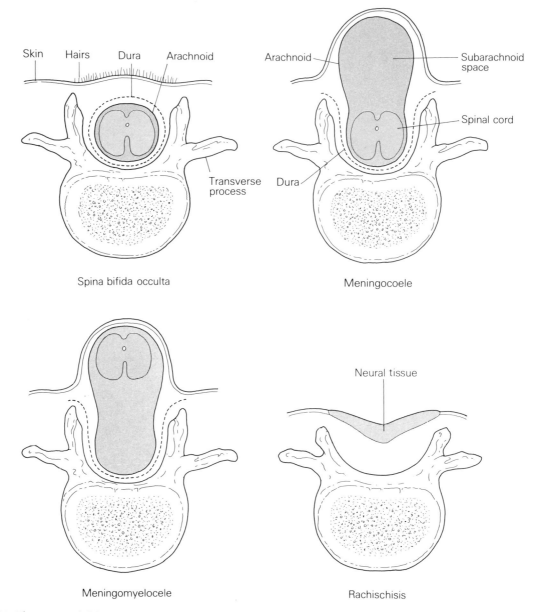

Fig. 11.5 *The structural defects of spina bifida.*

Spina Bifida Occulta

This is one of the commonest congenital anomalies and, because its prevalence is as high as one in ten, it is often regarded as a normal variant. It is most commonly sited at the L5–S1 level, less commonly at C2, D12 and L1 (Fig. 11.6). Fusion of the posterior elements does not

take place until the first year of life and is not complete until adolescence.

A local hairy patch, port wine stain, naevus, dimple, sinus, or fistula are cutaneous stigmata strongly associated with an underlying spina bifida occulta. Occasionally, minor degrees of motor loss, sensory deficit or alteration of bladder or bowel control coexist. Surgical

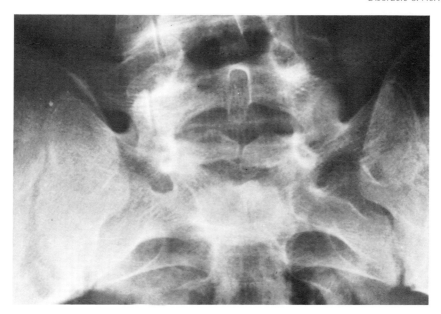

Fig. 11.6 *Anteroposterior radiograph of the lumbosacral region showing a spina bifida occulta of the first sacral segment.*

treatment is only necessary in a few selective cases where the neurological deficit is increasing, e.g. local spinal cord tethering.

Meningocele and Myelomeningocele

The incidence of 3 per 1000 live births in Britain, which is much higher than in the United States or Sweden, is fortunately falling due to the introduction of an amniotic fluid screening programme. It is slightly more common in females than males.

Clinical features

There is a definite family history, with an increased incidence in subsequent siblings if one child is already affected. The exogenous factor must be present in the first weeks of pregnancy, since neural tube closure is complete by the end of the fourth week. The higher the lesion, the less likelihood of neurological involvement.

The skin is almost always incomplete over the sac, and the central area of the sac is arachnoid which may be leaking cerebrospinal fluid. The meninges are normal above and below the lesion, but the dura fuses with the skin edges and a dysplastic cord is closely adherent to the undersurface. The spinal cord may be completely absent, or split, or it may be formed but cystic or cavitated. Neural tissue can be demonstrated by transillumination in a darkened room. The peripheral roots are not affected but may be hard to identify. The vertebral abnormality is principally an arrest of laminar development, with the pedicles alone being present, which can be detected both by palpation and antero-posterior spinal radiography.

Neurological examination

Peripheral neurological changes are noted, starting at the anus with determination of sphincter control, tone and reflex. Dribbling of urine accentuated by suprapubic pressure indicates loss of sphincter control. The degree of distribution of paralysis should be noted by careful repeated examinations so that a segmental level can be established. Lumbosacral lesions give rise to a flaccid paralysis whereas cervicothoracic lesions give rise to a spastic type of paralysis because of partial cord involvement. The precise level can be determined with reference to the segmental innervation of the lower limb muscles, reflexes, joint movements and consequent deformities (Fig. 11.3).

Associated congenital anomalies

These are present in one-third of patients and the most common are club foot, congenital hip dislocation, mega-ureter and hydronephrosis. Accordingly, pyelography and other urological investigations are imperative in the older child. Half of all patients have a congenital bony anomaly of the spine in the form of hemivertebrae or fusions higher in the spine than the laminar defect which may produce a progressive deformity above.

General Principles of Treatment

When an infant is born with a myelomeningocele, a serious ethical question has to be resolved: whether or not the child is to be treated. There are two possible approaches – positive 'aggressive' total care, or negative 'passive' encouragement not to survive. The initial assessment of such children, with particular reference to the neurological level and associated anomalies such as hydrocephalus and urinary problems, is critical in this respect so that the ethical question can be answered as objectively as possible. Many children with severe involvement do not respond to aggressive treatment and it is unrealistic to promote parental enthusiasm for treatment. Equally, many children relegated to the passive method survive.

The infant's management is best conducted in a multiple-discipline clinic, since many systems are involved. A combination of neurosurgical, orthopaedic, urological, paediatric, psychological and social work specialities is favoured.

Neurosurgical primary closure of the sac as an emergency provides a great sparing of nerve pathways and a lower eventual mortality. This, combined with the successful control of hydrocephalus, has decreased mortality from 90% to below 20%.

Orthopaedic Management

The most important musculoskeletal assessment is whether the child has the potential for walking, which requires that the child must have at least grade 4 quadriceps power and sufficient intelligence to mobilise. It is quite unrealistic to supply children who do not have walking potential with splints and frames just so that they can stand; they will eventually inevitably discard these in favour of the sitting position. It is far better to establish sound sitting stability in non-walkers, and this does not give the parents an erroneous impression of the potential of their child. On the other hand, if there is walking potential every effort must be made to maximise it, and the aim should be a child walking with aids by 18 months of age.

As a result of improved medical and surgical care, more children are surviving to adolescence with progressive deformities of the spine which, in turn, may jeopardise sitting stability or walking potential because of the pelvic obliquity they produce. The only indication for surgical stabilisation of such a spinal deformity is loss of sitting stability (Fig. 11.7) or walking potential due to the spine itself and not, for example, due to poor central control consequent upon a severe degree of hydrocephalus. Fixed adduction contractures of the hips may require surgical correction, to improve either mobility in the walker or toilet hygiene in the sitter. Tendon transfers tend to be unpredictable in the spina bifida child and the aim of surgery for foot deformities should be the provision of a reasonably-shaped foot to fit into conventional footwear. Spontaneous pathological and painless fractures are common in the lower limbs of spina bifida children but denervated bone fortunately unites rapidly. The ever-present threat of septicaemia arises from infection of pressure areas and, for both the sitter and walker, the load to the integument should be distributed as widely as possible by using a buffering material such as sheepskin.

DIASTEMATOMYELIA

This is a congenital malformation of the neural axis, with a sagittal division of the spinal cord by a piece of bone or fibrous tissue, attached anteriorly to the vertebral body and passing posteriorly through the spinal canal. Congenital scoliosis is often associated.

No neurological abnormality may be detectable at birth, but cutaneous stigmata similar to those associated with spina bifida occulta are commonly present.

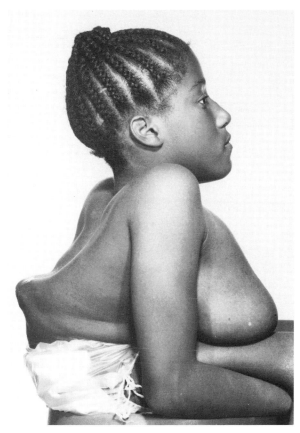

Fig. 11.7　*A severe thoracolumbar kyphosis in association with myelomeningocoele, with complete paralysis of the lower extremities. Sitting stability is only possible by using the hands, which therefore cannot perform their most important prehensile function.*

The neurological deficit is insidious and tends to develop with growth. Atrophy of one lower extremity, often with a limp and foot deformity, is very suggestive (Fig. 11.8).

Myelography confirms the diagnosis and directs surgical attention at the appropriate level so that the bony spur can be excised.

POLIOMYELITIS

This is an acute infectious disease caused by a neurotropic group of viruses initially affecting the gastrointestinal and respiratory tracts and subse-

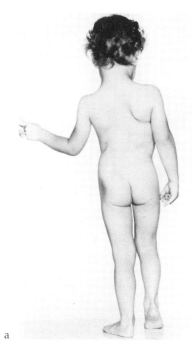

a

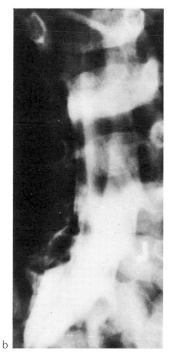

b

Fig. 11.8 (a) *Progressive weakness and wasting of one lower extremity in association with a diastematomyelia—a characteristic combination.* (b) *Myelography demonstrates that the dural sac has been divided into two components by an intervening septum.*

quently spreading, via the bloodstream, to the central nervous system. It has a special predilection for the anterior horn cells and certain of the brain stem nuclei. These cells undergo necrosis, with loss of function of the innervation of the motor cells they supply. There are three types of virus and there is no cross-immunity, thus reinfection is possible.

Damage to the anterior horn cells occurs particularly in the lumbar and cervical cord enlargements. This may be due either to the primary toxic effect of the virus or secondary oedema or haemorrhage in the supportive glial tissue. The motor-cell involvement causes a flaccid paralysis, varying from minimal injury with temporary inhibition of metabolic activity followed by rapid recovery to irretrievable cell destruction with replacement by scar tissue. The resultant muscular weakness is therefore dependent on the number of motor nuclei lost.

Disease Course

There are three phases to the course of this disease:

Acute phase

This is a period of acute illness lasting 5–10 days, with pyrexia. It is considered to last until the temperature has been normal for 48 hours. During this phase paralysis occurs.

Convalescent phase

This phase lasts up to 18 months following the acute phase. It is the period when any muscle recovery occurs, which is most marked during the first 3–6 months. During the early part of this phase, muscles are hypersensitive, tender, and often in spasm.

Residual phase

This encompasses the rest of the patient's life following the convalescent period.

Treatment

While the acute phase is basically a medical management problem, the prevention of deformity is an orthopaedic one. During the paralytic phase, the patient's limbs should be positioned in the correct anatomical alignment and gently moved through a full range of motion several times a day without overstretching muscles. 'Muscle spasm' is resistance to painful movement rather than true spasm, and may be eased by the application of moist heat. The paralysis is usually asymmetrical and each limb requires a different form of treatment.

During the convalescent phase the objectives are: to obtain the maximal recovery of individual muscles; to restore normal joint movement; and to prevent and correct any deformity. Partially paralysed muscle is rapidly fatigued and must not be forced as this will inhibit recovery. Muscle imbalance and increased stress produce deformity, and splintage is used to control deformities, together with active supervised exercises to integrate recovering motor units into the normal pattern of movement. Hydrotherapy is particularly helpful. Since this disease predominantly affects children, growth also greatly increases any deformity due to dynamic muscle imbalance.

In the residual phase, treatment is designed to obtain maximal function despite residual weakness. Passive stretching exercises are used to prevent or correct deformity, and hypertrophy exercises are used to increase the strength and function of weakened muscle. In this phase, orthoses may be required to support the patient in order to facilitate walking and prevent overstretching of weak muscles. Surgery, which is basically aimed at the correction of a paralytic deformity, includes release of tight soft tissues, tendon transfers, and bony surgery by osteotomies and fusions to correct deformity or stabilise positions.

The principles of tendon transfer are important. The transferred muscle must have adequate motor strength, and it should be remembered that one grade of motor power is lost on transfer. The range of movement should also be similar to that of the muscle for which it is being substituted. Furthermore, the loss of function due to a transfer must be balanced against the gain obtained. Most important, the joint affected must have an adequate range of passive movement. Treatment of joint deformities is often a combination of a tendon transfer for one joint, and the stability of a fusion for a nearby joint. In the upper limb, mobility is the desired result; in the lower extremity, stability of the major joints and a plantigrade foot are the surgical aims.

PERIPHERAL NERVE LESIONS

Certain peripheral nerves, during their course through tunnels or around bony prominences, are affected by a neurapraxia occasioned by pressure or repetitive frictional trauma. The anatomical structure of a peripheral nerve is important in this respect (Fig. 11.9). Axons are gathered into bundles – fasciculi – surrounded by a perineurial sheath, and there are several fasciculi in a peripheral nerve, gathered together by the outer supportive connective tissue framework – the epineurium. The fascicular pattern changes, however; in areas

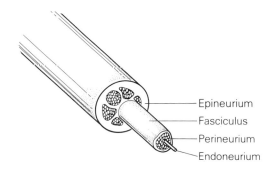

- Epineurium
- Fasciculus
- Perineurium
- Endoneurium

Fig. 11.9 *The anatomical structure of a peripheral nerve.*

where there are many fasciculi there is a maximum of buffering connective tissue and blood supply so that, in these sites, peripheral nerves are able to resist injury. Interestingly, in the places where peripheral nerves tend to be entrapped, e.g. the ulnar nerve behind the medial epicondyle of the humerus, the radial nerve in the spiral groove, the lateral popliteal nerve as it spirals round the neck of the fibula, there are a minimum of fasciculi and therefore a minimum amount of buffering connective tissue is present.

The Carpal Tunnel Syndrome

This syndrome is due to compression of the median nerve as it passes beneath the carpal ligament. The condition is regarded as being either primary or secondary to known related causes. Thus compromise of the dimensions of the carpal canal due to previous wrist injury, or rheumatoid synovium or myxoedema-

tous tissue, which may fill the canal, are established causes. However, the majority of cases are primary and it is speculated that local fluid overload may be an important factor. The passage of extracellular fluid from the extremity of a limb occurs during the day by the pumping action of local muscles. This effect is absent at night, when symptoms tend to predominate, and accordingly the canal is waterlogged. This may serve to explain the higher prevalence of carpal tunnel syndrome in other conditions associated with fluid retention, such as cardiac and renal failure and pregnancy.

Clinical features

Patients complain of painful paraesthesiae restricted to the median nerve territory of the hand (Fig. 2.4) which frequently wakes them at night and for which repetitive shaking of the affected hand provides relief. With diminished sensation of the radial three-and-a-half digits many fine prehensile activities are lost and patients complain of the inability to perform fine movements so that they notice clumsiness (Fig. 11.10). They are unable to recognise objects by feel, a facility termed tactile gnosis. In extreme cases they may burn themselves owing to marked sensory loss.

On examination there is weakness and wasting of the abductor pollicis brevis muscle, with hypo-aesthesia over the palmar aspect of the radial three-and-a-half digits and widening of two-point discrimination. The skin is dry and the nails may be atrophic.

Confirmatory tests

While the diagnosis can frequently be made on clinical grounds alone, the postmenopausal female often has associated cervical spondylosis. Differential diagnosis from root entrapment is therefore important. Electrophysiological determination of nerve conduction velocities is definitively diagnostic. The only other useful test is the tourniquet test, when symptoms are reproduced within one minute of applying an upper arm tourniquet inflated above systolic pressure.

Treatment

Diuretic therapy may be useful in pregnancy, or for those with fluid retention, but the definitive treatment for this condition is division of the carpal ligament. In

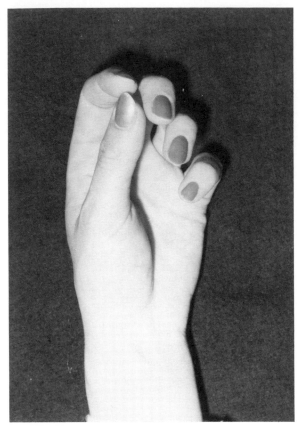

Fig. 11.10 *The thumb, index and middle fingers form a dynamic tripod of prehension—this function is markedly impaired with median nerve damage.*

the rheumatoid patient this provides an opportunity to remove the diseased synovium from around the flexor tendons, thus promoting their integrity.

Ulnar Neuritis

As the ulnar nerve passes behind the medial epicondyle of the humerus, it may suffer from frictional trauma or a bowstringing tension neurapraxia. This is more common in females, who have an increased carrying angle, and in those with previous elbow injury which has caused a cubitus valgus deformity.

Clinical features

Painful paraesthesiae are restricted to the ulnar one-and-a-half digits (Fig. 2.4), but may spread proximally up the forearm. There are few other sensory symptoms, however, as the ulnar nerve is not important for the sensory aspects of prehension. On examination the hand may appear clawed, particularly on the ulnar side, with hyperextension of the metacarpophalangeal joints and flexion of the interphalangeal joints (Fig. 1.31). This is due to paralysis of the intrinsic muscles which would normally place these joints in the opposite position. There is weakness of abduction and adduction of the fingers and, in particular, the first dorsal interosseus is wasted and weak. The ulnar nerve behind the medial epicondyle may be tender to palpation, and pressure may reproduce the sensory symptoms. Nerve conduction studies confirm the diagnosis and there are no other valuable tests.

Treatment

Resiting the ulnar nerve anterior to the medial epicondyle removes the bowstringing effect and readily relieves symptoms, although motor power seldom recovers fully.

Cervical Rib Syndrome

Pain may occasionally present in the arm from compression of the first thoracic nerve root as it arches over an additional rib or fibrous band arising from the seventh cervical vertebra (Fig. 11.11). Symptoms are localised to the distribution of the first thoracic nerve with paraesthesiae along the medial border of the arm exacerbated by carrying a load in the ipsilateral hand. Wasting and weakness of the small muscles of the hand also occurs, as in an ulnar nerve lesion (Fig. 1.31).

Radiographs demonstrate the abnormal rib or may show a large transverse process to which the band is attached. Surgery is indicated only if conservative measures such as shoulder elevation exercises and the avoidance of carrying heavy objects do not improve the discomfort. The operation consists of relieving the pressure on the nerve by excising the rib or fibrous band.

Radial Nerve Palsy

As the radial nerve passes distally from the axilla to the elbow it traverses the spiral groove of the humerus. It is

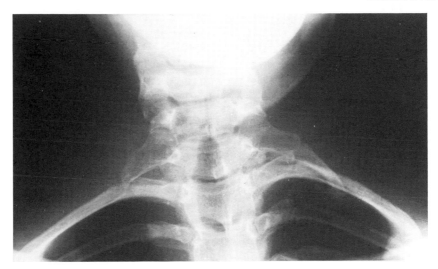

Fig. 11.11 *Anteroposterior x-ray of the cervicothoracic junction showing bilateral cervical ribs coming off the seventh cervical vertebra.*

therefore vulnerable to injury in humeral shaft fractures. This may occur either at the time of fracture or when the nerve subsequently becomes involved in callus formation locally.

The classical clinical features are wrist drop and inability to extend the fingers. Treatment should be expectant as the great majority are only temporary neurapraxias and recover completely with time. Only if recovery is negligible and nerve conduction studies confirm the level should surgical decompression of the nerve be considered.

Meralgia Paraesthetica

The lateral cutaneous nerve of the thigh becomes superficial as it passes between the lateral attachment of the inguinal ligament and the anterior superior iliac spine. It supplies the skin over the anterolateral aspect of the thigh. Compression of the nerve in this area results in pain or paraesthesiae over its cutaneous distribution. It may also be due to external compression, e.g. from the pelvic part of a spinal brace. Persistent symptoms can be relieved by exploration and decompression of the nerve as it passes beneath the inguinal ligament.

Common Peroneal Nerve Palsy

As the common peroneal nerve spirals round the neck of the fibula, it is particularly vulnerable to local pressure. Although this can occur through ganglion formation referable to the superior tibiofibular joint, extrinsic pressure is a much more common cause, usually from a splint or plaster. Common peroneal nerve palsies typify neurapraxias with a motor loss far in excess of the sensory deficit. There may be a complete foot drop, whereas the autonomous sensory zone is only a postage stamp over the dorsum of the first web. Treatment is always expectant but recovery is frequently a long time coming and nearly always incomplete. In the interim, the functional position should be maintained, using a lightweight plastic right-angle ankle splint.

MUSCLE DISORDERS

Duchenne Muscular Dystrophy

This is a progressive inherited muscular dystrophy of childhood which is a sex-linked recessive disorder, affecting 2 per 10 000 boys. It is usually first noted as a muscle weakness as the child starts to stand and walk. At this point he is usually referred, with a waddling gait and frequent falls, to an orthopaedic surgeon.

As the child gets older he has to use his hands to push himself up onto his legs from the sitting position because of weakness of the muscles of the pelvic girdle; he also acquires a broad-based stance and gait with an increase of the lumbar lordosis. Later, contractures of the hip flexors and calf muscles frequently develop; at this stage immobilisation is harmful as it adds to the weakness and causes further contractures of the muscles. Muscle weakness and contractures soon make walking impossible, and the patient spends the remainder of his few years in a wheelchair. A patient with Duchenne muscular dystrophy rarely reaches the age of 20. Death is due to cardiac and respiratory complications.

Management

Duchenne muscular dystrophy is incurable. Management consists of regular physiotherapy to encourage mobilisation, and night splints to correct deformities. Later on, simple release of contractures at the ankle, knee or hip, with continued physiotherapy and the fitting of calipers and braces are necessary (Fig. 11.12), until finally the child loses his mobility.

Facio-scapulo-humeral Muscular Dystrophy

This dystrophy, also inherited, is an autosomal dominant whose prevalence has been estimated at three per million of the population. Classically, weakness is first noticed during the teens or early twenties; the patient is unable to close his eyes completely or to whistle, and there is weakness of the muscles of the shoulder girdle, producing winging of the scapula.

An infantile form of facio-scapulo-humeral dystrophy presents in the first two years of life and in these cases the child is usually wheelchair-bound by the age of ten.

Management

Two orthopaedic problems occur with this dystrophy: pes cavus and winging of the scapulae. Pes cavus can be treated by a number of bony operations and, whilst

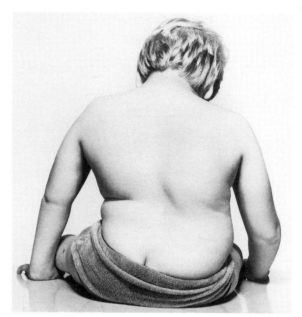

a

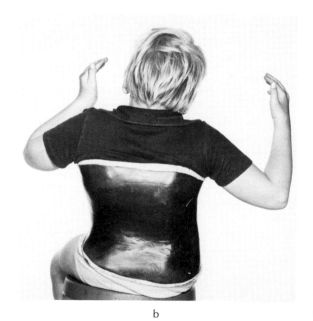

b

Fig. 11.12 *Duchenne muscular dystrophy. (a) The collapsing spine has caused pelvic obliquity and the hands are necessary to maintain sitting balance. (b) After fitting a simple block leather torso support, sitting stability has been restored and the hands are now free for prehensile function.*

winging of the scapula is mainly a cosmetic defect, fixation of the scapula to the fourth and fifth ribs can assist in stabilising the shoulder.

Congenital Muscular Dystrophy

It is important to diagnose this form of muscular dystrophy by muscle biopsy as it is a non-progressive condition presenting with numerous musculoskeletal deformities. It is usually first noticed at birth as generalised muscular weakness together with difficulty in swallowing. Later, such children present at orthopaedic outpatient clinics with dislocation of the hips, talipes equinovarus, and scoliosis.

Management

Because the condition is non-progressive, early diagnosis and correction of the deformity is all-important, as this can enable the child to lead an essentially normal life.

LOWER MOTOR NEURONE DISORDERS

Spinal Muscular Atrophy

This is an autosomal recessive disorder, with an incidence of 1 in 10 000 live births, in which there is degeneration of the anterior horn cells of the spinal cord and of the motor nuclei of the cranial nerves.

Three main groups can be found:

Severe

There is weakness of all muscles, with head lag, absence of arm movement, weakness of respiratory muscles, and a frog-leg position. The child is unable even to sit unsupported and, because of the breathing and swallowing difficulties, the child eventually dies from inhalation or hypostatic pneumonia.

Intermediate

In this group, the onset is usually in the first year of life and, following a period of progressive weakness, the disease may remain thereafter static. These children have facial and respiratory muscle weakness but are able to lift their head and move their limbs and can stand for brief periods of time. As they get older, the deformities become more apparent, most commonly as scoliosis and contractures in the upper and lower limbs (Fig. 11.13).

These children survive into early adult life.

Mild

This group is usually detected between 5 and 15 years, presenting with difficulty in walking. Proximal muscle groups are more frequently affected, particularly the thigh muscles. The disease progresses slowly and the patient continues to walk up to about the age of 30, when weakness of the shoulders and arms compounds

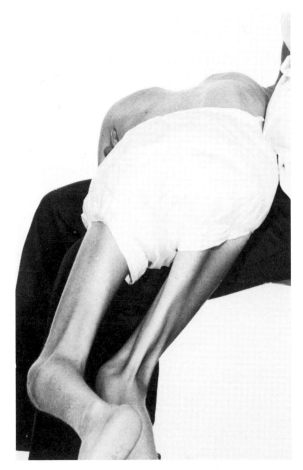

Fig. 11.13 *Severe knee contractures in a child with advanced spinal muscular atrophy.*

their problem and they then become confined to a wheelchair.

Management

For severe cases there is little to offer other than lightweight supporting braces.

In the intermediate group, early active treatment in the form of bracing, and later operative management of scoliosis with correction of contractures around the hips and knees, enables the child to maintain his mobility for the maximum amount of time and finally to sit comfortably in a wheelchair.

There is little need for active orthopaedic interven-

tion in mild cases other than the correction of contractures if they develop.

Peroneal Muscular Atrophy

This disorder is also inherited as an autosomal dominant and there is both motor and sensory impairment. The child presents in the first decade of life with an abnormal gait, pes cavus and foot drop.

Management

The foot deformities may be corrected by soft tissue and tendon operations or by bony procedures.

12

Amputations and Prostheses

Eighty per cent of amputations are carried out for vascular disease and diabetes, and three-quarters of these are in patients over sixty years old.

Amputation is distasteful to the surgeon and alarming to the patient; the decision to amputate electively is often difficult, but amputation of an irreparably diseased or damaged limb is the first step in returning the patient to more normal life. Amputation performed as an emergency, however, e.g. after injury, can often be life-saving and the decision is usually not difficult.

INDICATIONS FOR AMPUTATION

1. a dead limb;
2. a dangerous limb;
3. a troublesome limb.

A Dead Limb

A limb, or part of it, may be dead because of:

a. severe trauma, where major blood vessels have been involved, or where there has been irreparable damage to large parts of the limb

b. vascular occlusion, usually of the lower limb, due to arteriosclerosis, embolism or thrombosis

c. gangrene, due to pyogenic infection, peripheral vascular disease, or diabetes.

A Dangerous Limb

A limb may be dangerous due to:

a. malignant tumour

b. severe infection, particularly gas gangrene

c. severe crush injury.

A Troublesome Limb

A limb may be troublesome because of:

a. pain

b. chronic infection as in chronic osteomyelitis with sinuses

c. flail as a result of paralysis due to either poliomyelitis or peripheral nerve lesion

d. deformity, particularly severe congenital deformities and acquired deformities, such as those caused by poliomyelitis and those due to stiffening of joints so that the affected part severely interferes with normal function.

TYPES OF AMPUTATION

Provisional

This is performed where re-amputation may be necessary when it is anticipated that primary healing will be unlikely or delayed, usually because of infection. The amputation is performed as far distally as possible, leaving skin and muscle flaps open.

Definitive

There are two types of definitive amputations:

Endbearing

These are lower limb amputations where the weight is taken on the stump. The scar therefore needs to be situated anteriorly or posteriorly. Examples of endbearing stumps are Syme's amputation above the ankle joint, and amputations through the knee.

Non-endbearing

These are the commonest variety. All upper limb amputations are of this category. In the lower limb, examples of non-endbearing stumps are an above-knee amputation and a below-knee amputation.

SITES OF AMPUTATION

In the past, amputation through specific levels was necessary for proper fitting of a prosthesis. Although modern modular design prostheses still demand certain lengths of stump, the level of amputation is more often determined by surgical considerations.

Sites of Election (Fig. 12.1)

Traditional sites of election for ideal stumps are:

for above-knee amputations, 25–30 cm from the greater trochanter;
for below-knee amputations, 14 cm from the knee;
for above-elbow amputations, 20 cm from the acromion;
for below-elbow amputations, 17 cm from the olecranon.

Amputation Other Than at Site of Election

Lower limb

Hindquarter amputation: this operation is performed for malignant disease.

Disarticulation of the hip: also usually for malignant disease.

At the knee: The classical amputation is the Gritti–Stokes, i.e. attaching the patella to the end of the femur, but the disadvantage of this is that a standard modular

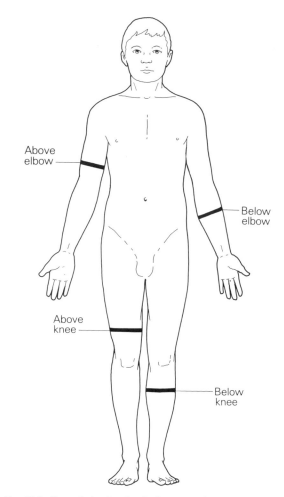

Fig. 12.1 *Sites of election for limb amputations.*

prosthesis cannot be used. Simple through-knee disarticulation may be useful for patients who are already bed-bound or chair-bound, and for children in order to allow maximal growth of the femur.

Above the ankle: Syme's amputation can be difficult to perform correctly; it is an endbearing stump and the vascularity of the end flap must be preserved very carefully.

At the foot: partial amputations have the disadvantage that the tendo achillis tends to pull the foot into equinus. Sometimes, however, these amputations can be very satisfactory, e.g. Lisfranc's amputation through the tarso-metatarsal joint.

Amputation of a single digit or an entire ray is often useful in treating infection, and amputation of a single toe may be used in treating deformities.

Upper limb

Forequarter amputation: this operation is a major procedure and is only performed in an attempt to eradicate malignant disease.

Disarticulation of the shoulder: this is rarely performed. The cosmetic appearance is much improved if the head of the humerus together with 3 cm of humerus can be left in place.

Below elbow: the shortest stump upon which a prosthesis can easily be fitted is 3 cm below the flexed elbow.

Amputations of the hand: single digits can be amputated, in the case of the index to ring fingers, leaving a short stump of proximal phalanx if possible. With the little finger, however, the whole finger can be amputated along with an oblique amputation of part of the fifth metacarpal producing a very acceptable cosmetic result. These amputations are usually carried out for tumours and severe deformities which interfere with the function of the rest of the hand. Every attempt should be made, however, to preserve at least the proximal phalanx of the thumb.

Modern techniques of prosthetic manufacture, however, now allow preservation of maximal length consistent with surgical judgement in upper limb amputations.

Preoperation Procedure

The patient's haemoglobin should be measured and the blood be cross-matched. Any infection should as far as possible be brought under control, as should diabetes, and appropriate antibiotic therapy started where indicated.

Operative Procedure

Meticulous attention to basic surgical principles is important. The aim is to provide a well-healed, non-tender stump which can be satisfactorily fitted with a prosthesis.

Postoperative Care

The patient requires general supportive measures, particularly analgesia and sedation. Where necessary, antibiotics should be given.

The stump should be firmly bandaged, placed on a pillow or a well-padded splint; with the lower limb in particular, measures should be taken to prevent contractural deformities developing. Physiotherapy should be started as early as possible to encourage the regaining of muscle power.

Complications of Amputations

Complications special to amputations are:

a. haemorrhage
b. infection
c. delay in healing of the wound and necrosis of the skin flaps
d. painful neuroma
e. phantom limb
f. osteomyelitis
g. callosities, ulceration, and adherence of the scar.

PROSTHESES

Most prostheses are now made from pre-built modules but modern techniques enable a prosthesis to be made for almost any stump. The prosthesis can be fitted as soon as the stump is well healed and the scar is stable.

Upper-limb Prostheses

At the present time, upper-limb prostheses are unable to provide delicate or controlled movements of the upper limb. They usually consist of a socket prosthesis with a harness to which various mechanical devices for gripping can be fitted (Fig. 12.2).

Lower-limb Prostheses

In order to give as normal a gait as possible, the prosthesis should be attached to the patient by the simplest possible means. The most acceptable method is the suction socket which can be applied to an above-knee amputation (Fig. 12.3), and a similar near-total contact socket which can be fitted to a below-knee amputation (Fig. 12.4). For amputations at the foot, the limb can be fitted with normal footwear with simple packing of the shoe or, above the ankle, with a prosthesis in the form of a high boot. Disarticulations and hindquarter amputations require a socket that fits the pelvis, combined with cushion seating under the ischial tuberosity for a disarticulation, and a similar socket in which weight is transmitted in a hydraulic fashion by the abdominal contents for a hindquarter amputation.

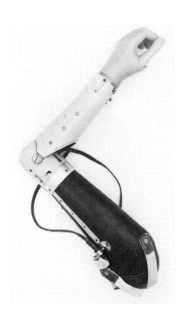

Fig. 12.2 *A complete upper limb prosthesis—various devices are attached for gripping purposes.*

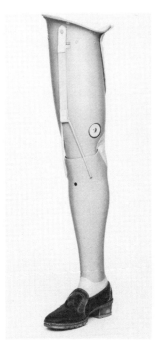

Fig. 12.3 *Lower limb prosthesis for above-knee amputation.*

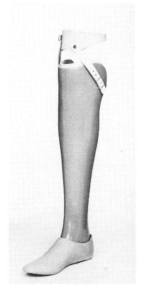

Fig. 12.4 *The lower limb prosthesis for a below-knee amputation.*

13

Osteoarthritis

INTRODUCTION

Vertebrates are distinguished from invertebrates by possession of an internal skeleton. The invertebrate exoskeleton also provides protection for the internal tissues, but the rigidity of this system allows only very stereotyped movements. In contrast, man and other vertebrates have a complex system of synovial and other joints between the parts of the endoskeleton which allows a wide range of movements. Wear and tear damage – osteoarthritis – may develop, following absolute or relative over-use of synovial joints, and has become one of the major causes of disability in our society. Some authors use the term osteoarthrosis to emphasise the wear aspect of the disease, while others prefer osteoarthritis in deference to this inflammatory component. The terms are usually synonymous.

THE BIOLOGY OF THE SYNOVIAL JOINT

A typical synovial joint consists of two articulating bony surfaces covered by hyaline cartilage. The joint is enclosed in the capsule, which is lined by the synovial membrane, and within the joint is a small volume of viscous synovial fluid. Ligaments, tendons and muscles may surround the joint and provide additional support. Despite its complex structure, the healthy synovial joint possesses low frictional properties – as low as the best of engineering joints.

Within the hyaline cartilage there is a meshwork of collagen fibres (Fig. 13.1). These fibres have high tensile strength. Near the articular surface they lie approximately parallel to the surface, but deeper down they lie at

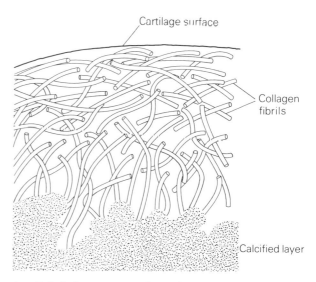

Fig. 13.1 *Collagen structure in cartilage.*

right angles to it and are attached to the subchondral bone. They interlace to form a tight meshwork, in the interstices of which lies the cartilage matrix. The metabolic turnover rate of collagen fibres is slow so that the cartilage has only a limited capacity for repair.

The cartilage matrix contains cells (chondrocytes) and proteoglycan aggregates. The chondrocytes are relatively sparse in normal adult cartilage; they do not divide although they are metabolically active.

The aggregates consist of long filamentous cores of hyaluronic acid to which are attached numerous side-chains of proteoglycan (Fig. 13.2). These attachments are stabilised by a small binding fraction. Each proteoglycan molecule contains a central protein core with glycosaminoglycan side-chains of chondroitin sulphate and keratan sulphate. The enormous proteo-

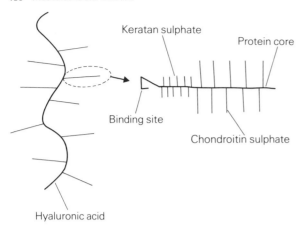

Fig. 13.2 *Proteoglycan aggregate.*

glycan aggregate macromolecules become entangled within the meshwork of the collagen fibres. They attract fluid by osmosis and swell, stretching the collagen meshwork, and are largely responsible for the turgidity and load-bearing properties of the articular cartilage.

The articulating surface of the cartilage is not smooth; there is a system of irregularities and shallow hollows of greatly varying sizes. At first sight this might seem to be incompatible with free joint movement but we now believe that these surface irregularities contribute significantly towards the low frictional properties of synovial joints. Synovial fluid is highly viscous because it contains hyaluronic acid. It is believed that, under load, synovial fluid becomes trapped between the joint surfaces, and particularly in these hollows and irregularities. Water may be able to escape, while the larger molecules remain in increased concentration, forming a lubricating gel between the surfaces. During movement, deformation of the surfaces by load could squeeze this thick gel-like material out in front of the contact area and facilitate lubrication.

PATHOLOGY — AGEING AND OSTEOARTHRITIS

A clear distinction must be drawn between the pathological changes of joint degeneration and the clinical syndrome of osteoarthritis. Examination of the joints of older people will reveal almost universal evidence of joint wear and tear, and yet the clinical problem is far less common. Even in those with clinical osteoarthritis, flares may occur intermittently with symptom-free intervals despite the continued presence of these pathological features.

The process of cartilage ageing must be distinguished from the pathological changes of osteoarthritis. Softening, splitting and fragmentation of the articular surfaces commonly, but not invariably, accompanies ageing, developing in normal subjects from the third decade onwards. Characteristically these features occur in the non-contact areas of joints, which suggests that normal joint use will protect against the development of age changes. Such features may not progress to the more advanced forms of osteoarthritis.

In osteoarthritis itself, the principal damage occurs in the load-bearing parts of the joint, with larger areas of split and fragmented cartilage, deep cleft formation and thinning of the surface layer occur until, ultimately, bone is exposed. There is loss of glycosaminoglycan from the cartilage matrix, and necrosis of the chondrocytes, particularly in the superficial layers. Sometimes clusters or nests of chondrocytes develop in the deeper layers of the cartilage.

The subchondral bone becomes increasingly dense or sclerotic. This results from the healing of fractures of the trabeculae. If the cartilage is totally worn away, bone is exposed and becomes increasingly sclerosed and eburnated. Cystic lesions may appear in the subchondral region. The articular surface becomes remodelled, with formation of new bone and regression in other areas, so that eventually the whole joint may appear distorted. In particular, bony outgrowths or osteophytes appear around the edge of the joint. In teleological terms, they appear to enlarge the joint surface, diminishing the stresses on any individual area, and they also splint the joint, thus limiting motion and the risk of further damage.

The synovium may appear relatively normal, but it sometimes develops mild inflammatory changes, which may be due to recurrent trauma following mechanical instability or to small fragments of debris from the joint surfaces acting as an inflammatory stimulant. Crystals of calcium hydroxyapatite have been identified within synovial effusions from osteoarthritic joints but it remains uncertain whether they can be responsible for the mild inflammatory features or simply accompany severe joint damage. In the late stages, fibrosis of the capsule will restrict motion and produce contractures.

PATHOGENESIS

Osteoarthritis should be regarded as a form of articular failure that occurs when the stresses on the joint exceed its capacity to accommodate them. Analogies may be drawn with cardiac, respiratory and renal failure. Excessive load on the joint may be absolute, or it may be relative, e.g. when a previously damaged joint is unable to withstand relatively normal stresses.

The principal classification of osteoarthritis is into secondary forms, which may be related to some predisposing problem, and primary disease when there is no obvious cause (Table 13.1).

In the former group, damage may be due to trauma; this may relate to a specific incident or to repetitive over-use, as in various occupational forms of the disease. Joint malalignment, instability or incongruity may lead to secondary osteoarthritis. Examples of this follow congenital dislocation of the hip, hip dysplasia, or previous joint injuries. It is now known that meniscectomy for a torn knee meniscus leads to an increased risk of osteoarthritis by the same mechanism. Previous joint infection, or inflammation such as rheumatoid arthritis, may damage the cartilage and lead to secondary osteoarthritis in later years. The cartilage may be damaged in ochronosis or chondrocalcinosis with widespread osteoarthritic changes.

Primary osteoarthritis often affects multiple joints in a characteristic pattern. By definition there is no recognisable cause, although there is a strong genetic component and it usually develops in middle-aged or elderly females. It may be that increased bone stiffness leads to excessive cartilage stresses and damage, or simply that physically active people are more likely to develop osteoarthritis and to have denser bones.

Absolute or relative over-use of the joint leads to failure, but the exact sequence of changes remains uncertain (Fig. 13.3). The collagen meshwork may be damaged, allowing the large proteoglycan aggregates to escape. There may be failure to form the large proteoglycan aggregates. The smaller molecules can diffuse out of the collagen network more easily and so are readily lost. Repeated stress may damage the chondrocytes, releasing degradative enzymes which destroy the cartilage matrix around them.

There is a compensatory increase in matrix synthesis rate, but this is insufficient to match the loss. The reduction in proteoglycan concentration leads to

Table 13.1

Classification of Osteoarthritis

1. Primary
    Primary generalised osteoarthritis

2. Secondary
    Joint damage   trauma
                     occupation
                     deformity, e.g.
                         congenital dislocation
                           of hip
                         joint dysplasia
                         malalignment
                     meniscectomy
                     previous infection, inflammation
    Metabolic disorders of cartilage
                     ochronosis (alkaptonuria)
                     chondrocalcinosis (pyrophosphate
                       arthropathy)

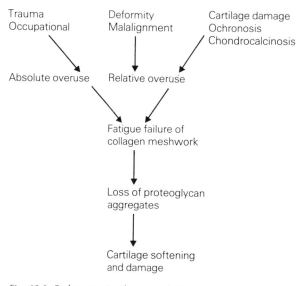

Fig. 13.3 *Pathogenesis of osteoarthritis.*

reduced osmotic pressure and softening of the cartilage so that it is less able to withstand stresses. Eventually abrasion and permanent cartilage loss develops.

Small fractures occur in the trabeculae, perhaps due to excessive local concentrations of stress consequent on the joint damage. The healing of these fractures leads to local increased bone density and the development of bone sclerosis.

MECHANISMS OF PAIN PRODUCTION

The relationship between the pathological changes of osteoarthritis and clinical symptoms is poor. Some patients may have gross radiographic disease and yet be functionally normal, while others have only trivial objective changes and yet suffer severe symptoms. In part this can be related to pain threshold in that the level of noxious stimulus required to produce the sensation of pain varies between individuals and can be related to the severity of problems in patients with osteoarthritis. Anxiety, mental stress, distraction and other factors alter the pain threshold and may well play an important role in determining the severity of symptoms in any individual.

The source of the symptoms is uncertain. There are no nerves in the synovium or the articular cartilage and these structures are insensitive, but the capsule and ligaments are richly innervated and very sensitive to stimulation. Mechanical stresses in the osteoarthritic joint could well lead to acute episodes of pain. Transient minor inflammatory episodes are not uncommon. They may be a form of crystal-induced inflammation, perhaps related to calcium hydroxyapatite or pyrophosphate if there is chondrocalcinosis. Debris in the joint may be trapped between the moving surfaces, or a synovial fringe may be trapped between the joint margins. Increased blood flow and pressure in the epiphyses is believed to be responsible for the deep aching pain felt by some patients.

EPIDEMIOLOGY OF OSTEOARTHRITIS

Pathological and radiological evidence of osteoarthritis is remarkably common, although many subjects do not suffer significant clinical problems. Sixty per cent or more of both males and females over 35 years old have osteoarthritic changes in at least one joint but the prevalence varies widely in different populations. Occupational factors may play a significant role, e.g. textile workers show an increased risk of developing changes in the hands. Racial and genetic factors may account for some of the differences between various population groups and particularly seem to influence the distribution of primary generalised osteoarthritis.

CLINICAL FEATURES

The term 'primary osteoarthritis' is used when there is no identifiable predisposing cause. It often involves multiple joints and is then termed primary generalised osteoarthritis (PGOA). It is more common in females and usually develops after the age of 50. There is often an increased prevalence in female relatives but with no clear genetic pattern of inheritance.

In the hands, PGOA characteristically affects the distal interphalangeal joints, less often the proximal interphalangeal joints, and rarely the metacarpophalangeal joints. Another characteristic site on the hand is the carpo-metacarpal joint of the thumb. Other joints commonly involved in PGOA include the first metatarsophalangeal joints, the knees, the hips and the apophyseal joints of the spine. Secondary osteoarthritis can develop in any joint which has previously been damaged (Fig. 13.4).

Gross osteoarthritis may be present with few or no symptoms, but the patient may be upset by the resulting deformity. A common problem in the hands is the bony swellings on either side of the dorsal surfaces of the distal interphalangeal joints (Heberden's nodes), perhaps with flexion or ulnar deviation of the terminal phalanges. Similar bony swellings occur at the proximal interphalangeal joints (Bouchard's nodes) or around the carpo-metacarpal joint of the thumb, producing a squared appearance to the hand. In the feet, bony swellings of the first metatarsophalangeal joint may be associated with lateral deviation of the great toe (hallux valgus) leading to the familiar bunion. This deformity may produce considerable difficulty in finding comfortable shoes and rubbing of the enlarged and deformed joint may lead to ulceration of the skin. Osteoarthritis

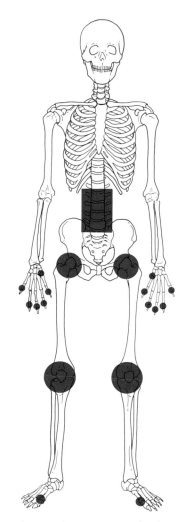

Fig. 13.4 *Distribution of primary generalised osteoarthritis.*

of the knee may affect the patello-femoral or tibio-femoral joints. In the former case, pain is felt behind the patella during flexion and extension and is often at its worst when climbing or descending stairs. In the hip, stiffness on movement leads to pain and difficulty in walking and, particularly, in putting on shoes and stockings. The typical deformity is fixed flexion and adduction producing apparent shortening of the involved limb so that the subject walks with a pelvic tilt, a lumbar scoliosis, and a flexed contralateral knee which may as a result develop further problems.

Pain and crepitus develop in and around the involved joint. These symptoms develop predominantly on joint use. They are aggravated by exercise and are worse towards the end of the day. In contrast to inflammatory arthritis, they are relieved by rest and show little or no element of morning stiffness on first waking, although some patients find that their joints 'gel' after sitting or lying in one position for a long period and may take a few seconds to get going.

Occasionally there may be more acute episodes of pain. These may be due to a transient inflammation in the joints, perhaps related to debris in the joint fluid; instability leading to minor trauma; strains on ligaments or joint capsule; or the trapping of synovial fringes between the articular surfaces.

Examination of the joint may reveal deformity and swelling, and palpation indicates this to be of bony origin or perhaps due to a small effusion. However, there is little evidence of synovial thickening as occurs in inflammatory arthritis. It is frequently possible to identify tender areas in the joint capsule or surrounding ligaments which may be treated locally. The range of joint movement may be limited with a fixed flexion deformity and it is usually possible to feel and sometimes hear the crepitus or grating occurring at the articular surfaces during joint movement. Any instability of the joint should be noted. There may be weakness and wasting of the muscles moving the joint. This is most obvious in the quadriceps muscle of the knee.

The examination is not complete without observing function, e.g. the use of hands for power and fine pinch grip, ability to walk, to get out of a chair, to climb stairs, etc.

Confusion between generalised osteoarthritis and inflammatory joint disease occasionally arises in some patients, usually middle-aged females, who develop evidence of osteoarthritis at the same time as mild inflammatory changes. There is often a marked element of morning stiffness, but investigations do not show any specific evidence of inflammatory joint disease other than a marginally elevated erythrocyte sedimentation rate (ESR). It remains uncertain whether these patients have developed osteoarthritis secondary to mild chronic inflammatory arthritis or whether two separate disorders are coinciding.

Investigations

There are no systemic features to osteoarthritis so that the ESR, plasma viscosity and blood count are normal.

There is no association with rheumatoid factor or other autoantibodies unless the joint damage is secondary to other disease. The radiological appearances will indicate osteoarthritis but sometimes it is possible to recognise this change as occurring secondary to previous inflammatory arthritis, malalignment, or other damage (Fig. 13.5).

Cartilage destruction leads to loss of the apparent joint space between the articulating bony surfaces. It is best detected by comparison with the contralateral unaffected joint and, in the lower limbs, on films taken during weight-bearing. The joint space is occupied by the radiolucent cartilage and narrowing is an index of

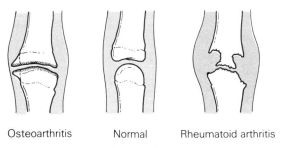

| Osteoarthritis | Normal | Rheumatoid arthritis |

Fig. 13.5 *Appearances of osteoarthritic, normal and rheumatoid joints, e.g. interphalangeal joints.*

cartilage loss. However, this change occurs in arthritis of various causes including inflammatory arthritis and is not specific evidence of osteoarthritis.

Osteophytes appear as sharpening of the joint margins followed by bony outgrowths forming a frill around the edge of the joint. In the fingers they may appear as isolated periarticular ossicles at the joint margins, and in the knees as 'sharpening' of the tibial spines.

Sclerosis develops in the subchondral bone, and small cysts may be seen close to the articular surface. These cysts have a sclerotic margin, in contrast with the bone cysts of rheumatoid arthritis which are surrounded by osteoporotic bone.

In late disease there may be gross deformity and destruction of the joint, perhaps with subluxation of the bone ends. Loose bodies may been seen, which probably represent fragments of bone from the destroyed articular surfaces.

MANAGEMENT OF OSTEOARTHRITIS

Although the pathological changes of osteoarthritis, once established, are permanent, it is usually possible to control the symptoms, relieve acute exacerbations of pain and disability, and to minimise progression of the disease. With relief of the acute symptoms, patients can usually lead a relatively normal life within limits dictated by the extent of joint damage.

The first task is to identify, and if possible to correct, factors leading to the development of secondary osteoarthritis. Valgus or varus deformities of weight-bearing joints produce abnormal stress distributions with osteoarthritic changes. A corrective osteotomy may prevent the progress of this problem. Inflammatory and infective arthritis must be treated promptly, not only to minimise the direct damage that may result, but also to prevent secondary osteoarthritic changes.

Occupational factors must be assessed and, if particular jobs are identified as being responsible for the development or exacerbation of osteoarthritis, the task should be altered accordingly. One example is the carpet-layer's knee, where the stress of banging the carpet-stretcher with one knee leads to precocious degenerative changes in that joint.

Although the relationship between obesity and osteoarthritis in general is not clear, there does seem to be an association with osteoarthritis of the knees and, in patients with osteoarthritis, being overweight will exacerabate the problem. Appreciation by the patient of the need to minimise stresses on the weight-bearing joints is essential if he or she is to lose weight successfully.

Patients should be advised to live within their tolerance limits. Over-use of an osteoarthritic joint will exacerbate the symptoms and increase the progression of the joint changes. In general terms, the use of an osteoarthritic joint is encouraged to the limit dictated by the onset of pain, but pain should be regarded as the warning sign that further use will produce damage. At the same time, however, the patient should be encouraged to protect the joint by minimising stress upon it. Use of a walking aid such as a walking stick will reduce the load upon an osteoarthritic hip or knee and may enable the patient to walk in reasonable comfort. Aids must be tailored to the individual patient and instruction on their use is provided by the physiotherapist. As an example, a walking stick should be held by the hand contralateral to the osteoarthritic hip or knee and not on the same side.

Physiotherapy is often prescribed, yet much of what is offered is of dubious value. Many forms of treatment offer only temporary palliation of symptoms without any long-term benefits. In particular, the many applications of heat, e.g. infra-red, short-wave diathermy, mud packs, etc., and of cold, e.g. ice packs, relieve pain only at the time of application and for a short while thereafter. These measures alone are of no value but they are sometimes combined with other measures as a preliminary to relieve pain before other forms of treatment.

A major problem in osteoarthritis is the wasting weakness of the muscles controlling damaged joints. This weakness, contributing to further instability, and difficulty in joint use, exacerbates the problem. Exercises are directed at restoring and maintaining muscle function. Quadriceps exercises for the osteoarthritic knee are particularly useful. Isometric exercises are used and forced movements of painful joints are avoided. As much benefit is gained by doing exercises at home, recording progress in a diary and returning for review as by attending the physiotherapy department for this regime.

The physiotherapist has an important role in patient education and advice. The patient will be taught how to get out of a chair, climb stairs and perform other tasks within the limits dictated by the severity of the symptoms.

Drug Therapy

Non-steroidal anti-inflammatory drugs and pure analgesics are used in much the same way as in inflammatory arthritis. There is frequently a mild inflammatory element in osteoarthritis so that on the whole the former group are the more helpful.

Some patients will only respond to a pure analgesic such as paracetamol or stronger analgesics such as dihydrocodeine. There is no indication for narcotic analgesics, as these drugs readily produce addiction, particularly in patients who are likely to suffer recurrent problems.

There is no place for the use of systemic corticosteroids in the management of osteoarthritis.

Injections

In selected patients, local injection of a long-acting corticosteroid may be helpful. They are used particularly when there is a flare of symptoms in one joint and expecially if there is evidence of an inflammatory component to the problem. Examples include injection into the knee or into the carpo-metacarpal joint of the thumb. Injections should only be given when the diagnosis is certain and not if there is any possibility of an infected joint. Scrupulous asepsis is mandatory to avoid the risk of introducing infection. The preparations used are sparingly soluble crystalline forms of corticosteroids which are slowly absorbed and have a prolonged effect. They may well prove adequate for controlling an acute exacerbation of the pain but they do nothing to alter the long-term course of osteoarthritis. Occasionally an acute exacerbation of pain may follow immediately after the local injection. This appears to be due to the crystalline nature of the preparation and will subside within a day or two. Repeated injections may accelerate degenerative changes and should be avoided.

Palpation of the osteoarthritic joint will often indicate that the pain arises from the soft tissues around the joint and particularly from the capsule and ligaments at the joint margin. If a focal area of tenderness is identified as being responsible for the symptoms, it is often well worth treating this area by local infiltration with corticosteroids, usually mixed with local anaesthetic. In this case the joint space is not punctured.

Surgery

Surgery is not indicated for the great majority of patients with osteoarthritis. When there is severe disability, however, and particularly when pain is unrelievable by conservative means, surgery is indicated. Total joint replacement has revolutionised the management of severe osteoarthritis of the hip and has provided mobility for thousands who would otherwise have been relegated to a wheelchair existence. However, although total joint replacement is the most commonly performed procedure for osteoarthritis, it is only part of the surgical armamentarium for these patients and is particularly favoured when the joint is severely destroyed in the older individual. When the joint is less severely damaged it can be amenable to osteotomy, while in the younger patient a severely damaged joint may be best arthrodesed.

Osteotomy

This is commonly performed at both hip and knee. The purpose of an osteotomy is to alter the mechanics of the joint so that local stresses are reduced or applied more symmetrically.

The neck of the femur makes an obtuse angle with the shaft, placing the longitudinal axis of the lower extremity well to the side of the centre of gravity of the body. This produces a lever arm effect across the hip joint which exacerbates local discomfort and renders the patient more susceptible to symptoms during load-bearing, a problem which may be reduced in the short term by the use of a walking stick. If the upper femur in the trochanteric region is divided and the distal fragment displaced medially, then the lever arm is reduced and the longitudinal axis of the lower extremity moves closer to the centre of gravity (Fig. 13.6). In addition to the mechanical effect thereby produced,

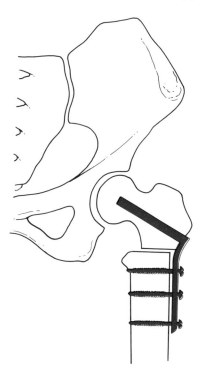

Fig. 13.6 *Trochanteric osteotomy redistributes joint load by reducing the lever arms across the hip.*

there is also evidence that symptoms may be ameliorated by the alteration of blood flow in the head and proximal neck of the femur consequent upon osteotomy. Such procedure may also promote the development of fibrous tissue over the denuded joint surfaces.

At the knee, osteoarthritis is seldom symmetrical; the medial or lateral joint spaces are much more severely involved. This is particularly true after menscial damage on one side of the joint. When the lower extremity is load-bearing, the side of the joint already damaged takes more stress, with the development of a painful valgus or varus deformity. Osteotomy is designed to redistribute load so that continued wear of the narrowed side can be minimised. A triangular wedge of bone is removed from the upper tibia just below the knee joint surface so that the extremity will be straight on weight bearing. With an osteotomy performed in the metaphyseal region of the tibia there is an abundance of cancellous bone here and union is rapid.

Arthrodesis

Before the very good long-term results of hip joint replacement became apparent, arthrodesis of the hip joint was favoured, particularly in the young who were thought to be at risk with total joint replacement because of the unknown effects of such a procedure with time. There are, however, still firm indications for this procedure. When a joint has worn out due to pre-existing disease, such as Perthe's disease or necrosis of the femoral head as a result of previous trauma or infection, and the patient is a young, heavy-weight, active individual, arthrodesis of the hip joint is still the procedure of choice. The excellent results of total hip replacement in the light-weight elderly are not reproduced in an individual such as a young farmer. Excision of the damaged joint surfaces and fusion of the hip in a fuctional position of abduction and flexion provide painless stability with little local risk. Unfortunately, because the load is transferred to nearby articulations, the lumbar spine, and the knee, premature wear here may occur consequent upon hip fusion. Indeed, many years after hip arthrodesis, if back or knee pain are significant symptoms, the fusion can be taken down and a total joint replacement inserted when the patient has gone through the greater phase of active working life.

Unfortunately the results of total knee replacement

do not match those of the hip, and arthrodesis of the knee is still a useful procedure. Again the younger, more active, male is the candidate of choice and the procedure is specially indicated in haemophiliacs with knee arthropathy, in whom the uncertainties of joint replacement could not be recommended. The knee joint surfaces are excised and fusion is achieved in 20° of flexion. Unfortunately, as with the hip, fusion tends to produce earlier-than-normal wear in the joints above and below.

Total joint replacement

Charnley has dramatically improved the prognosis for severe hip osteoarthrosis by his low-friction arthroplasty, which replaces the acetabulum with high-density polyethylene, and the femoral head with a stainless steel spherical head with an intramedullary stem passing down the femoral shaft (Fig. 13.7). This is the basis of all models of total hip replacement and has superseded the prosthesis of McKee which loosened early because both components were made of metal.

Although the procedure still enjoys its best indication in the elderly with severe joint disease, its wide margin of safety has led to its use in younger individuals who are not prepared to accept the limitation of arthrodesis. Its success rate of over 90% is attributable to its marked pain-relieving effect rather to any improvement in mobility, which is often difficult to demonstrate. The most prevalent local postoperative problem is infection, and such procedures should be performed in an ultra-clean-air environment to minimise this risk. Dislocation of the components also occurs in 1% of patients during the course of the first year or two, but loosening, particularly of the femoral component, probably occurs in more than 5% of cases. The prostheses are fixed in position using methyl methacrylate cement and it is at this cement–bone interface where loosening is liable to occur. After a period of excellent pain relief and improved function, a dull thigh ache occurs, particularly on weight-bearing. Heel percussion or leg telescoping reproduces the symptoms. It is important to ensure that the loosening has not occurred in the presence of low-grade infection, and the ESR is the most important indication of this. Treatment, however, remains the same, which is removal of the loose component along with all cement and other debris and the insertion of a fresh prosthesis.

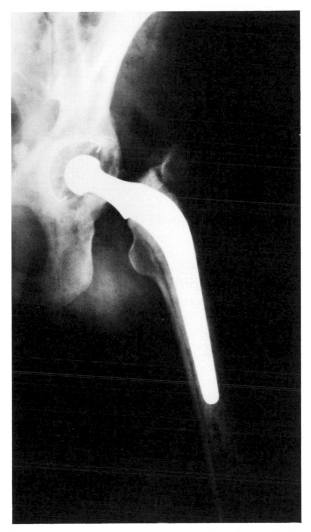

Fig. 13.7 *Anteroposterior x-ray of hip. Charnley total hip replacement has markedly improved this patient's quality of life.*

The operation of total hip replacement is, however, a major one and has the morbidity and mortality to be expected from the ageing population on which it is performed. Undiagnosed hypertension and diabetes are the most potent causes of morbidity, together with deep venous thrombosis and cardiac arrhythmias, which are particularly liable to occur when the constituents of methyl methacrylate enter the bloodstream during cementing of the components.

Total knee replacement does not enjoy the same success and this is because the anatomy of the knee joint is more complex from the mechanical point of view. In particular the cancellous bone of the tibial plateau is vulnerable to stress when the harder sub-chondral bone is removed for a replacement to be fitted. When the femoral and tibial components of the new joint are attached to each other, the joint is described as constrained and stresses are transferred from the site of the hinge mechanism to the femur above and below. This leads to loosening. When the components are unconstrained, there is freedom of movement between the articulating surfaces of the two components. The joint therefore depends, for stability, upon intact surrounding ligaments. Loosening does not occur with the same prevalence but fixation to the soft tibial plateau still remains a problem. Unconstrained prostheses are therefore favoured, and an elderly light-weight female patient is preferred. In younger, heavier, more active males there is an unacceptable rate of loosening and complication.

Excision arthroplasty

This is essentially a salvage procedure. Although, before the advent of the total joint replacement, it was popular for a severe hip joint arthritis, it is now reserved for those who have severe disability as a significant local complication of joint replacement, or for a situation such as old congenital hip dislocation where a prosthesis could not be inserted in the first place. The joint surfaces (artificial or real) are excised, and a period of traction in bed enables fibrous tissue to fill the resultant gap. There is often a good degree of pain relief with mobility, but loss of stability necessitates the wearing of a lower extremity splint and a raise on the ipsilateral shoe.

14

Polyarthritis

INTRODUCTION

The most common diagnosis in a patient with inflammation in several joints is rheumatoid arthritis (RA), but polyarthritis features in many other syndromes; individually these are much less common but collectively they pose a major exercise in differential diagnosis. The term 'syndrome' is used because we are concerned with conditions which are recognised as entities by distinctive clusters of clinical features rather than by clearly-defined aetiologies.

A feature of many cases of RA is the presence in the serum of antiglobulins, loosely referred to as rheumatoid factor(s), and this is the basis for a broad division into seropositive and seronegative polyarthritis. Not all cases of RA are positive, nor are quite all of the rest negative, and we have to be sure in aberrant cases that the clinical features conform with those generally accepted as characteristic of the two types.

Several subgroups of seronegative arthritis can be separated because the individual syndromes which compose them share certain features. One of these common denominators is chronic disease of the gut, another is the combination of sacro-iliitis with a specific genetic marker. There is some overlap between subgroups, but they provide a useful working classification in default of precise knowledge of aetiology.

In the diagnosis of these syndromes much can be learned from the age and sex incidence, the distribution of affected joints, the pattern in time – acute or insidious onset, persistent, recurrent or self-limiting – and the ultimate presence or absence of irreversible joint damage. There may also be features in other tissues or organs which aid diagnosis. Some of these features, particularly the pattern of joint involvement, are summarised in the skeleton figures: bright red patches show the joints most often involved, paler red indicates those next most commonly affected, and those only occasionally involved are indicated by a grey patch.

Rheumatoid arthritis will be described first; much of what can be learned from studying it is pertinent to other syndromes and some comparisons with RA will be made when these are considered.

RHEUMATOID ARTHRITIS

Rheumatoid arthritis is usually a symmetrical polyarthritis which starts most often in the small joints of the hands but soon spreads to the metatarso-phalangeal joints and, to a lesser degree, the knees and ankles (Figs 14.1 and 14.2). Later almost any joint may be involved, including those of the neck but rarely the terminal finger joints.

Inflammation tends to wax and wane spontaneously so that periods of activity alternate with remissions. Joint destruction in progressive cases leads to characteristic deformities. About three women are affected for every two men and the prevalence in the UK population is in the region of 1%. The peak age of onset is in the fourth and fifth decades, but cases are so numerous throughout adult life that age is of little value in diagnosis. RA in children will be considered in a separate section.

Pathology, Clinical and Radiographic Features

The easiest way to interpret the clinical and radiographic features is to combine them with a mental

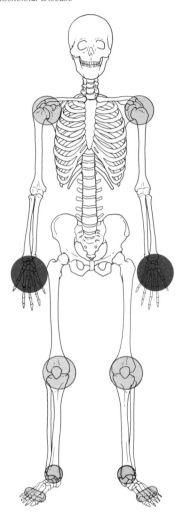

Fig. 14.1 *Rheumatoid arthritis—onset.*

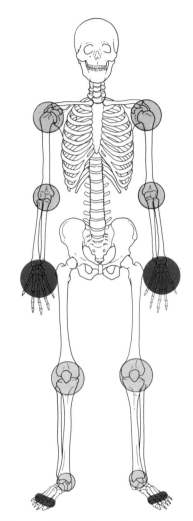

Fig. 14.2 *Rheumatoid arthritis—early.*

picture of what is happening inside the joints, and so all three will be described in parallel. The reader must keep the following points in mind: a joint is a bearing which permits movement of two bones in relation to each other in one or more planes; frictional resistance is minimised by a coating of hyaline cartilage on the opposing bone surfaces and by the lubricant action of synovial fluid; movement beyond normal limits is constrained by the capsule and ligaments; and muscles contribute stability as well as powering movement. Some or all of these attributes are impaired by arthritis.

Synovitis (Fig. 14.3) is the first abnormality; as in all types of inflammation, blood flow in the synovial membrane increases and cells migrate into it from new vascular loops. At the same time the synovial surface cells proliferate, forming villous projections and increasing the thickness of the membrane. After a brief migration of polymorph leucocytes, lymphocytes and monocytes predominate and form a dense infiltrate in the synovium, with many congregating into lymphoid follicles, occasionally with germinal centres. Excessive amounts of synovial fluid, excreted into the joint cavity, is less viscous than normal synovial fluid because the hyaluronic acid in it is poorly polymerised. Despite the predominance of lymphocytes in the synovial tissue, the cells in the joint fluid are mainly polymorphs.

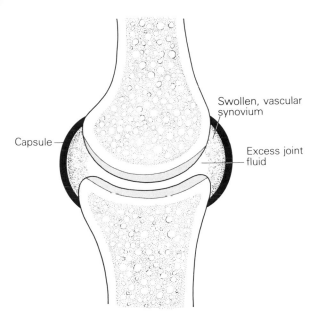

Capsule

Swollen, vascular synovium

Excess joint fluid

Fig. 14.3 *RA—synovitis.*

From all this it follows that the joint will be swollen because it contains an increased volume of fluid as well as a bulky synovial membrane, it will be warm to the touch because of the increased flow of blood and it will be painful and tender. The intra-articular pressure may rise in a joint which has to accommodate an increased volume of fluid and synovium. Pressure changes during movement are maximal in full flexion and minimal in partial flexion. High pressures cause pain because they stretch receptors in the capsule, which is why a patient will often keep a joint partially flexed. Reluctance to flex a joint fully under these conditions does not amount to permanent loss of movement, nor is the adoption of a position of partial flexion a fixed deformity. Both symptoms disappear if pressure is reduced, either by treatment or by a spontaneous remission, but may become permanent, because of secondary changes, if pressure is allowed to persist. High pressures, which may reach 1000 mmHg, are likely to be found in joints which still have a firm capsule and strong muscles. To find the true range in such a joint, very gentle passive movements are needed. Brusque movement immediately elicits a stretch reflex, which is already exaggerated in these painful joints, thus checking movement. Fine crepitus may be felt in a joint which contains an effusion but has its bearing surfaces as yet undamaged;

it is caused by fluid streaming through a constricted channel during movement.

Radiographs at this stage may show loss of density in the bone on either side of the joint, but give little additional information. Bone and cartilage appear otherwise unaffected, and the contours of the bones forming the joint are unaltered, as is the 'space' between them (not a true space, but occupied by joint cartilage which is radiolucent). The films may show swelling of soft tissues but this should be visible clinically.

The configuration of a joint is determined by the thickness of the capsule at various points around the joint, notably the position of the strengthened bands which form ligaments. The proximal interphalangeal joints bulge sideways, giving the digits the shape of a spindle, while swelling of the metacarpophalangeal joints protrudes at either side of the overlying extensor tendons. Synovitis in the carpus is often accompanied by inflammation in the sheaths surrounding the tendons which pass over it. At the front, swelling is constrained by the strong flexor retinaculum and is usually recognised by palpable tenseness rather than by visible swelling. Swelling on the dorsum is easily seen, and extends up to the boundaries of the extensor sheath. In the elbow, swelling is seen most easily between the olecranon and the back of the medial epicondyle; the olecranon bursa may also be distended. In the shoulder, it is difficult to be sure whether there is an effusion within the joint; visible swelling usually indicates subacromial bursitis. The hip joint lies deep, and is surrounded by muscles and a strong capsule, so that synovitis is hard to establish clinically; very occasionally a related psoas bursitis is visible in the groin. In the knee, a small effusion is diagnosed most readily by stroking it away from the medial side with the back of the hand and seeing the swelling wave return when the lateral side of the joint is pressed. Larger effusions fill the suprapatellar pouch and bulge out at each side of the patella. The back of the knee should be examined for a popliteal cyst, produced by fluid under pressure moving posteriorly through a narrow one-way communication. Rupture of such a cyst produces sudden pain and swelling in the calf, often mistaken for a deep vein thrombosis. Alternatively, a cyst may balloon out into a thin-walled calf cyst, sometimes extending as far down as the ankle. If the ankle is inflamed, there will be swelling below the malleoli and perhaps around the tendo Achillis. Swelling of the metatarsophalangeal joints is not easy to recognise unless the related bursas protrude into interdigital clefts. As a rule it is not easy to be sure how much of the swelling in a joint is due to fluid and how much to synovial thickening although, in the knee, the latter can be estimated by pinching the suprapatellar pouch between finger and thumb.

There are more than 180 synovial joints and none is immune to RA. Many are clinically important but a few are inaccessible to examination, though some produce signs and symptoms peculiar to their position and function. Thus RA in the small synovial joints of the cervical spine, particularly its upper end, causes instability, often with pressure on the medulla or cord, though there may be no neurological signs of damage. Sometimes severe occipital headache gives warning. Sudden braking of a vehicle has been known to cause death in patients with an unstable neck. General anaesthesia is another hazard; radiographs of the neck should always be taken beforehand in patients with RA.

Arthritis in the crico-arytenoid joints causes hoarseness and, very occasionally, life-threatening respiratory obstruction. Involvement of the synovial joints of the middle ear is a probable cause of impaired hearing but this is hard to confirm, especially if the picture is complicated by treatment with a salicylate, which may also cause deafness. Arthritis of the temporo-mandibular joint is painful and may limit movement; this usually resolves, though some destruction of the condyle often remains and the bite may be altered.

Apart from the joints, patients usually show some systemic signs of an inflammatory illness. Fever is not common but there is often malaise, lassitude and sometimes depression. There may be some loss of weight. Anaemia appears as inflammation continues; it is normochromic and normocytic unless complicated by iron deficiency or some other factor. The serum iron is low and iron-binding either normal or reduced. The ESR is increased and other acute-phase reactions are positive – but these tests are not specific.

In its early stages, rheumatoid synovitis can resolve temporarily or permanently. Unfortunately, however, it often persists and begins to threaten the permanent structure and function of the joint. The threat first develops in the recesses where the synovial membrane is reflected off the inner surface of the capsule to clothe the bone up to the edge of the articular cartilage. In these recesses, synovial inflammation generates a nest of vascular granulation tissue capable of damaging both cartilage and bone. Articular cartilage is normally avascular and reacts badly to contact with vascular granulation tissue. The destructive enzymes hitherto locked in the lysosomes of cartilage cells are activated by the increased oxygen concentration, and other enzymes probably also play a part. The matrix of the cartilage is lost, initially at its edge; although at this stage there is nothing to show clinically that destruction of cartilage has begun, it should be suspected if synovitis is persistent. Insidious destruction may, however, occur in the absence of florid synovitis. There may be local tenderness where there is early marginal cartilage damage but, as the full thickness of cartilage is still preserved, a radiograph will show no decrease in joint space.

For a short time, loss of cartilage matrix is reversible; soon, however, the collagen fibres embedded in it are destroyed and regeneration is no longer possible. By this stage a thin layer of granulation tissue or 'pannus' is advancing across the surface of the cartilage (Fig. 14.4), leaving defects which can only be replaced by undifferentiated fibrous tissue which is ill-suited to take over the specialised function of hyaline cartilage as a low-friction bearing surface. Invasive granulation tissue attacks bone in much the same way, with destruction

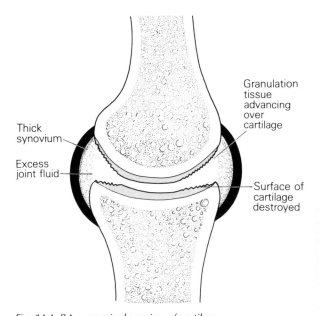

Thick synovium

Excess joint fluid

Granulation tissue advancing over cartilage

Surface of cartilage destroyed

Fig. 14.4 *RA—marginal erosion of cartilage.*

again starting close to the synovial reflection. The earliest lesions develop just outside the edge of the articular cartilage and are easily seen on radiographs as juxta-articular erosions (Fig. 14.5).

As destruction of cartilage progresses, leaving only remnants (Fig. 14.6), the denuded end plate of the bones becomes dense and polished (eburnated). Two eburnated surfaces moving across each other produce a distinctive, coarse, creaking, eburnation crepitus which can often be heard as well as felt, particularly when the two surfaces are pressed together by the muscle contraction of active weight-bearing movement. It may be much less apparent during passive movements with no loading. Movements of a joint in this state will be stiff. A radiograph at this stage will readily reveal loss of joint space.

By this time, marginal erosions have grown larger and subarticular pseudocysts may have appeared. These are round translucent areas in the metaphysis (Fig. 14.6) which result from synovial fluid and granulation tissue being driven by a high intra-articular pressure through small defects in the bony end plate. Sometimes the joint surface collapses into a large lesion of this kind. Osteoporosis of bone adjacent to the joint facilitates these lesions and is probably a factor in arthritis mutilans, a variant of RA in which substantial lengths of bone on either side of the joint disappear.

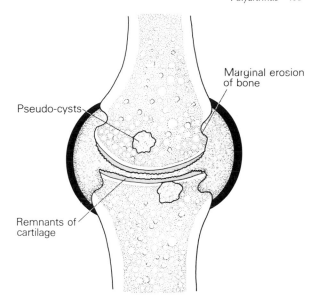

Fig. 14.6 *RA—advanced destruction of cartilage.*

Destruction of cartilage and its replacement by fibrous tissue causes still more trouble if two such areas of scarring meet across the joint line and fuse. Tenuous connections (adhesions) will restrict movement, but if they mature and thicken the result is fibrous ankylosis and movement is reduced to no more than a jog. Fibrous bridges may ossify, producing bony ankylosis with trabeculae (clearly seen on radiographs) running in unbroken continuity from one bone to another across what was once the joint space. This is rare but, when it occurs, no movement is left and the joint is pain-free.

Deformities and Instability

A tense effusion can inhibit full flexion and induce a patient to keep the joint slightly flexed at the most comfortable angle. At later stages, several factors produce more permanent deformity and instability. All the elements which make a normal joint stable are vulnerable to the inroads of RA. The congruity of joint surfaces, already impaired by loss of cartilage, may be affected more dramatically by collapse into areas undermined by pseudocysts or weakened by osteoporosis. In the knee, for example, valgus or varus deformity may result from collapse of the lateral or medial tibial plateaux respectively. Such deformities are unstable

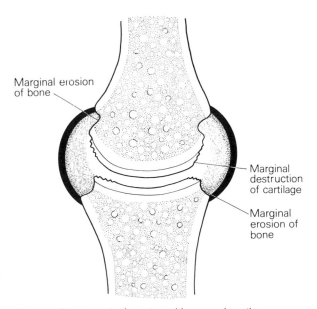

Fig. 14.5 *RA—marginal erosion of bone and cartilage.*

because collapse leaves a slack collateral ligament on the same side; they can be seen while the patient is standing, but may disappear when there is no load. Joint capsules become lax after repeated stretching by effusions and synovial hypertrophy combined with inflammation spreading from the synovium.

Weak muscles also contribute to instability; an imbalance between antagonist groups may allow the more powerful flexors to pull the joint into flexion deformity. The hands are particularly susceptible to deforming forces since they depend so much on a complex balance between the long flexors and extensors, supplemented by the intrinsic muscles and their attachments. The fibrous extensor capsular hoods over the joints, so important functionally, are vulnerable to the effects of inflammation underneath. Slight changes in the alignment of metacarpals and phalanges change the direction of pull of flexor tendons, turning them into powerful deforming forces. Flexion deformity and ulnar drift are common at the metacarpophalangeal joints and are disabling when it is no longer possible to touch the tips of the medial digits with the thumb. Two kinds of deformity occur at the proximal interphalangeal joints. Loss of extension (the boutonnière deformity) is due to softening of the extensor hood. The contrasting and more disabling ('swan-neck') deformity is hyperextension, combined with flexion at the distal interphalangeal joint.

Stiffness in the fingers, perhaps with some loss of extension, can be due to flexor tenosynovitis rather than arthritis, while nodules in flexor tendons cause triggering. At the metatarsophalangeal joints, hyperextension is the usual deformity, together with flexion at the interphalangeal joints. The thick pad which normally lies under the metatarsal heads is drawn away distally so that the heads come to lie immediately under the skin, which becomes calloused. Such feet are very painful, and the patient feels as if he is walking on pebbles.

If two bones move out of alignment so that they cease to be contiguous – partially in subluxation, wholly in dislocation – there is yet more disruption of stabilising ligaments and muscles and still more deformity. At the wrist, the lower end of the ulna is often displaced dorsally. This is not only painful but carries the threat of attrition rupture of extensor tendons, particularly those of the fourth and fifth digits and especially if there is ulnar drift at the wrist. Combined

with flexion deformity at the wrist, this makes for a very weak hand. Rupture of tendons is another cause of deformity; it most often involves extensors, and the significance of drooping fingers should not be missed. Flexor tendons rarely rupture, but rupture of the long head of biceps is not infrequent. Many other deformities also occur.

Laboratory and Radiographic Investigations

The most useful laboratory tests are those which detect serum antiglobulins loosely referred to as rheumatoid factors(s). There are several techniques: the sheep cell agglutination test (SCAT), its variant the differential agglutination test (DAT, or Rose–Waaler test), and the latex test. About 60% of patients with RA have a positive result in a single random test, and about 70% will have at least one positive result if tested repeatedly. The antiglobulins detected by these tests are not specific for RA but their presence adds useful weight to the diagnosis if there are already enough clinical features. Swings between positive and negative results are common, and slow-acting drugs such as gold (see below) often reverse a positive. The terms 'seropositive' and 'seronegative' refer to the results of these tests.

Antibodies which react with nuclear material are common in serum from RA, but activity specifically against native DNA – a feature of systemic lupus erythematosus – is not found.

The cell content of synovial fluid is important in distinguishing between RA and infective arthritis, though the findings overlap. As a rough guide, a total count of up to 20 000 cells/mm^3, with 80% or more polymorphs, is usual in RA. In infective arthritis, counts in excess of 50 000 are usual. Fluid from RA may be turbid; fluid from infected joints will certainly be. Normal joint fluid contains fewer than 100 cells/mm^3 and is clear and viscous. Crystals should be sought in joint fluid if there is a possibility of a crystal deposition disease.

The ESR and other acute-phase reactions are most useful for following the progress of the disease and its response to treatment. They are of some value in distinguishing between RA and non-inflammatory arthropathies such as polyarticular osteoarthrosis, but must not be relied upon too heavily.

The important radiographic changes have already

been noted. They are rarely important in early diagnosis except in helping to distinguish between RA and polyarticular osteoarthrosis. In the hands, the distinction is not always easy, but a finding of erosions in the metatarsophalangeal joints, which are rarely affected by osteoarthrosis except for the first, leave the diagnosis of RA in no doubt. Erosions here may also exclude 'simple' metatarsalgia. Serial radiographs are valuable in assessing the tempo of the disease when prosthetic replacement of a joint is being considered.

Diagnosis

A list of criteria, devised by the American Rheumatism Association, is used for codifying the diagnosis of RA and is useful in ordinary clinical practice. Five criteria are used for a diagnosis of 'definite' RA: one point is scored for morning stiffness, a second if any joint is tender or painful on movement, a third if one joint is seen to be swollen, a fourth if another joint is seen to be swollen and a fifth if there is symmetrical swelling with simultaneous involvement of the same joint on both sides of the body. In the case of the small joints of the hands and feet, any joint is accepted as symmetrical with any other in the same row on the other side. The signs and symptoms must have been present for at least six weeks – a wise provision which prevents some misdiagnoses. These five criteria are those most often satisfied, but several others that can be used to make the required total of five include positive serology, subcutaneous nodules, radiographic abnormalities – ranging from juxta-articular osteoporosis to erosions – and others, such as a positive biopsy, which are less often available. 'Definite' satisfies most clinicians but there is another category, 'classical' RA, for which seven criteria are required. If only three or four criteria are satisfied, a diagnosis of 'probable' RA is allowed. As well as the presence of these positive criteria, certain listed features, or negative criteria, must be absent because they point to a different diagnosis; these will emerge when we consider other types of polyarthritis. There is a fourth category, 'possible' RA, for which less demanding criteria are required; such cases rarely develop more convincing evidence of RA as time goes by unless they are seropositive. Morning stiffness, although it is a prominent feature and useful in diagnosis if severe, is certainly not specific for RA.

Most cases of RA conform with the definition of a symmetrical polyarthritis which starts insidiously in the small joints of the extremities, but there are some notable exceptions which broaden the field of differential diagnosis, e.g. cases in which RA remains confined to one joint for months or years and in which alternative diagnoses such as tuberculous arthritis or pigmented villonodular synovitis must be entertained. Episodic RA, characterised by a succession of acute monarticular attacks, is a far more common variant, in which attacks last for 48 hours or less, during which pain is of immobilising severity. Attacks in the shoulder are common and, if careful enquiry is made, it will be found that one or more acute attacks of this sort figure in the early history of one-third of patients with the familiar polyarthritic pattern. Often, acute attacks soon become less severe and last longer until the process loses its episodic character. In other cases, acute attacks continue for years, often as periodic salvoes, with no symptoms in the intervals. Serological tests are helpful; these cases are seropositive as often as those with typical RA. Differential diagnosis includes crystal arthropathy, but this does not settle so quickly.

Course and Prognosis

It would be misleading to paint a picture of steady and inexorable progression through clearly-defined stages to inevitable severe destruction. The disease is, in fact, both variable and unpredictable. Synovitis may disappear without residua and may or may not recur in the same joint; it may persist in one joint after settling in the remainder. Severe cases are easy to recognise but at the other end of the scale there may well be cases so mild as to escape notice. Of patients who seek medical advice, about 10% are eventually severely handicapped, a similar proportion suffer no more than mild discomfort, and the rest progress slowly over the years but are never more than moderately disabled.

Complications

Nodules

Subcutaneous nodules over bony prominences, such as the subcutaneous border of the ulna just below the elbow, and the smaller intracutaneous nodules often seen on the fingers, are integral features of RA rather than complications; they are found in 20% of cases. An ulcerated sacral nodule, however, complicates management by producing an intractable bed sore, and nodules in internal organs introduce their own problems, as will be seen shortly. Nodules are composed of a central focus of necrosis surrounded by elongated histiocytes arranged radially as a palisade.

Nervous system

Neurological lesions include nerve entrapment, other peripheral neuropathies, and the lesions of the medulla and cord associated with cervical instability. The most common entrapment is of the median nerve in the carpal tunnel. This produces pain and paraesthesiae distal to the wrist and also pain in the elbow and shoulder, symptoms which must be distinguished from those due directly to arthritis since they can be very effectively treated by surgical decompression. There are two other types of peripheral neuropathy: one, which tends to improve with time, is sensory, symmetrical, occurs predominantly in the legs, and often starts with a sensation of coldness; the other, more serious, type is asymmetrical and involves motor as well as sensory fibres in one or more nerve trunks.

Respiratory system

Apart from nodules in the pleura, which are sometimes hard to distinguish from a lung tumour, the respiratory complications of RA include pleural effusions and fibrosing alveolitis; the latter is suspected if there is increasing dyspnoea and fine ('Velcro') crepitations, usually with clubbing of fingers. Coalminers with rheumatoid arthritis may develop multiple, well-defined round opacities in the lungs. These are spread throughout the lungs, with some concentration in the periphery. Background pneumoconiosis is slight. This is known as Caplan's syndrome, and may also be found in rheumatoid patients in other occupations carrying a pneumoconiosis risk. All these respiratory complications are commoner in men than women.

Cardiovascular system

The commonest sign of vasculitis is a crop of micro-infarcts in the form of tiny brown or black spots around the finger nails and sometimes on the summit of intracutaneous nodules on the fingers. They are most common in severe cases of RA. A more serious symptom is occlusive disease of large digital arteries, responsible for Raynaud's phenomenon or even gangrene. Still worse is the type of diffuse necrotising vasculitis which resembles polyarteritis nodosa; it causes asymmetrical neuropathy, deep and painful leg ulcers, and occasionally infarction of internal organs.

In the heart, nodules may cause conduction defects or, occasionally, aortic incompetence. The commonest lesion here is pericarditis, very frequently found at necropsy but less often diagnosed in life.

Haemopoietic system

Anaemia is common, as has already been noted. Leucopenia with splenomegaly, leg ulcers, and susceptibility to infection constitutes Felty's syndrome, a variant of RA rather than a distinct disease. The platelet count in RA is often raised; a low count, like leucopenia, may be an adverse effect of a drug.

Lymphatic system

Diffuse and sometimes massive enlargement of lymph nodes may be found. Enlargement of the spleen is common and not necessarily accompanied by other features of Felty's syndrome.

Ophthalmic

The commonest complication in the eye is keratoconjunctivitis sicca, in which reduced secretion of tears causes gritty discomfort and sometimes corneal ulceration. It is often accompanied by a dry mouth and this 'sicca syndrome' together with RA constitutes Sjögren's syndrome (see Chapter 17).

Next in frequency is episcleritis or scleritis and most serious is perforation of the eyeball by a scleral nodule: scleromalacia perforans. Iritis is not a feature of RA.

Superimposed infection of joints

Unless diagnosed and treated very promptly, this is a serious complication. Diagnosis is not always easy, as the signs of inflammation may not be obviously more severe than those of exacerbations of RA. The only prudent policy is to aspirate any joint which has suddenly become more acute and to send the fluid for culture. Fluid from an infected joint usually has a low glucose content as well as a high cell count but only isolation of an organism can clinch the diagnosis.

Amyloidosis

RA is now the commonest cause of amyloidosis in the UK. It should be considered as a probable cause of proteinuria and nitrogen retention unless these can be ascribed to pyelonephritis or a reaction to a drug. Failure of infiltrated arteries to retract when damaged may result in bleeding from the gastrointestinal tract or bladder.

Aetiology

The aetiology of RA is uncertain but the most favoured concept is a sequence of events triggered by an unidentified microbiological agent. This causes tissue damage which elicits a harmful immunological reaction, causing further tissue damage and thus perpetuating the process. There is strong evidence of genetic susceptibility, either to the microbiological agent or to the harmful type of immune reaction which it initiates. The best of this evidence comes from genetic markers of the HLA system first used in tissue-typing and particularly from the DR locus. In Caucasians and some other ethnic groups there is an association with DR4, but in patients from the Indian subcontinent and those of Ashkenazi origin the link is with DR1. There is also a negative association with some other DR antigens, suggesting that these may be protective. It is possible that the DR antigens themselves do not play a part in increasing susceptibility to RA but that the locus for increased susceptibility is closely linked to the DR locus.

Treatment

The essence of treatment is a three-pronged attack: relieving pain and stiffness; preventing or correcting deformity; and modifying the natural course of the disease. Many drugs alleviate pain and stiffness (see p. 198); there are also valuable physical methods such as complete immobilisation of acutely inflamed joints combined with static exercises to maintain muscle bulk.

Prevention of deformity is an early and pressing task. Resting splints for wear at night check flexion deformity at the knees, ankles, wrists and fingers. They should keep the wrist in a neutral position and the fingers slightly flexed. The knee should be straight but not uncomfortably hyperextended. Flexion deformity of the knees that has already developed can often be corrected by a series of splints. The first is applied with the patient prone and relaxed; the joint should not be forced into greater extension as the weight of the lower leg often undoes a few degrees of flexion if a support in front of the ankle is slowly lowered. After several days, and when the leg has settled comfortably into the splint, a second splint is applied with a further gain in extension. These cylindrical or cuffed splints are replaced by removable rest splints after maximum correction has been attained. Work splints are particularly useful for guarding a painful wrist, while allowing the fingers to function better.

Surgery for Rheumatoid Disease

It is useful to consider the scope of surgery in three broad categories according to the stage of the disease process.

Stage of acute synovitis

There is no place for surgery in this early stage of the disease. Treatment is entirely conservative, with anti-inflammatory analgesics and joint splintage as the fundamental basis.

Stage of soft tissue destruction

If the disease is aggressive and does not respond to conservative measures, the harmful synovitis will persist in joints and around tendons and jeopardise the integrity of these structures. Synovectomy is the procedure of choice at this stage, which seeks to remove the damaging synovium before it can rupture tendons or weaken ligaments. This is particularly useful in the knee and elbow but synovectomy is not effective in the finger joints. Frequently, by the time surgical attention is drawn to the synovitis around tendons, the latter have ruptured or become significantly attenuated, and then tendon reconstruction becomes a part of the synovectomy procedure. An early effect of synovitis is attenuation of the ligamentous support for the head of the ulna and, rather than attempting to repair these flimsy structures, the ulnar head, which is relatively unimportant in wrist function, can be excised. Synovectomy is less effective in the foot.

Stage of bone and joint collapse

When the disease process is particularly aggressive or advanced, the effect of persistent synovitis is to destroy the joint surfaces, when it is manifestly too late to perform a synovectomy and some form of joint reconstruction (arthroplasty) is frequently necessary. Total hip and total knee replacement are particularly useful procedures, but replacement of the shoulder and elbow are still being developed and the results with current designs are poor. In the peripheral joints, where disease tends to start and has its most devastating effect, excision arthroplasty is the predominant procedure. Joint deformities in the foot, often with overlying pressure areas, are particularly amenable to simple excision. In the hand, the disease tends to affect the metacarpo-phalangeal and proximal interphalangeal joints. The former are best treated by joint replacement, using small silicone rubber prostheses, while the proximal interphalangeal joints are best dealt with by fusion in a position of function.

DRUG TREATMENT OF INFLAMMATORY ARTHROPATHY

The treatments of the rheumatic disorders have much in common. A summary of current regimes may be helpful.

Specific Drugs

For infective arthritis the appropriate antibiotic, determined by the culture and sensitivity of the organism, must be given as soon as possible. Acute gout can be brought under control by indomethacin or phenylbuta-zone (colchicine is largely reserved for preventing acute attacks during long-term therapy). Reduction of serum uric acid or, 'interval treatment', as it is sometimes termed, is accomplished by uricosuric drugs, such as probenecid and sulphinpyrazone, or the enzyme-blocking agent, allopurinol, which prevents the formation of uric acid. There is no specific treatment for rheumatoid arthritis or osteoarthritis.

Analgesics

Drugs which are purely analgesic, such as paracetamol, are used where there is little or no inflammatory component. They are, therefore, used particularly in degererative joint disorders. It is important not to use drugs of addiction in a chronically painful state.

Non-steroidal Anti-inflammatory Drugs (NSAIDs)

These agents, of which there are many, appear to exert their analgesic action by an anti-inflammatory mechanism, although they do not affect the basic disease and do not alter objective measures of inflammation such as the ESR, or C-reactive protein. They are the first line of treatment in rheumatoid arthritis, and are also commonly used in osteoarthritis, because of the inflammatory component in that disease.

Before one drug is abandoned and another tried, the preparation should be given in adequate dosage. The cheapest, and one of the most effective, is aspirin. This is usually given either as a soluble preparation or in an enteric coating to minimise the gastric side-effects. In a few patients, haematemesis or melaena may result from gastric erosions. Dyspepsia is more common. Tinnitus and deafness frequently cause the patient to stop the drug. The commonly recommended dose is 1.2 g 6-hourly. At this high dose, however, many patients experience side-effects, and even at the lower dose of 900 mg four times daily, the rheumatoid patient frequently has CNS side-effects. Benorylate, which chemically combines paracetamol and aspirin and which does not break down until the drug is absorbed, has been used to minimise gastric side-effects, and to lower the incidence of tinnitus and deafness. Other efforts to minimise the gastric side-effects have included a preparation which does not dissolve until it reaches the alkaline medium of the small intestine (aloxiprin), and a salicylate surrounded by a coating of paracetomol granules. A less common side-effect is the precipitation of acute asthma in a sensitive subject. A list of other NSAIDs is shown in Table 14.1. Since these all act by inhibition of the cyclo-oxygenase pathway of prostaglandin synthesis, they have similar gastric side-effects.

Indomethacin is one of the most widely-used preparations. It may produce a silent gastric ulcer, and care must be exercised in its long-term prescription. In some patients, a throbbing headache occurs, especially if a high dose is administered from the start. The headache disappears on withdrawal of the drug. A slow-release preparation has proved effective and, given at night, a dose of 75 mg is particularly useful in alleviating morning stiffness. To minimise gastric side-effects, suppositories have been used, although it should be noted that not all such side-effects are due to direct contact and the circulating levels of indomethacin may also be damaging.

Phenylbutazone is a powerful agent, but has the propensity to retain fluid (as indeed all this group have to some extent) and therefore may precipitate cardiac failure. Its most dangerous side-effects are agranulocytosis and aplastic anaemia. Of all the cases of blood dyscrasias from this drug that were reported to the Committee on Safety in Medicine, half died. Women over the age of 50 seem to be particularly at risk. Oxyphenbutazone, a derivative of this, also suffers from the same drawbacks. Another attempt to overcome the gastric problem has been to use a pro-drug, which does not dissolve into its active component until it has been absorbed. Benorylate is an example of this; another is fenbufen, and there are many more propionic acid derivatives that can be tried. Some patients respond better to one drug than another, and it is reasonable to try more than one.

Physicians have been keen to reduce the frequency of dosage, since this increases patient compliance. This is accomplished by having a drug with a relatively long half-life. Several preparations can now be administered twice daily (such as naproxen), and some can be given once daily (such as piroxicam). The disadvantage of any drug with a long half-life is that, if side-effects occur, they are likely to persist for longer. Elderly patients are particularly at risk because of the their poorer renal function and reduced serum albumen (most of these preparations are highly bound to protein). Although polypharmacy is deprecated, in reality many of these patients take more than one preparation. It is logical, if this is necessary, to take preparations from different groups.

Corticosteroids

The corticosteroids were isolated in the USA from adrenal glands as a result of the rumour during the

---

Table 14.1

Classification of NSAIDs based on those available in the United Kingdom

---

Aspirin family (salicyclic acids)
  Soluble aspirin
  Effervescent aspirin
  Slow release aspirin or enteric-coated aspirin

Relatives of aspirin	Benorylate
	Salsalate
	Choline magnesium salicylate
	Diflunisal
	Aloxiprin

Indomethacin family (indole and indene acetic acids)
  Indomethacin
  Sulindac

Phenylbutazone family (enolic acids)
  Phenylbutazone
  Oxyphenbutazone
  Azapropazone
  Feprazone

Other acidic drugs

Anthranilic acids	Mefenamic acid
	Flufenamic acid
Arylpropionic acids	Ibuprofen
	Flurbiprofen
	Ketoprofen
	Naproxen
	Fenoprofen
	Indoprofen
	Carprofen
	Fenbufen
	Tiaprofenic acid
Arylacetic acids	Diclofenac
	Fenclofenac
Heteroaryl acetic acids	Tolmetin
Oxicams	Piroxicam

second world war that Luftwaffe pilots were using the drug to improve their performance. It was this meagre store of cortisone that Hench used to treat rheumatoid arthritis with such dramatic effect. Only later was it realised that the side-effects of these drugs were considerable. Almost all the organs in the body may be affected. A moon face develops, and the skin becomes thin and bruised, particularly in women. Striae appear, and a fatty pad over the upper dorsal region gives a 'buffalo hump'. Dyspepsia may occur (particularly if NSAIDs are also given), and a peptic ulcer may bleed or perforate. Osteoporosis is frequent, and crush fractures of the vertebrae also occur. Hypertension, glycosuria and psychosis may all be precipitated by these drugs. With the earlier members, such as cortisone and hydrocortisone, fluid retention, combined with sodium retention and potassium loss, were frequent. With the newer preparations, such as prednisone, prednisolone, triamcinolone and betamethasone, this is not so frequent. A proximal myopathy occurs (particularly with triamcinolone), and cataracts and glaucoma may appear after prolonged administration. Adrenal function is suppressed, and it is vital for a patient on steroids to carry a card giving the name of the preparation, the dose, and the duration of treatment, together with the name and address of the family doctor. Such a card carries instructions to the patient not to stop the drug suddenly and to report to the doctor if indigestion occurs. The additional value of the card is if the patient is involved in an accident and brought into the Casulaty Department unconscious. It also alerts the anaesthetist that supplementary steroids may be needed during surgery. Steroids reduce inflammation non-specifically, and infection (such as pneumonia or peritonitis) may be masked. Tuberculosis may be reactivated and, in a patient with any suspicion of active tuberculosis or healed lesions which could be reactivated, concomitant antituberculous therapy is given. There must be, therefore, well-defined indications for the use of systemic steroids. These are:

1. Some connective tissue disorders, e.g. polyarteritis nodosa with renal involvement. In a patient with temporal arteritis, serious damage such as blindness may be prevented.
2. Fulminating progressive rheumatoid arthritis that has not responded to other measures, including in-patient therapy.
3. Acute rheumatoid arthritis in the elderly.
4. Where socioeconomic factors demand alleviation of symptoms. Examples are the breadwinner of the family who has been off work for some time or whose job is threatened, and the busy housewife with many duties to perform.
5. Some physicians would give a small dose of steroids at night to alleviate severe morning stiffness, although this can often be achieved by a high dose of a NSAID, e.g. indomethacin 100 mg, given with a glass of milk before retiring.

Slow-acting Anti-rheumatoid Drugs

Gold has been in longest use for this purpose. It requires about six weeks to take effect and is given as an intramuscular injection of sodium aurothiomalate in a dose of 50 mg weekly to a total of 1 g. If the patient has responded, maintenance therapy is continued at monthly intervals. The inflammation is frequently brought under control, which is evidenced by a fall in ESR and other acute phase reactants. The titre of rheumatoid factor also decreases. Before each injection, the urine must be tested for albumen, and regular blood testing is necessary since thrombocytopenia and agranulocytosis occasionally develop. A rash appears quite commonly; the drug should be stopped if itching occurs, since continued administration may produce exfoliative dermatitis.

D-penicillamine is another slow-acting anti-rheumatoid drug. It is given first in a small dose of 125 mg daily, commonly increasing to 500 mg daily, and less frequently to as much as 1 g per day. The urine and blood must be checked, as with gold. If haematuria occurs, the drug must be stopped immediately because of the danger of potentially fatal Goodpasture's syndrome, in which pulmonary and renal haemorrhages occur. Hydroxychloroquine or chloroquine are less effective than gold or D-penicillamine, but they are safer in that no deaths have been reported from their use, and they do not give blood dyscrasias. However, the drug may be deposited in the cornea, producing haloes of light, an effect which is reversible on stopping the drug. An irreversible retinopathy may also develop, in which the patient experiences tunnel vision. Patients should be tested ophthalmologically before the drug is begun and 6-monthly thereafter; no more than a total of 200 g should be given. The drug is administered in a dose of chloroquine 250 mg daily or hydroxychloroquine 200 mg daily.

Sulphasalazine, a drug which was originally synthesized for the treatment of rheumatoid arthritis, and whose value has been confirmed by recent studies in Leeds and Birmingham, is a useful preparation in this category. It has fewer side-effects than gold and D-penicillamine, whilst being of comparable efficacy. It is given in a dose of 500 mg daily, increasing to 2–3 g daily by increments of 500 mg weekly. Although given as an enteric coated preparation, it may still cause dyspepsia.

No programme of treatment is complete unless the patient is given the support of a physician who is willing to spend time listening to his worries and uncertainties and explaining the aims of treatment. Indeed a direct question may reveal that this is the main need rather than a prescription for a pain-relieving drug. Increasingly, too, patients have read or heard about adverse drug effects and their misgivings must be respected when deciding to embark on any form of treatment. Once confidence has been established, it must be nourished by regular follow-up visits at predetermined intervals and not left to the patient's discretion.

ANKYLOSING SPONDYLITIS

This is a common type of polyarthritis which always involves the sacroiliac (SI) joints and usually the spine, but it is also an important cause of peripheral arthritis. It is a disease of young people, starting before puberty in 10% of cases and before the age of 40 in 70%. It affects males three times as often as females, in whom it tends to be milder. The prevalence in the UK population is about 0.1%.

Clinical Features

Figures 14.7 to 14.9 depict the pattern of joint involvement at three stages of ankylosing spondylitis (AS). Figure 14.7 shows the sites of origin of the earliest symptoms, as deduced from the history; Fig. 14.8 illustrates the average pattern when a patient first seeks

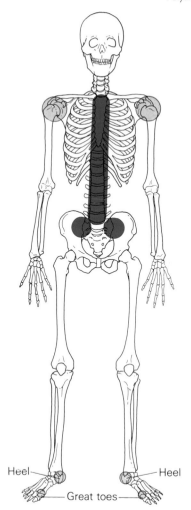

Heel — — Heel
— Great toes —

Fig. 14.7 *Ankylosing spondylitis—earliest symptoms.*

advice; and Fig. 14.9 gives the maximum involvement in progressive cases.

The onset is insidious and the earliest symptom is commonly aching pain and stiffness in the buttocks and the backs of the thighs – the classic symptom of sacroiliitis. Stiffness is particularly severe on rising in the morning but returns after any period of inactivity; patients quickly learn how to relieve it by exercise. Similar symptoms may be felt over any part of the spine and circumthoracic or manubriosternal pain may create problems in diagnosis. Lesions at ligamentous and muscular attachments to bone both around joints and elsewhere are an integral feature of the pathology of AS; these attachments are called entheses, hence

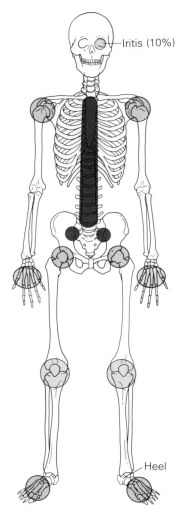

Fig. 14.8 *Ankylosing spondylitis—presenting features.*

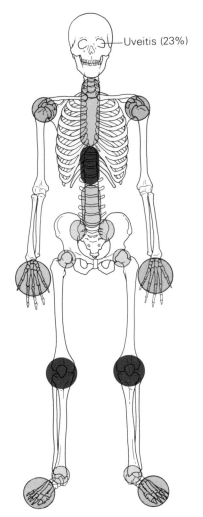

Fig. 14.9 *Ankylosing spondylitis—maximal involvement.*

'enthesopathy' designates the process. It is reflected clinically in pain and tenderness around the rim of the pelvis, over the greater trochanter, and in the heel. If the disease progresses, the lumbar curve is lost and movement of the lumbar spine becomes limited. This is detected by placing the thumb and middle finger over the upper and lower ends of the lumbar segment, asking the patient to bend down and observing how much the exploring fingers are distracted. Lateral movement is most easily assessed by marking the tips of the spinous processes with ink. Loss of extension also occurs early, and reduction of chest expansion is a useful sign, provided that account is taken of differences between men and women and the effects of

ageing or unrelated chest disease. Pain can often be elicited by stressing the SI joints. In advanced cases the entire spine may be rigid, and a characteristic posture is apparent: head craned forwards, a stoop from dorsal kyphosis, flat lumbar spine, hips flexed and knees bent to move the centre of gravity backwards. A severe dorsal kyphosis and a rigid neck restrict forward vision. AS sometimes affects peripheral joints before the SI joints, particularly in children, making diagnosis difficult. Joints most often involved are the knees, hips and shoulders and these are also frequently affected in more advanced cases. Early involvement of these joints is also a feature of many conditions yet to be discussed, but is unusual in RA.

Aetiology

There is ample evidence for genetic predisposition in a high familial aggregation of AS together with the fact that nearly all patients possess the HLA antigen B27. Presumably there is also an environmental factor but none has as yet been conclusively identified.

Associated Conditions

Sacroiliitis or the full picture of AS, indistinguishable from the idiopathic form, occurs more often than would be expected of a chance association with psoriasis, Reiter's syndrome, ulcerative colitis, Crohn's disease and possibly Whipple's disease. AS may antedate bowel symptoms in the last three by several years. An association with HLA B27 has been found in all these conditions except Whipple's disease, for which there are insufficient data. Each of these conditions may also be accompanied by a type of peripheral arthritis distinct from AS, not associated with B27, and known as enteropathic arthritis (see below).

Laboratory Tests and Radiographs

There is no specific test for AS, but a number of tests may be needed to exclude alternative diagnoses. The ESR is raised in the early stages but this is not a reliable guide to activity. Tests for rheumatoid factor are no more often positive than in the general population. Tissue-typing is indicated only in special circumstances. As 6–8% of the white population of the UK belong to the B27 type, a positive result may be misleading when the clinical evidence for AS is only equivocal.

Radiography plays a more important role in early diagnosis of AS than in RA, and often confirms a clinical suspicion of sacroiliitis. The earliest abnormality seen in the SI joints is poor definition at the lower margins, sometimes with apparent widening. Later, marginal erosions make the articular surfaces irregular and ragged, with a zone of sclerosis outside them, especially on the iliac side. Finally the joints may disappear, leaving only a thin line of sclerosis. The SI joints in adolescence are normally wide and irregular, however. In the spine, fine bony bridges (syndesmophytes) between vertebral bodies are often seen first at the dorsolumbar junction. In very advanced cases, the bridges extend over the whole length of the spine, producing the 'bamboo' picture. Feathery formation on new bone, which is the radiographic expression of enthesopathy, may be seen around the rim of the pelvis and on the greater trochanter. The appearances in peripheral joints are much as in RA but with less erosion and more frequent ankylosis.

Radiographs taken primarily to investigate bowel disorders yield good views of the SI joints and lumbar spine and may be informative.

Diagnosis

Symptoms often antedate abnormal signs by a considerable period; on average, the diagnosis is not made until three years have elapsed in men and ten in women since the first symptom. Early diagnosis rests heavily on the correct interpretation of early symptoms, but a family history of AS is very helpful. Radiography of the SI joints is the most important investigation. Many alternative causes of back pain must be considered, notably disc lesions. The most common misdiagnosis is sciatica, but this is rarely bilateral and, though pain in AS may be aggravated by coughing, there are no root signs. Restriction of lateral movement in the lumbar spine favours AS rather than a disc lesion. Sclerosis of the SI joints occurs in paraplegia and also in polymyalgia, but this involves an older age group. RA rarely affects the SI joints or the spine below the neck, whereas AS may extend upwards to affect the entire spine. Tuberculosis of the SI joints is usually unilateral. Hyperparathyroidism and fluorosis affect the spine but spare the SI joints. Brucellosis mimics some of the features of AS. The coarse osteophytes of spinal osteoarthrosis and the lesions of ankylosing vertebral hyperostosis differ from the fine syndesmophytes of AS.

The problem of diagnosis when peripheral joints are affected first has already been mentioned. Finally, it should be remembered that iritis may be the earliest sign of AS.

Complications

These include iritis, aortic incompetence, heart block, apical infiltration of the lungs, atlanto-axial subluxation, secondary amyloidosis, and fracture by minor trauma of a rigid and brittle cervical spine.

Treatment

The two main objectives are to minimise disability from flexed spine and hips and to alleviate pain and stiffness. The patient should spend part of each day lying prone and should sleep on a firm mattress with a low pillow. He should be instructed in back extension and breathing exercises. A fixed spine is less disabling than might be expected provided that an upright posture is preserved and that the hips retain some movement and do not become fixed in flexion. Drugs relieve symptoms and make exercises and postural precautions easier. Phenylbutazone, indomethacin and some other NSAIDs, such as naproxen, are effective. Where there is accompanying bowel disease, however, drugs most liable to cause gastrointestinal bleeding (e.g. phenylbutazone, indomethacin) or diarrhoea (e.g. fenamates) are best avoided. Intra-articular injections of a corticosteroid may be effective for peripheral joint synovitis, and oral corticosteroids are reserved for severe cases of iritis.

Surgical treatment may be required to replace severely-damaged hips; the results are generally as good as in RA, though ectopic bone is sometimes laid down around the joint. Spinal osteotomy has been used to correct crippling kyphosis, but this calls for exceptional expertise.

Some 85% of patients with AS are able to remain in gainful employment.

ENTEROPATHIC ARTHRITIS

This embraces the peripheral arthritis which sometimes complicates ulcerative colitis and Crohn's disease, but is not associated with sacroiliitis nor with HLA B27. It occurs at any time in the course of the bowel disease and may be accompanied by erythema nodosum. It rarely persists for more than one year, leaves no permanent damage in the joints, and is seronegative. It is more often monarticular than polyarticular, and picks out the joints shown in Fig. 14.10.

The joint symptoms of Whipple's disease have a

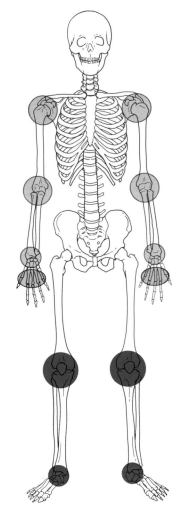

Fig. 14.10 *Enteropathic arthritis.*

rather different pattern, sometimes including short acute attacks which may antedate other features by many years; the only way to make the diagnosis at this stage is jejunal biopsy.

REACTIVE ARTHRITIS

This differs from enteropathic arthritis in that it complicates an acute bowel infection with an organism which can be isolated and identified, and in having a strong link with HLA B27. The infecting organisms include *Salmonella*, *Yersinia* and *Campylobacter*. The arthritis is usually self-limiting, but some patients develop sacroiliitis and it is not entirely clear whether reactive arthritis should rank as an entity distinct from Reiter's syndrome. Reactive arthritis associated with salmonella infection must be distinguished from septic arthritis in which the organism penetrates the joints.

REITER'S SYNDROME

This is a recurrent, non-suppurative polyarthritis which starts one to three weeks after an attack, often a mild one, of nonspecific urethritis (NSU) or dysentery. The pattern of joint involvement and other features are shown in Fig. 14.11. Fever is common in the early stages,

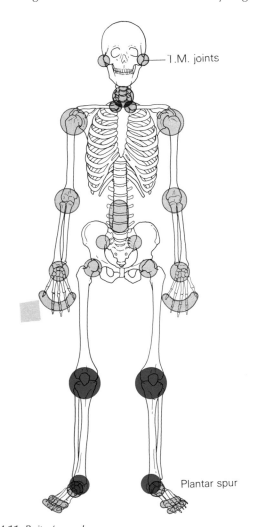

Fig. 14.11 *Reiter's syndrome.*

and the ESR is often very high. There may be urethritis in the dysenteric form and diarrhoea in the NSU variety. In many cases the joints escape permanent damage, though recurrences of synovitis are frequent, often after years of freedom from trouble; in other cases, deformities develop in the feet and occasionally in the fingers. Sacroiliitis is common and some patients develop the full picture of AS. Tests for rheumatoid factor are negative and radiographic changes are confined to progressive cases in which there may be signs of sacroiliitis, the spinal changes of AS, and erosions and loss of joint space at the periphery, notably in the metatarso-phalangeal joints. Other radiographic features are large, fluffy plantar spurs and periostitis along the small bones of the feet. Conjunctivitis is often so mild as to escape notice. There is a strong correlation with HLA B27, especially if there is sacroiliitis. Pustular psoriasis and the keratoderma blenorrhagica of Reiter's syndrome may be impossible to differentiate.

NSU is usually treated with a tetracycline but it is doubtful whether this has any effect once arthritis has started. The symptoms of arthritis are relieved by drugs (see p. 198). Wasting of muscles is apt to progress quickly and calls for resisted active exercises.

BEHÇET'S SYNDROME

The original triad of oral and genital ulceration with relapsing iritis has, over the years, been expanded to include skin lesions (notably erythema nodosum and pyoderma), other lesions of the eyes, involvement of the CNS, thrombophlebitis migrans and arthropathy. The last occurs in some 60% of cases and usually takes the form of intermittent effusions in the knees, ankles, elbows or wrists. Arthropathy may be persistent but is not destructive, though involvement of the SI joints has been reported.

ARTHRITIS AND PSORIASIS

Several patterns of arthritis are seen in patients with psoriasis, of which two are distinctive. The first of these predominately affects the terminal joints of fingers and toes, often with psoriatic lesions of the adjacent nail. It is more unsightly than disabling. The second is widespread and disabling with much more destruction and deformity than is usual in RA and has a greater tendency to ankylosis. In the early stages cylindrical swelling or dactylitis may be seen in one or two digits, often with dusky red discolouration of the skin. Both of these types are seronegative.

Apart from these two varieties with features specific for the association with psoriasis, there are at least two more patterns which are less distinctive. The first is indistinguishable from AS as seen in patients who do not have psoriasis and is one of the intriguing group of overlapping syndromes, some of which have been noted above, which cluster round the central pivot of the HLA B27 tissue type. The second resembles uncomplicated RA; some patients are seropositive, may have nodules, and are probably victims of two common diseases occurring quite fortuitously in the same individual. The relationship between skin and joint disease is less clear in seronegative cases. In yet another pattern, less well-established as a separate entity, only a single joint, or a small number, may be affected.

The diagnosis is easily missed if a careful search is not made for psoriasis lurking under the scalp hair, in folds of skin or limited small lesions in or around the umbilicus. Psoriatic lesions of the nails may help, being more common in the presence of arthritis than in uncomplicated psoriasis. The diagnosis may be delayed if arthritis precedes the first lesions of psoriasis. The terminal digital variety has to be distinguished from Heberden's nodes (see p. 182). Acute episodes of monarticular arthritis resembling gout occur in some patients with arthritis and psoriasis, but the serum uric acid is usually normal.

The arthritis usually responds to treatment with NSAIDs. Steroids are seldom used since they may destabilise the skin condition. Gold injections (sodium aurothiomalate) may be used as in the treatment of RA if a second-line drug is required, although their value is not proved. Skin rashes are no more common as a complication of crysotherapy than in RA, but chloroquine or hydroxychloroquine are avoided because in a few patients they promote exfoliation. Immunosuppressive agents (e.g. Methotrexate, azathioprine) are used in resistant cases. The skin lesions are treated separately and on their own merits. Successful treatment of skin lesions does not influence the course of the arthritis.

JUVENILE CHRONIC POLYARTHRITIS

This is a useful term encompassing a variety of clinical patterns, 'juvenile RA' being best reserved for just one of these. Children are not immune from types of polyarthritis which occur in adults, but one clinical pattern, Still's disease, is almost entirely confined to children. It is seronegative and seen most often in young children, when it is equally common in boys and girls; in older children it becomes more frequent in girls. Three modes of onset can be distinguished: systemic, polyarticular and pauciarticular. The systemic type is characterised by high swinging fever, rash, enlargement of lymph nodes and spleen and polymorph leucocytosis. The rash, small morbilliform macules, is often evanescent and seen only with the evening peak of fever. Polyarthritis, which may not be present at first, later causes permanent joint damage, often including fusion of upper cervical vertebrae and severe disruption of the hip. General or local retardation of growth is common and micrognathia and disproportionate shortening of some digits are characteristic. The pauciarticular pattern, affecting four joints or less, has its own distinctive features: usually seen in young children, especially girls, it affects particularly the ankles, knees and elbows. There is a high incidence of antinuclear activity in the serum but no antibody to native DNA such as is found in SLE. Growth changes, both retardation and acceleration, may be seen in affected joints. The most important complication of this pauciarticular variety of Still's disease is a chronic, insidious iridocyclitis which carries a threat to vision. The end result in bad cases is a band of opacity running right across the cornea. As there may be no symptoms, this is easily missed and it is wise to arrange for skilled ophthalmic examination of every child with pauciarticular arthritis every three months.

Seropositive RA may start as early as five years of age but is more common after 10. It is usually polyarticular from the start, and is persistent and liable to damage joints severely. Twenty per cent of patients have nodules.

The pattern of AS in children is different from that in

adults. It is the only variety of juvenile chronic polyarthritis (JCP) with a predilection for boys and usually starts between the ages of 3 and 15 as a monarthritis in a hip, knee or ankle. Several years may elapse before sacroiliitis or limitation of back movement reveal the diagnosis and during this period the best evidence may come from a family history of AS or possession of the B27 tissue type. As in adults, the characteristic ophthalmic complication is an acute iridocyclitis; this is clinically overt in contrast to the insidious eye lesion of pauciarticular Still's disease. Again, as in adults, AS in children may be associated with disorders of the gut.

Arthritis associated with psoriasis is not common in children. It tends to start at the age of 10 or thereabouts and to continue into adult life more often than other types of seronegative JCP. If arthritis precedes psoriasis, early clues to diagnosis may be given by pitted nails or a family history.

Amyloidosis is a potentially fatal complication of all types of JCP except for persistently seronegative monarthritis. It is most frequent in the seropositive RA group but is common in systemic Still's disease.

Many conditions have to be considered in the differential diagnosis of JCP, including some more acute polyarthritides. Before it declined in frequency, rheumatic fever was the classical cause of 'flitting' polyarthritis, in which inflammation in one joint begins to settle as it starts in another. Nowadays the commonest causes are leukaemia and Henoch–Schoenlein purpura – in which there may be no purpuric element. Rheumatic fever was never common below the age of four. Postdysenteric arthritis is encountered in children, and other diagnoses to be considered include SLE, hypogammaglobulinaemia, Clutton's joints (in congenital syphilis), osteomyelitis, and osteochondritides.

The management of JCP cannot be reviewed in detail here but some reactions to treatment which are peculiar to childhood are worth mentioning. Immobilisation of an inflamed joint is much more likely to produce rapid loss of movement than it is in an adult; daily administration of a corticosteroid is liable to stunt growth and alternate-day treatment may be preferable; salicylates are effective, but it is wise to check blood levels as tinnitus is less reliable as a warning of high levels than in older patients. The logical approach to the treatment of amyloidosis is to control the arthritis; this may not be easy, though cytotoxic drugs have shown some promise.

MISCELLANEOUS ACUTE POLYARTHRITIDES

Rheumatic Fever

Once a major scourge in children and young adults, this is now a rare disease except in very poor communities. The cardinal features are fever, flitting arthritis and carditis, but there may be no fever, and only minimal synovitis, yet severe damage to the heart. Other manifestation include chorea, small subcutaneous nodules, and erythema marginatum, which are temporary symptoms of importance only in diagnosis. Fever is sustained, in contrast to the swings of systemic Still's disease, though both will respond to a salicylate. Pharyngeal infection with β-haemolytic streptococci precedes the fever by about 19 days (between 7 and 37 days). An immune response is induced by the streptoccus, which shows a higher antibody level in patients who go on to develop rheumatic fever. Recurrences after a first attack, and the risk of further damage to the heart, can be minimised by prophylactic doses of a sulphonamide or penicillin.

Erythema Nodosum

Some 75% of cases develop arthritis; the distribution and some of the associated diseases are shown in Fig. 14.12. The arthritis is self-limiting and not destructive, usually settling in less than six months. Sarcoid produces an entirely different type of arthritis with infiltration of the synovium. It may also infiltrate the bone.

Arthritis in Viral Infections

The features of rubella arthritis are shown in Fig. 14.13, from which it will be seen that the joints involved are much as in RA. It usually starts a few days after the rash, but may precede it, and lasts 2–28 days. Compression of the median nerve in the carpal tunnel is frequent. Arthritis also occurs after rubella inoculation.

Arthritis also occurs in mumps, in infective hepatitis, and probably in other viral infections.

Other Arthritides

A migratory polyarthritis occurs in type 2 hyperlipoproteinaemia and should be suspected in the presence of xanthomata and premature arcus senilis. Joint pain and morning stiffness and possibly a mild but persistent synovitis may be associated with the type 4 variety.

Other causes of synovitis include familial Mediterranean fever, sickle-cell disease and the Stevens–Johnson syndrome.

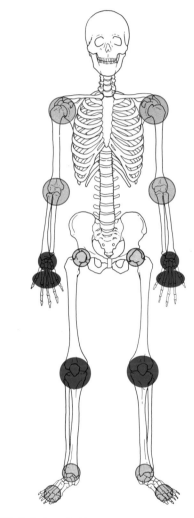

Fig. 14.13 *Rubella arthritis.*

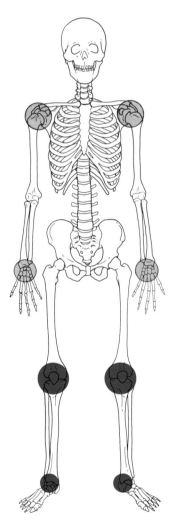

Fig. 14.12 *Erythema nodosum.*

15

Diffuse Disorders of Connective Tissue

AETIO-PATHOGENESIS OF CONNECTIVE TISSUE DISEASES

Classification and Concepts

Genetically determined diseases of connective tissue have a primary abnormality of the components of connective tissue, e.g. collagen or proteoglycans, which leads to manifestations of disease. This group of disorders includes such conditions as Marfan's syndrome, Ehlers–Danlos syndrome, pseudoxanthoma elasticum and the mucopolysaccharidoses. These rare diseases are not considered further in this chapter, which deals mainly with *acquired conditions* in which inflammatory reactions in connective tissue in and around blood vessels are observed and are associated with prominent immunological phenomena.

The original term, 'diffuse collagen disease', arose from the finding of prominent hyaline deposits in tissues termed 'fibrinoid'. This material shows affinity for the same dyes as fibrin and was assumed to be altered collagen. It was subsequently shown that fibrinoid included immune complex material and necrotic tissue. In these diseases, disorganisation, particularly necrosis, of connective tissue is frequent, and is due to the combined effects of vascular insufficiency and extracellular enzymatic digestion. In view of the prominent involvement of blood vessels some use the term 'collagen–vascular diseases' as a more appropriate description. However, both the vessels and connective tissues simply act as passive structures which are the site of immunopathological processes. The alternative term, 'multisystem autoimmune disorders' has also been used.

Diagnostic criteria

Since the diffuse disorders of connective tissue are of unknown aetiology, their division into disease entities is based on the recognition of distinct clinico-pathological patterns. The diagnosis resides in the conjunction of more than one feature of high sensitivity and specificity. A feature of high sensitivity is frequently positive in patients with the disease and therefore has a low proportion of false-negatives. High specificity means that the feature is disease-specific and absent in populations without the disease. Such a feature is therefore associated with a low proportion of false-positives. In general, highly specific individual features tend to have low sensitivity and therefore occur only in a proportion of patients. This may lead to some features being regarded as more significant than others (major criteria), in contrast to less specific but more sensitive criteria (minor criteria).

The American Rheumatism Association (ARA) has been particularly active in defining criteria and those for SLE are shown in Table 15.1. It has been suggested that

---

Table 15.1

ARA Preliminary Criteria for SLE*

Non-deforming arthritis	Photosensitivity
Butterfly rash	Alopecia
Discoid lupus	Haemolytic anaemia/leukopenia/ thrombocytopenia
Pleurisy/pericarditis	LE cells (+ve ANA)
Raynaud's phenomena	False positive tests for syphilis
Oral/nasal ulcers	Proteinuria > 3.5 g/day
	Cellular casts

* 4 or more criteria—at least four features required.

Table 15.2

Laboratory Tests for Autoimmunity in Diffuse Disorders of Connective Tissue

Autoantibody/test system	Antigen	Usual methods of detection	Clinical significance/General remarks
I. Rheumatoid Factors (RF)	Fc portion of heavy chain of IgG		
(a) IgM class	Rabbit IgG	Sheep cell agglutination (SCAT, DAT and RAHA) Latex agglutination	Raised titres (SCAT or DAT > 1:32 in 'seropositive' RA). Increased positivity, especially of latex tests in elderly, transiently in SBE and viral infections (e.g. infectious mononucleosis), leprosy, kala-azar, sarcoidosis, cirrhosis of the liver, Sjögren's syndrome, SLE, fibrosing alveolitis, industrial diseases of the lung, etc.
(b) IgA class		Solid phase immuno-radiometric (SPIRA) or enzyme-linked (ELIZA)	Ubiquitous in low titres; high levels in IgM-positive RA, especially in patients with complicating vasculitis.
II. Antinuclear Antibodies (ANA)	Nuclear antigens		
(a) LE cell test	DNA histone	Defibrinate blood and make and stain smear	LE cell is a polymorph with a phagocytosed basophilic intracytoplasmic inclusion. This consists of nuclear-antigen–antibody complexes formed by interaction of nuclear debris and serum ANA
(b) Immunofluorescent (IF) patterns			
(i) Homogeneous	DNA histone DNA and others	Indirect immunofluorescence using rat liver cryostat or single cell suspensions	> 1:10 (usually > 1:1000) titre in SLE. Also occurs in RA (40%), juvenile RA, drug-induced lupus, Sjögren's syndrome, immune liver and lung diseases and less commonly in some infections, normal relatives of SLE patients and laboratory workers. SLE, overlap syndromes (e.g. MCTD) polymyositis, scleroderma, Sjögren's syndrome.
(ii) Speckled	Ribonuclear protein (RNP) and Sm		
(iii) Nucleolar	7S nuclear RNA		Scleroderma, other CTD.
(iv) Peripheral (Rim)	DNA		Rare pattern, usually SLE.
(v) Centromere	Chromosomes	Dividing cells	CREST (scleroderma) syndrome
(c) Defined antigens			
(i) DNA	Polynucleotides and 'back-bone' (? several antigens)	Farr Assay (IF) antibody binding to kinetoplast of crithidia luciliae	High levels in active SLE (approx. 60% of patients), low levels in most SLE. Less common in: RA, polymyositis, Sjögren's syndrome, chronic active hepatitis and 'overlap' syndromes
(ii) RNP	RNase and trypsin sensitive antigen in soluble extracts of nuclear antigens (ENA)	Haemagglutination, counter immunoelectrophoresis, immunodiffusion	SLE, polymyositis and scleroderma especially in patients with overlap features (MCTD). Raynaud's syndrome a common feature
(iii) Sm	RNase resistant, trypsin sensitive	Haemagglutination, counter immunoelectrophoresis, immunodiffusion	Specific for SLE but only occurs in 25–40% of patients
(iv) SS-A (Ro)	Antigen in soluble extracts of spleen and nuclei of EBV-transformed cells	Precipitins	SLE (40%); 'rare' ANA-negative SLE, keratoconjunctivitis usual feature
(v) SS-B (La)	Antigen in soluble extracts of thymus and EBV cells	Precipitins	Primary sicca complex, Sjögren's syndrome, SLE
III. Smooth muscle	Actin, other cyto-skeletal filaments	IF, stomach and rat kidney	SLE, chronic hepatitis, RA
IV. Skeletal muscle			
(a) Myosin	Various	IF, haemagglutination	Common in polymyositis but with poor diagnostic specificity
(b) Motor endplate	Acetylcholine receptor	IF, radioinhibition assay	Myasthenia gravis – spontaneous and induced by penicillamine

the diagnosis can be considered 'definite' when four or more criteria are present in the individual patient. Individual features seen in different disorders of connective tissue are often common to many and are not in themselves diagnostic.

Autoimmunity

Autoimmunity is the expression of specific immunological reactivity against 'self' antigens.

Laboratory tests for autoimmunity

A large number of immunological techniques have been employed to demonstrate autoantibodies in the blood of patients with connective tissue disease. The autoantibodies that are found are directed against antigens that are ubiquitous in many tissues (i.e. non-organ specific). These include antibodies directed against antigenic determinants on IgG (rheumatoid factors), nuclei (antinuclear antibodies), smooth muscle and skeletal muscle (see Table 15.2).

Cellular basis of autoimmunity

Tolerance. The immune system possesses the unique quality of being able to distinguish between 'self' and 'non-self'. The basis of the lack of reaction against self antigens ('tolerance') is poorly understood at present and a variety of mechanisms are thought to be involved.

Autoimmunity: According to current theories, autoimmunity may result from one of the following mechanisms:

1. Emergence of 'forbidden clones' in a person in whom self-reactive clones have been previously deleted.
2. It is suggested that the immune system is continually exposed to certain autoantigens and this leads to a situation in which T cells are tolerised (e.g. by deletion) but B cells remain undisturbed. If such a split-tolerant state were to exist, the B cells would remain dormant since the participation of T cell 'help' is obligatory for the synthesis of antibody. Under certain circumstances, however, the toler-

ance mechanism dependent on T cells is bypassed as shown in Figs 15.1 and 15.2.

3. Autoimmunity may also result from the breakdown in the regulation of normal cellular mechanisms. The mechanism of production of autoreactive anti-lymphocyte antibodies is unknown, but is a feature of certain virus infections.
4. Finally, the production of autoantibody requires exposure of the B cell to autoantigens. Possible

1. *In health*

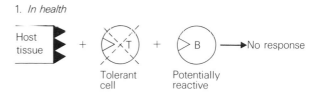

2. *Following exposure to cross-reacting extrinsic antigen*

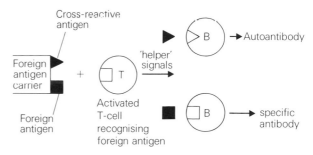

Fig. 15.1.

candidates for autoimmune diseases or reactions occurring in this manner include autoimmunity observed to cardiac antigens following infarction or surgery and autoimmunity diverted against the lens of an eye, testicular tissues and brain tissue.

Pathogenetic Mechanisms and Tissue Injury

Experimental investigations have revealed a number of ways in which immunological mechanisms mediate tissue damage and many of these mechanisms are now thought to be involved in the production of autoimmune diseases. These include the following:

Immune complex mediated tissue damage

By analogy with experimental studies of serum sickness and the Arthus reaction (Type III reaction), it has been

1. *In health (T suppression exceeds help)*

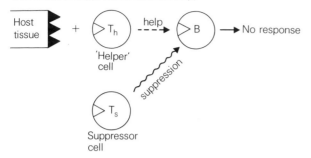

2. *In autoimmunity (T help exceeds suppression)*

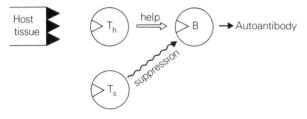

3. *In autoimmunity polyclonal B cell activation may occur and be independent of T help*

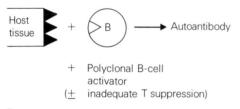

Fig. 15.2.

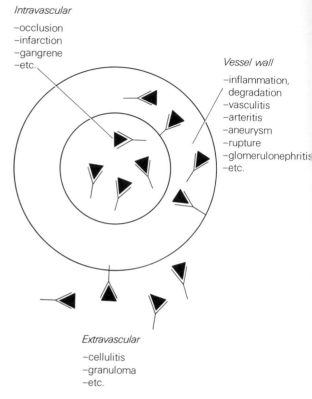

Fig. 15.3.

suggested that the localisation of circulating immune complexes in and around the vessel wall is an important event leading to damage in diffuse disorders of connective tissue. The sequence of events is shown in Fig. 15.3.

Circulating immune complexes have been demonstrated in patients with connective tissue diseases such as SLE and RA with extra-articular disease manifestations. Vasculitis of various types is believed to be associated with circulating immune complexes, although the possibility has been raised that in some of these syndromes immune complexes are formed locally in the vessel wall by sequential trapping of antigen followed by antibody.

Antibody mediated cytotoxicity

Cytotoxic damage mediated by antibody and comple-

ment (Type II reaction) is thought to be involved in the depletion of circulating haematopoietic cells, which is a feature of some connective tissue diseases. This mechanism may account for haemolytic anaemia (with a positive Coombs' test), leukopenia (associated with anti-polymorphonuclear and anti-lymphocyte antibodies) and thrombocytopenia (associated with anti-platelet antibodies).

Anaphylaxis

Autoantibodies belonging to IgE class can be demonstrated in SLE and RA patients. Although their functional role in tissue damage is not fully understood, they may be important in initiating the localisation and pathogenic effects of immune complexes by virtue of their binding to basophils and platelets, which are reservoirs of vasoactive amines. They may also be involved in pathogenic effects in the respiratory tract.

Lymphocyte mediated mechanisms

Under certain conditions, specifically sensitised lymphocytes against the host cell tissue may be shown to produce damage.

Aetiology

The aetiology of diffuse disorders of connective tissue is obscure. As shown in Fig. 15.4, three main factors are involved.

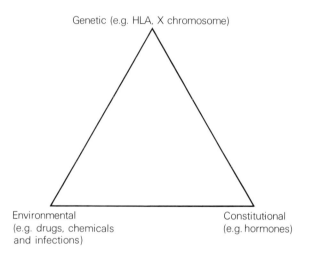

Genetic (e.g. HLA, X chromosome)

Environmental
(e.g. drugs, chemicals
and infections)

Constitutional
(e.g. hormones)

Fig. 15.4.

Genetic factors

These have been established by epidemiological studies which show an increased prevalence of disease in first degree relatives compared with controls.

Environmental factors

A lack of better concordance of disease in identical twins, or genetically similar siblings, and increased incidence of autoimmunity in genetically dissimilar individuals in the same environment has provided evidence for the involvement of environmental factors in some connective tissue disease. A number of factors are suspected or known to be involved and include drugs, e.g. procainamide, hydralazine and penicillamine, in the production of lupus-like syndromes,

chemicals and dusts such as silica in fibrotic disorders, and penicillamine and sulphonamides in vasculitis. Exposure to viruses and ultraviolet light have been implicated in the production of SLE.

Constitutional factors

Constitutional factors are also involved, and the most important may be hormonal. There is a marked female sex predominance in the connective tissue diseases and it is suggested that this partly due to the effect of hormones on the immune response. Male hormones can be shown to encourage the normal maturation of immune cells and the ability of lymphocytes to produce IgG class antibodies whereas oestrogens delay this process and may favour immune-dysregulation.

SYSTEMIC LUPUS ERYTHEMATOSUS

SLE is a chronic inflammatory disease with multi-system involvement. Characteristic features include arthritis, cutaneous manifestations, vasculitis, glomerulonephritis, haematological abnormalities, pleurisy, pericarditis and central nervous system disease. Almost all patients show the presence of antinuclear antibodies and the LE cell test is positive.

Epidemiology

It is estimated that the incidence of the disease in the United Kingdom is 1–2/100 000 per year and the prevalance is 6–8/100 000. Substantially higher figures are reported in some studies in the USA, where regional differences have also been noted. Over the past few decades an increased incidence of the disease has been reported. Such figures should be interpreted with caution, since increased awareness of the disease, and wider availability of laboratory tests for antinuclear antibodies, may have contributed to these differences. The increased prevalence may also be related to the increased survival of patients with this disorder. Survival is currently estimated to be about 90% over 10 years. The disease is four times as common in women as men, and marked ethnic variations in populations resident in the same area have been reported. The interaction between ethnic and geographical factors is demonstrated by the observation of a very high incidence of SLE amongst blacks in the Carribean when compared with a low incidence amongst West Africans with the same genetic background.

Aetiology

The aetiology of SLE is unknown but is believed to be multifactorial. There is an increased incidence of SLE in identical twins and other features of autoimmunity, especially the presence of autoantibodies, are found in families of patients with SLE. In some studies certain HLA markers are reported to occur more frequently, especially in sub-sets of SLE characterised by shared clinical and antinuclear antibodies, e.g. HLA B8-DW3 in patients with prominent cutaneous lesions and membranous nephropathy. The importance of genetic and environmental factors is best demonstrated in drug-induced SLE, such as that provoked by hydralazine. Exacerbation of SLE symptoms following exposure to UV light, intercurrent infections, and following parturition is well recognised. It has been considered that the common denominator in these situations may be tissue injury leading to release of nuclear antigens.

Infective agents have been implicated in the initiation of SLE, but data are inconclusive.

Other environmental aetiological factors include diet. Recent work with SLE in New Zealand mice has suggested a protective role for polyunsaturated fats.

The increased incidence of SLE in females of child-bearing age, and exacerbation during pregnancy, has suggested that hormonal factors may be of importance.

Pathogenesis

Many of the tissue lesions in SLE are believed to be mediated by immune complexes. In the kidney, spleen and skin, antinuclear antibodies (especially DNA antibodies) complexed with their antigens have been demonstrated. One of the unexplained paradoxes is the widespread presence of immune complexes in apparently non-lesional tissues, e.g. skin and choroid plexus. It is suggested that this may be related to heterogeneity of immune complexes in these patients,

some being non-pathogenic. The pathogenicity may, in part, be related to their ability to fix complement and thereby mediate hypersensitivity reactions. The haematological features of SLE may be related to the cytotoxic effects of complement-fixing autoantibodies.

Widespread defects of lymphocyte and mononuclear phagocytic function have been reported in SLE.

Pathology

Bone and joint changes

The synovitis of SLE is characterised by hyperaemia and infiltration by lymphocytes. Exudation of fibrin on the surface of the membrane is also observed. Unlike rheumatoid arthritis, increased cellularity of the lining layer and plasma cell infiltration are not usual. However, the synovial membrane changes may be indistinguishable from those seen in rheumatoid arthritis. Pannus formation is uncommon and erosion of bone and cartilage are rare. If synovitis occurs, it resembles Jaccoud's arthropathy of rheumatic fever. Damage to the capsule of joints occurs, as well as tenosynovitis. Osteonecrosis (avascular necrosis) is seen in some patients and typically involves the head of the femur and humerus. It has been suggested that steroid treatment or vasculitis may be responsible for this complication.

Skin changes

These are characterised by hyperkeratosis, follicular plugging, necrosis of the basophil layer and hypertrophy or atrophy of the prickle cell layer. Perivascular and subdermal infiltration by lymphocytes is prominent. In patients with cutaneous vasculitis, necrotising vasculitis involving small blood vessels may be seen. In some patients, fat necrosis (panniculitis) is prominent. By immunofluorescent microscopy, immunoglobulin, complement factor C3, components of the classical (C1a, C4, C2) and alternative pathway (factors B and D) have been demonstrated in 'granular' deposits at the dermo–epidermal junction. These changes have been observed not only in biopsies of 'lesional' skin but also in clinically normal skin. In up to a third of skin biopsies immunoglobulin appears to be fixed to the epidermal cell nuclei.

Kidney involvement

Clinical and pathological changes in the kidney are observed in up to 50% of patients with SLE. It has been claimed that up to 100% of patients show the presence of immune complexes in the glomerular tufts when tissue sections are examined by immunofluorescence or electron microscopy. At the light microscope level, three main types of lesions are recognised:

   i. Focal glomerulonephritis;
   ii. Diffuse glomerulonephritis;
   iii. Membranous nephropathy.

Blood vessels

Necrotising vasculitis involving medium and small-sized arteries is observed in some patients. In others there is a prominent perivascular inflammation. Vascular occlusion may be observed.

Other organs

Lymph nodes may show necrosis and appear acellular. There is marked reticular hyperplasia. The spleen may be enlarged and a characteristic finding is the 'onion skin' lesion, consisting of concentric perivascular fibrosis involving medium-sized arteries. Central nervous system changes include vasculitis and localised brain infarcts. Pericardial abnormalities are reported in the majority of cases of SLE, characterised by chronic inflammatory cell infiltration, fibrinoid degeneration, and laying down of the fibrin. Similar changes are described in the pleura. Myocardial involvement is less common but an increasing number of patients with SLE appear to show coronary arterial occlusive disease. Small vegetations on the mitral valve were originally described by Libman and Sacks but this form of endocarditis is rare. Some patients with SLE show characteristic changes of polymyositis.

Clinical Features

SLE may present in a variety of ways and, in early stages, patients may pose a diagnostic conundrum. The diagnostic criteria for SLE according to the ARA are shown in Table 15.1. To diagnose definite SLE requires the fulfilment of four or more of the features. The clinical patterns predominantly fall into two groups: firstly, patients with prominent renal disease and, secondly, 'non-renal' SLE. Although patients show multi-system features, involvement of one or two organs (or systems) may be prominent. The disease is characterised by exacerbations and remissions, and periods of disease activity in one patient may not always follow a similar pattern. Thus, in an individual patient, joint involvement may be common during one episode whereas renal disease may be the main feature on a subsequent occasion. The following clinical features are noteworthy:

General: Fatigue, weight-loss and fever are prominent. Fever may be intermittent and give rise to the suspicion of a systemic infection. Infections may coexist with active SLE and can be extremely difficult to diagnose and distinguish from the underlying disease. However, it is vital to exclude the possibility of infection, which may be fatal since patients with SLE are immunosuppressed either as a part of their disease process or as a consequence of drug therapy.

Musculoskeletal symptoms: Polyarthritis, often of a transient nature, is common. In some patients tenosynovitis is seen. In many patients, painful joints are not associated with clinical signs of arthritis although pain and disability are severe. Muscle weakness, especially of the proximal muscle groups, due to a myopathy or polymyositis, may be seen. Severe pain in joints with loss of function may result from osteonecrosis.

Cutaneous involvement: The typical erythematous scaly eruption on the face in a butterfly distribution is seen in the majority of patients with active SLE. This appearance is characteristic and the term 'lupus' (Latin, wolf) is due to a resemblance to the facial markings on a wolf. More widespread cutaneous lesions, such as erythematous macules and papules, occur. Other patients show urticaria, purpura, cutaneous infarcts and ulcers. Livido reticularis is seen in many patients with active disease. Photosensitivity of exposed areas of the skin is a prominent feature, and alopecia is frequent.

Vascular changes: Vascular changes, characterised by Raynaud's phenomenon, periungual erythema, telangiectasia and gangrene of the extremities, may be seen.

Pleurisy and/or pericarditis are frequent. Pericardial constriction has been described. Patchy (non-infective) pneumonia, lung infarcts and diffuse interstitial pneumonitis (fibrosing alveolitis) with 'shrinking lungs' occur.

Renal disease: Clinically this is characterised either by asymptomatic proteinuria, by nephrotic syndrome or by chronic renal failure. Red-cell and hyaline casts in the urine and microhaematuria are a feature of active renal disease. The progress of the disease is characterised by intermittent variation in renal function, with a tendency to steady deterioration. There is a marked difference in progression depending on renal histology.

Haemotological abnormalities: Anaemia is common in active disease, and is usually normocytic and normochromic. However, in some patients autoimmune haemolytic anaemia is present. Many patients with active SLE show leukopenia due to diminution in all types of leucocytes, with lymphopenia being particularly prominent. Thrombocytopenia associated with anti-platelet antibodies is frequent in active disease.

Central nervous system disease: Seizures, focal cerebral cortical lesions, cervical myelopathy, cranial nerve lesions, aseptic meningitis, psychiatric syndromes (especially depression, mania and confusional states) occur in patients with SLE with great frequency. Up to two-thirds of patients may manifest such changes at some stage of their disease.

Other clinical features include hypertension, cardiac failure and eye manifestations, e.g. haemorrhages and exudates (cytoid bodies) in the retina and xerophthalmia as part of Sjögren's syndrome. Hepatomegaly, splenomegaly and lymphadenopathy may be present. Abdominal pain is sometimes seen in active SLE and may be due to serositis, vasculitis or pancreatitis.

Laboratory and Clinical Investigations

The aim of carrying out investigations is to establish a diagnosis, assess the extent of organ involvement and disease activity, predict outcome, and guide therapeutic intervention.

Plasma proteins

Abnormalities in plasma proteins are common, and include increased levels of IgG, IgM and IgA. Depressed serum albumin is seen in active disease and in patients with renal disease. Surprisingly, acute phase reactants, such as C-reactive protein, are normal in patients with active disease. In patients with SLE who have intercurrent systemic infections a significant rise in C-reactive protein may occur.

Haematological

Anaemia, leucopenia and thrombocytopenia are found with active disease. Bleeding associated with a prolonged prothrombin time and KCCT is seen in a few patients due to autoantibodies against clotting factors.

Renal function

Proteinuria of varying amounts, associated with a diminution in glomerular filteration rate and an associated rise in blood urea and creatinine, may be observed in patients with renal SLE. The presence of casts is an indication of active renal involvement. The extent of proteinuria does not correlate with a particular histological type of involvement and may persist in patients in whom other parameters indicate that the disease has been suppressed.

Immunological tests

Nearly all patients with SLE show the presence of antinuclear antibodies. It is usual for patients to show antibodies with specificities to various nuclear antigens, for example, double-stranded and single-stranded DNA, DNA histone, Sm, RNP, SS-A and SS-B. High levels of ds-DNA antibodies and Sm antibody show diagnostic specificity (see Table 15.2). Some antibodies correlate with particular disease features; e.g. ds-DNA with renal and cutaneous disease, anti-RNP with Raynaud's phenomenon and myositis, anti-Sm with membranous nephritis, photosensitivity and cutaneous manifestations and anti-SS-A and SS-B with features of Sjögren's syndrome.

Patients with active SLE frequently show changes in serum complement levels. Total serum complement haemolytic activity (CH50) is lowered and is due to a diminution in individual complement components of the classical and alternative pathway. Most laboratories are able to measure C3 and C4 components.

The simultaneous measurement of DNA antibodies and complement levels offers a means of monitoring disease activity in many patients with SLE.

The majority of patients with SLE in the active stage of disease show the presence of circulating immune complexes. The clinical value of these tests has not yet been established.

Organ imaging

X-rays of the chest in SLE frequently show the presence of pleural effusions, pleural adhesions (tenting of the diaphragm), cardiac enlargement due to pericardial effusion or heart disease, and various forms of lung parenchymal disease, including patchy pneumonic consolidation and diffuse interstitial pulmonary fibrosis.

The liver and spleen may be enlarged and CAT scans of the brain may be abnormal in patients with central nervous system involvement. X-rays of joints show subluxations without significant erosions of cartilage and bone. Osteonecrosis is observed in some patients.

Liver function tests may show a raised alkaline phosphatase and serum transaminase in some patients, possibly associated with disease activity or as a result of therapy with aspirin.

Other organ function studies: Physiological lung function tests frequently show abnormalities of a restrictive type, and mild diminution in gas transfer in the absence of prominent radiological signs. EEG may be abnormal in patients with CNS disease. The CSF protein levels may be elevated and there may be a pleocytosis.

Treatment and Prognosis

The natural history of SLE appears to have altered in the last few decades. This may be due to better diagnosis, and to the use of steroids and antibiotics. Patients with severe multi-system disease, especially associated with diffuse glomerulonephritis and central nervous system involvement, may die within one year of onset but, on the other hand, 90% of patients survive more than ten years. Common causes of death include overwhelming infection (including infection with opportunistic agents such as fungi, pneumocystis and viruses), renal failure, cerebral disease and vascular occlusive disease (possibly related to prolonged steroid therapy).

Patients with renal involvement show a prognosis related to the type of renal lesions, e.g. patients with diffuse glomerulonephritis have the worst prognosis, whilst patients with focal and membranous glomerulonephritis have an intermediate or benign prognosis.

Drug treatment of SLE is determined by the pattern of disease.

1. *Non-steroidal anti-inflammatory drugs* are indicated for symptomatic treatment of joints, muscles, and vasculitis. In many patients, no other drug treatment may be required.
2. *Corticosteroid therapy* is mandatory in patients with severe multi-system SLE, and may be life saving. The dose of steroids is determined by the extent and severity of symptoms, e.g. prednisolone in the range of 0.2 mg/kg to 1 mg/kg body weight. In some patients, pulses of up to 1 g of methyl prednisolone intravenously daily for three days may be beneficial. Initially the steroid dose is commenced at a high level; after a period of 2–3 months or weeks, or when clinical response (monitored by laboratory investigations) is seen, the steroids are gradually reduced to a maintenance level, usually between 7 and 15 mg per day. In such patients, steroids may be required for life. However, if the condition is very stable a reduction at the rate of 1 mg per month, to total withdrawal, can be attempted. Steroid side-effects are frequent in patients with severe SLE since high doses for prolonged periods appear to be required.
3. *Immunosuppressive agents.* Immunosuppressive drugs such as azathioprine, cyclophosphamide and chlorambucil have long been used in the treatment of SLE. Controlled clinical trials have at best shown marginal benefit although the heterogeneity of clinical expression and the rarity of the disease makes these trials difficult to conduct. It is the impression of units dealing with SLE that some patients with severe forms of SLE may benefit from short periods of treatment with cyclophosphamide, 2.5 mg/kg body weight. However, the toxic effects (especially alopecia, cystitis and bladder fibrosis, infertility and possible oncogenic effects) limit its use

seriously. Azathioprine appears to be a useful drug in some patients, especially in its steroid-sparing effect when very high doses of steroids appear to be required for maintaining a satisfactory level of suppression of the disease.

4. *Anti-malarials*. Chloroquine or hydroxychloroquine (200 to 400 mg per day) has proved to be of benefit in many patients with SLE, especially with cutaneous manifestations. This drug too is limited by its toxic effects, especially when used for prolonged periods, when dose-related irreversible retinal damage may be seen. It is therefore recommended that the drug should only be given under constant supervision of an ophthalmologist.

5. *Plasmapheresis*. The place of plasmapheresis is controversial in SLE. Claims have been made that it is beneficial in severely ill patients not responding to steroids and immunosuppressive drugs.

6. *Other measures*. Patients with SLE, like other patients with chronic diseases, require sympathetic support. Bed rest may be indicated during period of serious illness. Exposure to sunlight should be avoided, not only to prevent severe photosensitive reactions but also to prevent disease activity. Infections are a constant scourge for patients with SLE and need to be recognised early and treated vigorously with the appropriate antibiotics. In patients with prominent and chronic muscular and joint symptoms, the use of splints and exercise may be indicated.

SJÖGREN'S SYNDROME

Sjögren's syndrome is defined as the triad of dry eyes (xerophthalmia) leading to kerato-conjunctivitis sicca, dry mouth (xerostomia), and a connective tissue disease, the commonest ones being rheumatoid arthritis, SLE, primary biliary cirrhosis, scleroderma and polymyositis. In some patients, xerophthalmia and xerostomia occur in the absence of a connective tissue disease, and then the disease is referred to as the 'sicca syndrome' (primary Sjögren's syndrome).

Epidemiology

The incidence and prevalence of this disorder is unknown. Criteria of Sjögren's syndrome are satisfied in up to 15% of patients with RA and a similar proportion of patients with SLE.

Pathology

The classical lesion is characterised by an infiltration by lymphocytes and plasma cells around the acini of lacrimal, salivary and other exocrine glands (e.g. of the respiratory, gastrointestinal tracts and the vagina). The cellular infiltrate is associated with destruction and fibrosis and secondary changes may occur in the ducts. In some patients with Sjögren's syndrome, extraglandular features may be prominent, including vasculitis and chronic renal failure. The renal lesion is characterised by renal tubular acidosis, and histologically prominent lymphoid and plasma cell infiltration of the parenchyma of the kidney is seen. Lymphadenopathy is common and may be due to a benign pseudolymphoma or malignant lymphoma.

Symptoms and Clinical Features

Involvement of exocrine tissue

Patients complain of a dry gritty sensation in the eyes and are liable to recurrent attacks of conjunctivitis. This may be associated with damage to the cornea (keratitis). Patients who have permanent symptoms of a dry mouth may have difficulty in masticating and swallowing due to lack of saliva. Dental caries and disease of the gums is frequent. Secondary infections of the salivary glands may occur. Dryness of the respiratory tract may lead to difficulty in expectoration of sputum, especially during infections. A dry vagina may present with dyspareunia.

Connective tissue disease

Arthritis may be present; in some patients it has an oligoarticular distribution, and in others typical rheumatoid arthritis is seen. Transient arthritis may also be observed, and vasculitis presenting with nodules in the lower extremities or purpuric lesions is also seen. Severe proximal muscle weakness and tenderness may be seen and is due to associated polymyositis. Muscle weakness may be associated with electrolyte imbalance and be a consequence of renal tubular acidosis and nephrocalcinosis. Peripheral or cranial neuropathy may occur.

Complications include a high incidence of lymphomas, mainly involving the B cell, and may be associated with paraproteinaemia.

Clinical and Laboratory Investigations

Many normal individuals complain of dry mouth and gritty eyes unassociated with diminished tear secretion. A diagnosis of xerophthalmia requires objective demonstration of loss of tear secretion. This is performed by a Schirmer test: a strip of blotting paper is inserted in the lower conjunctival sac for five minutes and the amount of tears secreted is recorded in terms of the length of wetness of the paper. Less than 5 mm of wetness indicates dryness of the eyes. Staining of the cornea with Rose Bengal and examination with a slit lamp shows filaments and corneal changes typical of keratoconjunctivitis sicca. The salivary gland secretion may be measured by giving the patient gum to chew for a period of time and then measuring salivary volume.

Salivary scintigram using radioactive pertechnetate is used to show impaired uptake and excretion by the parotid glands. Lip biopsy allows examination of salivary exocrine tissue, and is claimed to permit histological confirmation of the diagnosis.

Hypergammaglobulinaemia, a raised ESR, cryoglobulinaemia and positive tests for circulating immune complexes are a feature in many patients. Antibodies to salivary duct antigens commonly occur, but they are not diagnostic since they are also found in patients with other connective tissue diseases. Rheumatoid factors and antinuclear antibodies are found in the majority of patients.

Treatment

The aim is to provide symptomatic relief. Ocular dryness is helped by the use of methyl cellulose eye-drops. Infective conjunctivitis requires appropriate local antibiotic eye-drops. Close dental care is beneficial and oral candidiasis may require antifungal drugs locally (e.g. nystatin). Infective parotitis requires sys-

temic antibiotic treatment, as do episodes of infective bronchitis.

Steroid and immunosuppressive drugs are of limited value in the treatment of exocrine gland dysfunction. However, they may be indicated in patients with severe extraglandular complications.

SCLERODERMA

Scleroderma is characterised by prominent thickening of the skin with loss of elasticity. Digital vasospastic and occlusive disease is usual. Visceral involvement occurs in many patients, typically of the oesophagus, intestinal tract, lungs, heart and kidneys. The term 'progressive systemic sclerosis' is used synonymously with scleroderma but is sometimes used to define patients with prominent visceral and cutaneous involvement. The criteria for diagnosis of scleroderma are shown in Table 15.3.

Table 15.3
Criteria for Scleroderma

Major
  Typical cutaneous involvement proximal to MCP joints
Minor
  Sclerodactly
  Digital pitting scars
  Basilar pulmonary fibrosis
  Colonic sacculations on barium enema
  Distal oesophageal hypomobility on barium swallow

Epidemiology

Scleroderma occurs three times more frequently in women than in men. All ages are susceptible and cases have been described in all ethnic groups. It is estimated that in the UK the incidence of the disease is 2/100 000 per year and the prevalence is 1/10 000 of the population.

Aetiology and Pathogenesis

The aetiology of scleroderma is unknown. There is a suggestion of increased incidence of the disease amongst workers chronically exposed to silica. Industrial exposure to polyvinyl chloride (PVC) in the manufacture of plastics leads to acrolysis, a condition radiologically similar to that seen in scleroderma, and a possible link with the condition of scleroderma has been proposed in some cases. The drugs methysergide and practalol have been implicated in retroperitoneal fibrosis and diffuse inflammatory fibrotic reactions involving viscera but, apart from the florid formation of collagen, do not resemble the clinical picture of scleroderma. A clinical similarity is, however, apparent in patients who develop graft-versus-host disease following transplants.

Increased formation of collagen in skin is believed to be mediated by autoimmune reactions. It has been suggested that lymphocytes infiltrating the skin are sensitised to connective tissue elements (e.g. collagen), and interaction between lymphocytes and collagen leads to the production of lymphokines. Lymphokines are believed to increase production of collagens by fibroblasts. The concept therefore envisages a cell-mediated autoimmune reaction. In some patients, circulating immune complexes are found and it has been suggested that the vascular changes may be mediated by interaction of immune complexes with complement or phagocytic cells.

In patients with scleroderma, small blood vessels are hyper-reactive to cold. This functional abnormality may indicate an abnormal physiological response to endogenous vasoactive factors and may be involved in the pathogenesis of the disease.

Pathology

Pathological changes in the skin depend on the stage of the disease. In early cases, there is little change observable by light microscopy although increased collagen around the hair follicles and sweat glands may be observed. Lymphocyte infiltration is clearly present, blood vessels may appear to be dilated, and tissue is oedematous. Later in the disease, there is a marked increase in dermal thickness due to bands of collagen being laid down and replacing dermal structures such as the hair follicles and sweat glands. The epidermis appears atrophic.

Joints

Ankylosis of affected joints, with prominent fibrotic reaction, is observed. In some patients a chronic synovitis resembling rheumatoid arthritis may be observed. Cartilage and bone erosion do not occur.

Vascular disease

The typical changes are observed in digital vessels and interlobular renal arteries. There is a bland internal hyperplasia leading to occlusion of the lumen. In renal vessels there may be fibrinoid degeneration and occasionally cellular infiltration. In renal scleroderma associated with malignant hypertension, 'onion-skin' perivascular fibrosis may be observed.

Gastrointestinal tract

The oesophagus is involved in the majority of patients with scleroderma and the distal part shows a combination of atrophy and fibrosis. Similar changes are present throughout the intestine, particularly in the duodenum and the large intestine. Dilatation of the second and third portions of the duodenum are typical, and in the large intestine widemouthed diverticula are seen. There is loss of the muscular mucosa and atrophy of the submucosa in the affected portions. These atrophic changes appear to be primary rather than secondary to vascular insufficiency.

Clinical Features

Scleroderma shows a variety of recurring clinical patterns. This may be regarded as a basis for considering that the disease exists in distinct sub-sets. The following main types are observed:

a. Symmetrical and diffuse cutaneous involvement of the extremities, with or without involvement of the trunk and face, without visceral involvement.
b. Localised scleroderma (sometimes referred to as morphea) involving any part of the body.
c. Cutaneous and visceral involvement.
d. CREST syndrome, an acronym for the main features, namely calcinosis, Raynaud's phenomen, (o)esophageal involvement, sclerodactyly and telangiectasia.

e. Visceral involvement without any significant cutaneous involvement.

Cutaneous involvement

This usually commences in the distal parts of the upper and lower extremities and, in the early phases, leads to oedema with puffy digits. Typical scleroderma changes occur later, consisting of thickening and loss of elasticity of the skin, loss of skin creases and hair, hyperpigmentation and – eventually – encasing of the affected part in leathery skin that restricts joint movement. These changes typically involve skin proximal and distal to MCP joints, in distinction to sclerodactyly occurring secondary to peripheral vascular disease (e.g. Raynaud's disease) which is distal in distribution. The skin of the proximal parts of limbs, the upper trunk, neck, and face may also be involved. When scleroderma involves the face there is loss of the normal skin-folds around the mouth and gradual diminution of the aperture of the open mouth, which appears fish-like and becomes puckered. Involvement of the skin around the eyes and nose may give rise to a masked appearance.

Raynaud's phenomenon

This is common and often antedates the appearance of scleroderma. In addition to the classical features on cold exposure, there may be signs of occlusive disease, e.g. ischaemic ulcers or gangrene involving the pulps of the digits which heal by leaving pitted scars and lead to pulp strophy. Shrinkage of the terminal phalanx may be observed.

Calcinosis

This may be prominent in some patients, especially in the digits. Calcareous or chalky material may be extruded. The coexistence of scleroderma and widespread calcinosis is known as the Thibierge–Weissenbach syndrome.

Joints

A symmetrical polyarthritis is sometimes seen, especially early in the onset of the disease. More usually there is restriction of joint movements due to overlying scleroderma change or ankylosis of the joints themselves. Contractures may occur. In many patients there is a characteristic crepitus, which is palpable and audible with a stethoscope as a rub.

Oesophageal symptoms

These occur in up to half of the patients. Patients complain of dysphagia, heartburn, or pains in the chest with acid regurgitation.

Gastrointestinal symptoms

Flatulence, a bloated sensation, and diarrhoea associated with steatorrhoea may be seen.

Respiratory involvement

Fibrosing alveolitis with prominent fibrotic reaction is frequent. However, in other patients, lymphocytic interstital pneumonitis may be observed, which is similar to that seen in idiopathic cases.

Renal disease

This is the most serious complication of scleroderma and may have fatal consequences. It occurs in a minority of patients with visceral involvement and frequently presents suddenly with features of malignant hypertension. There is rapid progression to renal failure.

Cardiac involvement

Heart failure due to cardiomyopathy may be seen in patients with scleroderma. Right-sided heart failure due to pulmonary hypertension is seen in others. Pulmonary hypertension is attributed to associated lung fibrosis, vascular disease in the pulmonary arteries, and hypoventilation due to involvement of the thoracic cage and skin of the thorax.

Investigations

X-ray investigations may be of value in diagnosis. Barium studies may reveal loss of mobility of the distal part of the oesophagus, dilated loops of the second and third part of the duodenum, and saccular diverticula in the large intestine. Chest x-ray shows miliary mottling and linear shadows compatible with fibrosing alveolitis. Cardiac enlargement may be apparent in patients with cardiomyopathy. X-rays may reveal subcutaneous calcinosis.

Urinary hydroxyproline levels are elevated in patients with scleroderma due to increased turnover of collagen.

Haematological and biochemical investigations are not significantly abnormal. Antinuclear antibodies are found in up to 60% of patients. By immunofluorescent techniques the nuclei show either a homogeneous or speckled or nucleolar staining pattern. Anti-RNP antibodies have been found in patients with scleroderma, especially when associated with polymyositis. Circulating immune complexes are found in some patients.

Prognosis and Treatment

The prognosis of patients with scleroderma is determined to a large extent by the distribution of the disease. In general, patients without visceral disease have only a slightly shortened life expectation. A significantly shortened life expectancy is found in scleroderma patients with visceral disease, the commonest causes of death being due to lung disease and renal involvement. The worst prognosis is in patients with renal scleroderma.

General measures in the management of scleroderma include suitable exercises to maintain full mobility of joints, skin care, and protection against exposure to cold.

The following specific measures have also been attempted:

1. *Vascular symptoms*. Vasodilators have been used for Raynaud's phenomenon without much success. Sympathetic blocking agents such as reserpine have been used with some benefit. Infusions of high-molecular-weight dextran are advocated for patients with severe ischaemia of the digits with threatened gangrene. Infusions of prostaglandin-E have been used experimentally with benefit.
2. *Skin involvement* may respond to treatment with penicillamine. Beneficial effects from the use of colchicine have been reported.

3. *In patients with dysphagia* and other oesophageal symptoms, the regime followed for hiatus hernia may be beneficial (i.e. sleeping on a bed with the head end raised by 15–30 cm, avoiding liquids before retiring, and using antacids and metochlopramide). In patients with diarrhoea due to an overgrowth of organisms in the gut, the use of antibiotics such as tetracycline may be beneficial.
4. *Pulmonary and cardiac* involvement may occasionally respond to steroid treatment.
5. *Renal failure and hypertension*. The appearance of hypertension in scleroderma is a grave prognostic feature. It needs aggressive treatment with appropriate antihypertensive agents. Recent reports suggest that captopril may be beneficial and arrest, or even reverse, the deterioration in renal function.
6. *Immunosuppressive agents* have been used in scleroderma but it is doubtful if they are of significant value.

Specific treatment of scleroderma is unsatisfactory. No single regime can be recommended. Although penicillamine has been shown to be beneficial in cutaneous manifestations, it has no effect on the evolution of visceral involvement. Colchicine may be useful but its value is not yet established. Steroids and immunosuppressive agents are disappointing but are used in some patients especially when autoantibodies and circulating immune complexes are prominent.

OVERLAP SYNDROMES INCLUDING MIXED CONNECTIVE TISSUE DISEASE

Documentation of clinical patterns of autoimmune disorders involving connective tissue has lead to the recognition of certain well-characterised entities. These include RA, SLA, scleroderma, polymyositis, Sjögren's syndrome and fibrosing alveolitis. Whereas the majority of cases seen in clinical practice fit into the entities by existing criteria, a minority of patients defy classification, usually because they show coexistence of features of two or more of these well characterised entities. It is suggested that when such patterns recur in several patients they constitute distinct clinical entities, which are termed 'overlap syndromes'.

Mixed Connective Tissue Disease (MCTD)

This term is applied to patients who have coexisting features of SLE, scleroderma, polymyositis and fibrosing alveolitis. The condition is also claimed to be characterised by the presence of high titres of antibodies to nuclear RNP. Whilst the individual clinical features resemble those seen in patients with classical definable diseases, there are minor but subtle differences in the details of the features and their evolution. Thus chronic synovitis is rarely associated with erosions of articular surfaces. The digits show characteristic sausage-shaped swellings in the early stages and sclerodactyly develops gradually. Sclerodactyly is less pronounced than that seen in scleroderma and, it is claimed, unlike scleroderma it may be responsive to steroid therapy. Raynaud's phenomenon is found in practically all patients and is a prominent clinical feature. Proximal muscle weakness due to polymyositis is seen in the majority. Barium swallow shows dilatation and hypomobility of the distal part of the oesophagus, changes similar to those seen in scleroderma. Lung involvement occurs in a significant number of patients with the changes of fibrosing alveolitis. Rashes similar to that seen in SLE, fever, pleurisy, pericarditis, leukopenia and occasional renal disease have been documented. It is claimed that the characteristic serological finding in these patients is the presence of high titres of speckled ANA by immunofluorescence techniques. The reacting antibody has been characterised as being directed against nRNP in high titres. It is suggested that in these patients other ANAs are absent, especially antibodies to DNA and Sm. Several studies have now been published which cast doubt on the specificity of anti-RNP for MCTD.

Patients with MCTD are believed to have a better prognosis than those with SLE, scleroderma and polymyositis, and apparently respond to prednisolone therapy in the dose range 7–15 mg per day.

Other overlap syndromes have been described.

POLYMYOSITIS AND DERMATOMYOSITIS

Polymyositis is a diffuse inflammatory disease involving muscular tissue leading to loss of power. The predominant muscle groups involved are those of the upper and lower limb girdles, axial spine and pharynx. The following main clinical patterns are observed: primary polymyositis (uncomplicated form); primary dermatomyositis, usually seen in children but increasingly recognised in adults; polymyositis associated with connective tissue diseases such as SLE, Sjögren's syndrome, scleroderma, and RA; polymyositis or dermatomyositis associated with malignancy.

Epidemiology, Aetiology and Pathogenesis

The group of disorders is heterogeneous and rare; its incidence is probably about 3 per million population per year in the UK. The primary forms of polymyositis and dermatomyositis show a slightly increased predilection for females (female to male ratio of 2:1).

Aetiological factors are poorly understood at present; claims have been made for a viral aetiology, and for the involvement of *Toxoplasma* on the basis of raised antibody titres in patients, but the organism has not been isolated from tissues. There is substantial evidence for the involvement of cell-mediated autoimmune damage to muscle cells in polymyositis.

Clinical Features

Polymyositis

This usually presents as symmetrical weakness of limb girdle muscles commencing in the lower limb girdle. The patient experiences difficulty in rising from a sitting position, going upstairs, getting in and out of a bath, and eventually getting out of bed. Axial muscle involvement, especially of neck muscles may become prominent and the patient has difficulty in raising his head from the pillow. Upper limb girdle weakness is characterised by difficulty in elevation of shoulders, e.g. doing hair and reaching for things on shelves. Muscle pain and tenderness are usually absent. Wasting of muscle groups may be prominent. In some patients there is asymmetrical wasting of muscles. Pharyngeal muscle involvement is sometimes seen, leading to dysphagia and choking when swallowing. Dysarthria may be prominent. In some patients respiratory muscle involvement may lead to respiratory failure.

The rash of dermatomyositis

The characteristic features of the rash in dermatomyositis are: prominent periungual erythema; scaly plaques leading to collodion patches on the knuckles; non-specific dermatitis with oedema and erythema sometimes in linear distribution, especially prominent on the upper limbs and the base of the neck; a periorbital oedema with lilac (heliotrope) discolouration of the upper eyelids.

Vascular manifestations

In many patients, Raynaud's phenomenon is prominent. It may be associated with obvious subcutaneous calcinosis of the type seen in scleroderma, especially in patients with childhood dermatomyositis.

Joints

Contractures of joints are common and are due to severe atrophy of muscle tissue with fibrosis. In some patients arthralgias and transient polyarthritis may be observed.

Associated features

Some patients with polymyositis show features of an associated connective tissue disease and others are associated with neoplastic disease, including carcinoma of the bronchus, prostate, ovary, uterus, breast, or large intestine. Occasional patients with lymphoma or thymoma have been described. The coexistence of malignancy is especially likely in patients with polymyositis or dermatomyositis presenting over the age of 40. Malignancy may be difficult to detect and may only emerge months or years after the onset of the connective tissue disorder. There are several reports of improvement in the polymyositis or dermatomyositis following the surgical removal of a malignancy.

Investigations

The key to the diagnosis of polymyositis rests on biopsy, measurement of muscle enzymes, and electromyographic findings. Satisfactory muscle biopsy can be obtained by sampling the quadriceps with a suitably modified biopsy needle. Characteristic findings include the demonstration of muscle necrosis, associated with prominent infiltration by lymphocytes or clusters of plasma cells and other mononuclear cells. Regeneration may be evident. The number of muscle cells with centralised nuclei increases. Immunofluorescent findings are not specific but immune deposits may be found in vessel walls. By electron microscopy, necrotic muscle tissue and occasional inclusion particles (suggestive of viruses) are visible.

There is characteristic elevation of muscle enzymes, especially creatinine phosphokinase, during active disease. Myoglobinaemia and myoglobinuria are sometimes seen.

Electromyographic findings may be helpful and characteristic features include spontaneous fibrillation and spike potentials, complex polyphasic potentials and repetitive high-frequency action potentials.

Many patients show evidence of hyperglobulinaemia. In a few patients, rheumatoid factor may be present (in the absence of rheumatoid arthritis), and antinuclear antibodies have been detected. A common antibody specificity is directed against nuclear RNP. In occasional patients, diminution of serum complement C3 level is observed. Antibodies to actin and myosin have been described, but are probably non-specific.

Treatment

The aims of the treatment are: (a) to suppress the inflammatory reaction; (b) to prevent disuse atrophy and contractures of muscles; (c) to provide adequate nursing care and supportive measures for the severely weak patient, who is especially liable to aspiration pneumonia, respiratory failure and inanition; and (d) to treat underlying malignancy when present.

In the severely affected patient the inflammatory reaction is suppressed by administration of corticosteroids (prednisolone in the dose range of 1–2 mg/kg body weight). Treatment is monitored with regular assessment of muscle power, locomotor function and blood levels of CPK. Treatment at this dose level may have to be maintained for several weeks, and side-effects are common enough to require expert evaluation and distinction of muscle weakness due to the disease or from steroid-induced myopathy.

It is usual to give steroids in doses (and for a duration)

determined by the severity of weakness and response to the individual patient. In life-threatening cases, or when steroid side-effects are a problem, cytotoxic drugs such as azathioprine and methotrexate may be added.

Passive movements of joints are required to prevent contractures and an exercise programme is instituted to maintain muscle strength after suppression of the disease. Splints for the wrists, knees and ankles may be required.

VASCULITIS

The clinical manifestations of vasculitis are protean. Diagnosis rests on the demonstration of an inflammatory reaction in (and around) blood vessels, with consequent production of localised signs of inflammation, constitutional disturbance and loss of function resulting from interference with the integrity of the wall of the vessel and blood supply to tissues. If the site of involvement is accessible to biopsy, a diagnosis is easily made.

The following main categories of vasculitis are recognised:

i. Necrotising vasculitis characterised by fibrinoid necrosis and mono- and polymorphonuclear cellular infiltration of vessel walls. This process gives rise to two main patterns arising from involvement of (a) medium- to small-sized muscular arteries with a well-defined internal elastic lamina as is typified by 'classical' polyarteritis nodosa or polyarteritis complicating cases of nodular and seropositive rheumatoid arthritis; and (b) arterioles, capillaries or venules as seen in conditions variously labelled as leucocytoclastic vasculitis or hypersensitivity angiitis or small vessel vasculitis.

ii. Granulomatous vasculitis, characterised by evidence of the formation of granulomas in and around vessel walls, in addition to a variable degree of necrosis, cellular infiltration and intimal thickening. This category includes: (a) giant cell arteritis (also called temporal or cranial arteritis); (b) Wegener's granulomatosis; and (c) allergic granulomatosis of Churg and Strauss.

iii. Inflammatory (extravascular) nodular disease, in which inflammation predominantly involves extra-vascular tissue as seen in: (a) erythema nodosum; (b) nodular panniculitis or Weber–Christian disease; and (c) inflammatory nodules associated with RA, rheumatic fever and SLE.

iv. Bland occlusive vasculopathy, seen in connective tissue diseases, although not strictly speaking a form of vasculitis (since histological features of inflammation are missing) is nevertheless included as another form of vascular injury possibly arising from similar pathogenetic mechanisms. This is seen in: (a) rheumatoid arthritis and (b) scleroderma.

Necrotising Vasculitis

Polyarteritis Nodosa (PAN)

A condition most often seen in men in middle life, it is characterised by necrotising nodular inflammatory lesions involving medium sized arteries. Whilst the majority of cases are of unknown aetiology, some are associated with persistent hepatitis B antigenaemia with circulating antigen–antibody complexes. Some patients with RA develop typical PAN, although renal involvement is rare.

Clinical manifestations

The onset is usually sudden and includes the following features:

i. Nonspecific features including fever, myalgia, arthralgia, and prominent weight-loss.

ii. Vascular occlusion leading to: (a) peripheral mononeuritis multiplex associated with a mixed sensory–motor neuropathy; (b) visceral infarction, which may present as an acute abdomen and be associated with infarction of the gut, the gall bladder or other viscera (cardiac and brain infarction also occur); (c) gangrene of the fingers or toes and of the acral parts of the face.

iii. Renal manifestations, including asymptomatic hypertension progressing to malignant hypertension, and proteinuria leading to chronic renal failure.

iv. Cutaneous manifestations may be prominent and include the development of painful inflammatory nodules along arteries. Purpuric lesions may be present.

Livido reticularis is usually prominent over the limbs and necrotic ulcers with sharp demarcated margins are characteristic. Ulcers also occur in the mouth and upper respiratory tract.

v. Peripheral vascular disease is common and, in some patients, may be the predominant feature. In such patients the features resemble Buerger's disease or premature arteriosclerosis. The concurrent presence of Raynaud's syndrome is characteristic of PAN.

vi. Pulmonary involvement may manifest as asthma, nodular infarcts in the lung, diffuse pulmonary infiltrates, pleurisy and pulmonary hypertension.

vii. Cardiac involvement is secondary to coronary occlusive disease. Patients may present with acute myocardial infarction or cardiac failure.

viii. Retroperitoneal fibrosis may be seen in some patients.

Investigations

Biopsy. A firm diagnosis ultimately rests on tissue pathology, which may be difficult to obtain. Biopsy of the sural nerve and associated arteries, epididymal tissue, liver, muscle and rectum may show evidence of arteritis. A renal biopsy may show typical arteritis and segmental glomerular necrosis.

Haematological abnormalities are common and include severe anaemia, persistent leucocytosis, eosinophilia and a very high ESR (usually in the region of 100 mm/hr).

Acute phase reactants such as CRP are raised.

Liver function tests may be abnormal, including a rise in serum transaminases and a moderate rise in alkaline phosphatase.

Blood chemistry may be abnormal in patients with renal involvement, reflecting the severity of renal failure.

Serum immunoglobulins tend to be marginally raised. Occasionally, serum complement C3 and C4 levels are decreased but they are generally normal and even increased. Tests for circulating immune complexes (e.g. cryoglobulins) may be positive in PAN associated with hepatitis B virus infection and rheuma-

toid disease, but in other patients these tests are consistently negative. In a few patients rheumatoid factor tests are positive.

Angiographic studies may be very helpful, especially with regional injection of the hepatic, coeliac and renal arteries. These may show typical aneurysmal dilatation of medium-sized arteries.

Careful urinanalysis may reveal microscopic haematuria, proteinuria and casts.

Treatment

The prognosis of this condition is uniformly bad. However, the course of the disease may be modified by the use of corticosteroids in high doses. Recent reports suggest that oral cyclophosphamide is beneficial; it may be used in a dose of 3 mg/kg body weight initially and then reduced according to the clinical and haematological response. Azathioprine and other immunosuppressive drugs have their advocates. In patients with hypertension, vigorous attention to control is required. Severe infections may occur and require early recognition and treatment.

Leucocytoclastic Vasculitis

In this category of vasculitides the best known example is Henoch–Schoenlein purpura in children and its counterpart in adults. The characteristic features include the following:

i. Palpable purpuric lesions on the extensor aspects of limbs, especially of the upper part of the lower limbs. Early skin lesions may be pleomorphic and include macules and urticaria. Subsequently the lesions tend to coalesce, ulcerate and heal by forming pigmented and pitted scars.

ii. Arthritis, which may be flitting in character, may involve several peripheral joints. Chronic arthritis with deformities does not occur.

iii. Abdominal pains of colicky nature with vomiting, haemorrhage and intussusception may occur.

iv. Renal involvement is seen in up to half of patients and may take the form of a transient nephritis with proteinuria and haematuria. Progressive renal failure is also recognised but, fortunately, is rare.

v. Fever frequently occurs and, in patients with prominent joint symptoms, may mimic rheumatic fever.

Pathogenesis and investigations

The clinico-pathological features of Henoch–Schoenlein purpura resemble acute serum sickness which is known to be mediated by circulating immune complexes. An antecedent history of upper respiratory infection is not unknown and suggests the possible source of the antigen. Circulating immune complexes have also been implicated in leucocytoclastic vasculitis associated with experimentally-induced allergic reactions, chronic infections with meningococcus, gonococcus and subacute bacterial endocarditis, hepatitis B virus infection, essential mixed cryoglobulinaemia and congenital complement deficiency of C2. IgA-rich complexes are particularly characteristic of Henoch–Schoenlein purpura and, in skin and renal biopsies, may be detected in the immune deposits in blood vessel walls and in the glomerulus. Within the glomerulus, the immune deposits are found in the mesangial region and in capillary loops. Light microscopy of skin biopsy shows necrosis and polymorphonuclear infiltration of small vessels in the superficial layers of the dermis.

Other laboratory investigations in patients with leucocytoclastic vasculitis may reveal elevated ESR, abnormal leucocytosis, proteinuria, microhaematuria and casts.

Treatment

Bed rest is usually indicated in the early stages of the illness, which usually lasts 4–6 weeks with complete resolution. Some cases show a tendency to frequent recurrences. Symptomatic treatment includes the use of non-steroidal anti-inflammatory drugs to control joint pains and fever, and splints for supporting painful joints. A short course of prednisolone may be indicated in severe cases, and is usually given a trial in patients with progressive renal disease, although evidence of convincing benefit is lacking. Other agents which have been tried in severe cases, with reports of benefit, include immunosuppressive drugs and dapsone.

Granulomatous Vasculitides and Polymyalgia Rheumatica

Giant Cell Arteritis (GCA)

In this condition, exclusively seen in patients over the age of fifty, the cranial blood vessels are predominantly involved by an arteritis characterised by mononuclear cell infiltration with multinucleated giant cell formation in the media, adventitial inflammation, disruption of the internal elastic lamina and intimal thickening associated with occlusion.

Clinical features

i. Pains in the upper limb girdle and neck with marked stiffness of neck and shoulder movements, especially on waking, with tenderness of muscles on palpation. This syndrome is termed polymyalgia rheumatica and may be the only presenting symptom of GCA.

ii. Headaches, especially over the temporal region, giving the synonym 'temporal arteritis' as a description of the condition. The patient may be aware of scalp tenderness and examination may show obvious thickening of the temporal arteries, loss of arterial pulsation, and signs of local inflammation. Occipital arteries may be similarly involved.

iii. Visual disturbances including loss of vision may occur, sometimes quite suddenly, and be the major presenting symptom.

iv. Severe constitutional symptoms and signs frequently occur and include fever, anaemia and loss of weight.

v. Although involvement of cranial vessels is the most widely recognised feature of the disease, all the major vessels arising from the aortic arch, as well as the arch itself and the iliac vessels, may be involved. Depending on the site of vessel disease, symptoms of vascular insufficiency are found and include cerebrovascular syndromes and claudication of the upper limbs, tongue and jaw. Involvement of the aortic arch may give rise to the clinical features of the 'pulseless syndrome', originally recognised as arising from arteritis of the aortic arch and affecting young women (Takayashu's syndrome).

Pathogenesis

This is a matter of speculation, although evidence of circulating immune complexes has been found in patients with GCA.

Investigations

i. In a patient suspected of GCA, an ESR of greater than 60 mm in the first hour is usual. Anaemia and leucocytosis may be present.

ii. A temporal artery biopsy is indicated and, if positive, is diagnostic. Multiple sections may need to be examined before a diagnosis of GCA can be excluded.

iii. The serum immunoglobulin levels, especially IgM, may be elevated. On protein electrophoresis the gamma- and alpha-2-globulin fractions may be increased.

iv. Tests of liver function may be abnormal, a mild to moderate rise in serum alkaline phosphatase being particularly noted. However, liver biopsy only shows minor abnormalities.

Treatment

If a clinical diagnosis of GCA is strongly suspected, and particularly in patients whom cranial vessel involvement seems likely and a rapid ESR is documented, immediate treatment with steroids is indicated. Prednisolone in an initial dose of 40 mg/day for up to 4 weeks, and then reduced to a maintenance level, is usually recommended. This is effective in suppressing the disease and may prevent a vascular occlusive episode, e.g. involving the ophthalmic territory. The risk of steroid toxicity has to be balanced against the benefit of preventing blindness and stroke.

Relationship of GCA to Polymyalgia Rheumatica

Polymyalgia rheumatica (PMR) is a syndrome characterised by pain and stiffness, especially after physical inactivity and bed rest, involving the pelvic and shoulder girdles, and associated with a raised ESR. Although the history suggests a primary muscle disorder, and indeed is often associated with muscle

tenderness and subjective weakness, objective evidence of muscle weakness and evidence of muscle necrosis as evidenced by a raised CPK or biopsy findings are lacking.

This syndrome may be the presenting feature of RA, although evidence of peripheral-joint polyarthritis usually easily distinguishes the two conditions from the outset. It has been previously noted that PMR may also form part of the clinical picture of GCA. In some patients in whom the clinical symptoms and signs are solely confined to the soft tissues of the limb girdles, and in whom no evidence of clinical arteritis is apparent, a biopsy of the temporal artery shows typical changes of GCA. This has led to the hypothesis that all patients with PMR may have underlying GCA which may be too localised to be clinically diagnosable.

The laboratory tests in PMR are essentially similar to those observed in GCA and response to prednisolone in the dose range of 20–30 mg is dramatic. When a good response is obtained, the dose can be rapidly reduced to 7.5 mg/day and therefore tapered to the lowest dose which suppresses clinical symptoms and ESR. In practice, an average dose around 5 mg/day seems to be required for 3–6 months before complete withdrawal. Continued supervision over prolonged periods is desirable since recurrences with clinical onset of GCA may supervene.

Wegener's Granulomatosis

Wegener's granulomatosis is characterised by the concomitant presence in a patient of granulomatous inflammatory and vasculitic lesions involving the upper respiratory tract (nose, sinuses, middle ear, etc.), lobes of the lung, kidneys, and occasionally a more widespread distribution. The patient may present with severe respiratory and/or renal symptoms, the latter progressing rapidly to renal failure. Response to steroids and cyclophosphamide is very impressive and may even reverse severe renal disease.

Other Forms of Vasculitis

Erythema nodosum

This condition is characterised by the sudden onset of painful subcutaneous inflammatory nodules, usually on the lower limbs, associated with oedema of the legs, arthralgia, oligoarthritis and fever. It typically affects young females and in Britain may be often associated with bilateral hilar lymphadenopathy due to sarcoidosis. It is a self-limiting disorder which usually lasts 4–6 weeks, and symptoms respond to non-steroidal anti-inflammatory drugs. Other underlying conditions include recent infection with beta-haemolytic streptococci, tubercle bacillus and reaction to drugs such as sulphonamides and the contraceptive pill.

Weber–Christian disease and other nodular conditions

In this very rare panniculitis, associated with inflammation in septa of fat lobules, the patient presents with inflammatory subcutaneous lumps.

Vasculopathy of rheumatoid arthritis and scleroderma

Bland intimal thickening and hyperplasia involving digital vessels and giving rise to nail-fold infarcts is characteristically seen in RA, although similar lesions also occur in SLE and scleroderma. In some patients necrotising arteritis may coexist. A histological lesion characterised by intimal proliferation and thickening involving renal arteries is also seen in scleroderma and may progress to severe malignant hypertensive change with fibrinoid necrosis of vessel walls and terminal renal failure.

16

Crystal Deposition Diseases

This chapter covers a group of joint diseases which result from the deposition of crystals in articular tissues. The group includes two common diseases: gout and pyrophosphate arthropathy, one rare curiosity: ochronosis (alkaptonuria), and one at present rather diffuse concept: hydroxyapatite deposition arthritis. The chapter will deal mainly with gout and pyrophosphate arthropathy. The other two are mentioned in order to complete the classification (Table 16.1).

In these diseases arthritis results, not from chemical irritation by the deposited material, but from the physical presence of microcrystals within the joint. The mechanism of this is discussed further in connection with gout.

GOUT

Definition

Gout is a joint disease in which a sustained elevation of uric acid in the plasma (hyperuricaemia) leads to deposition of urate crystals in articular structures. The resulting episodes of acute arthritis may later progress to chronic joint destruction and visible subcutaneous nodules of urate (tophi).

Hyperuricaemia and gout

Hyperuricaemia is the metabolic abnormality essential for the development of gout. Above a critical concentration, urate crystallises out into the tissues and, because of a predeliction for cartilage, arthritis results. For reasons which are not understood, transient hyperuricaemia (even when extreme) appears to be insufficient to produce gout, which requires plasma

levels of urate to be sustained over months or years. The aetiology of gout is clearly closely linked with the causes of hyperuricaemia. These are therefore considered below, before the clinical features of the disease.

Aetiology of hyperuricaemia

Uric acid is a weak divalent organic acid with the following formula:

Uric acid
(keto form)

Uric acid
(enol form)

pK 5

It has pKa values of 5.75 and 10.3. In acid urine it exists as uric acid, but it is deposited in the tissues as monosodium urate.

In man uric acid is the end degradation product of the two purines, adenine and guanine (Fig. 16.1). Uric acid therefore results from the breakdown of adenine and guanine bases in nucleic acids and in nucleotides. In lower animals this degradative pathway is taken one stage further, with the enzyme uricase converting uric acid to allontoin. Man has suffered an apparently deleterious mutation and does not possess uricase.

Table 16.1

Classification of Crystal Deposition Diseases

Disease	Type of crystal	Features
Gout	Urate	Acute and chronic arthritis of peripheral limb joints
Pyrophosphate arthropathy	Calcium pyrophosphate dihydrate	Acute and chronic arthritis of large limb joints
Ochronosis (alkaptonuria)	Derivatives of homogenitisic acid*	Chronic spinal arthritis
Apatite deposition arthropathy	Hydroxyapatite (the mineral of bone)	Uncertain

* Initially not a true crystalline deposition. Later calcification occurs.

Purines are building blocks of which the body requires a continuous supply. The metabolic pathway by which purines are synthesised, the interconversions by which a pool of purines is maintained, and the pathways by which intermediate degradative products are salvaged for reutilisation, are shown in Fig. 16.1. The size of the purine pool exerts feedback control on the rate of synthesis by inhibiting an early step in the synthetic pathway.

Renal handling of urate. In order to understand the consequences to man resulting from the loss of uricase, consideration of the renal handling of urate is necessary. Because it is a small molecule, bound lightly (if at all) to protein, urate enters the glomerular filtrate freely. From the tubule it is completely or almost completely reabsorbed back into the circulation. This reabsorption is an advantage in those animals which possess uricase; it prevents the relatively insoluble uric acid from

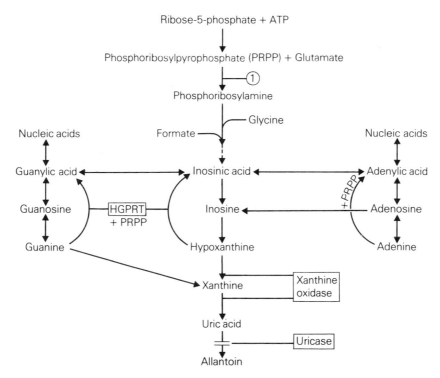

Fig. 16.1 *Purine metabolism pathways. Reaction (1) is brought about by the enzyme amidophosribosyltransferase, and is the site of feedback inhibition by purines. HGPRT, hypoxanthine-guanine phosphoribosyltransferase, the enzyme missing in Lesch–Nyhan syndrome. Man lacks uricase.*

travelling further, where the concentrated acid urine would favour crystallisation. In man, lacking uricase, elimination of uric acid takes place by secretion back from the plasma into the tubular lumen. The process is complex and not fully understood. It appears that some further reabsorption takes place distal to the site of secretion (postsecretory reabsorption). The end result of a lack of uricase is therefore that man has levels of urate in both the plasma and the urine which are uncomfortably close to the point at which spontaneous crystallisation occurs.

Both reabsorption and secretion of urate by the renal tubule are active transport processes. This pathway is shared with other weak organic acids, and it can be modified by certain drugs. Because the tubular transport is bi-directional, the same drug in different doses may produce opposite effects. Thus aspirin (a weak organic acid) in small doses causes urate retention, while in full doses (4–5 g daily) it is an effective uricosuric drug.

Plasma uric acid levels are highly sensitive to alterations in urate tubular transport. Thus starvation, through competitive blocking of the pathway by keto-acids, produces hyperuricaemia. Drugs such as thiazide diuretics and pyrazinamide have a similar effect, and prolonged administration of these may cause gout. Tubular damage due to lead poisoning, and chronic renal failure from any cause, may also cause hyperuricaemia. By contrast, drugs such as probenecid which produce more complete tubular paralysis, induce a net increase in urinary urate and can be used to lower plasma uric acid levels.

The level of uric acid in the plasma reflects the balance (Fig. 16.2) between the processes adding urate to the plasma (synthesis and dietary purines) and those removing it (renal and gut excretion – about 30% by the latter route).

The 'upper limits of normal' (males 420 μmol/l, females 360 μmol/l) depend on the laboratory and are arbitrary. Some men have levels greater than this, but never develop gout. However, above some critical level the solubility of urate in plasma is exceeded, and crystals of urate are deposited in the tissues, particularly in articular cartilage and in the renal parenchyma. Effective allopurinol therapy can reverse this process by lowering the level of plasma uric acid (Fig. 16.2).

Sex hormones appear to exert a modest but important influence on plasma urate levels. Up to puberty the

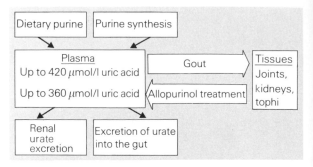

Fig. 16.2 *The level of plasma uric acid represents a balance between the rate at which urate enters and leaves the plasma. Above a critical level, urate crystallises out of the plasma into the tissues to produce gout. Effective therapy with allopurinol can reverse this process.*

sexes have similar levels. At puberty, males rise by about 50 μmol/l and this difference is maintained until after the menopause, when the female levels approach those of males. Significantly, primary gout is mainly a disease of postpubertal males and (occasionally) postmenopausal females. There is an interesting parallel with frontal baldness, another trait determined by an autosomal gene with sex hormones exerting a permissive influence on its expression.

Figure 16.2 provides a scheme for subdividing the causes of hyperuricaemia, and hence the types of gout. The two main variables influencing plasma urate levels are the rate of purine turnover and the rate of renal urate elimination. On this basis, gouty subjects can be subdivided into 'overproducers' and 'underexcretors'. Urinary urate output reflects the rate of purine synthesis. On a low purine diet (and in the absence of drug and other modifying influences) the 24-hour output does not normally exceed 3.6 mmol (600 mg).

A second subdivision is into 'primary' and 'secondary' gout. Secondary refers to cases in which a clear cause accounts for the hyperuricaemia. For example, myeloproliferative disorders such as myeloid leukaemia or polycythaemia rubra vera may lead to gross overproduction of purines, while chronic thiazide diuretic administration may produce marked underexcretion of urate. By contrast, primary gout tends to run in families and depends on an altered 'setting' for the regulation of purine synthesis or (more often) renal urate clearance.

In practice these distinctions are less clear-cut. Influences such as diet, obesity and alcohol intake are additive, and in most instances hyperuricaemia is multifactorial.

Clinical Features

Males are affected more often than females in a ratio of 10:1, and the onset is usually between 30 and 60 years. Only about 10% of cases are clearly 'secondary' and, amongst these, there is a lower male predominance. About 40% of gouty patients give a positive family history. The onset is almost invariably an attack of acute arthritis.

The acute attack

Gout is a disease predominantly of small peripheral joints and, surprisingly often, the initial attack involves the first metatarsophalangeal joint ('podagra'). A dull ache in the great toe – typically starting at night – builds up over 2–3 hours into what may be extremely severe pain. The affected joint becomes swollen and exquisitely tender, and the overlying skin red and dry. Walking is often impossible and there may be mild fever, leucocytosis and elevated ESR. If untreated, the attack may last a few days to a week or two. It then subsides, leaving a completely normal joint.

The initial episode is likely to be followed by further attacks at intervals of weeks, months, or years. Subsequent attacks may involve the same joint, the opposite great toe, or other peripheral limb joints. Hip, shoulder and spinal involvement is rare. Occasionally more than one joint is involved at the same time, and attacks may be provoked by trauma, surgical operations, alcoholic excess or – surprisingly – factors which lower the level of plasma uric acid.

In the more severe cases, there comes a stage when joints no longer return to normal between attacks, and the condition evolves into one of chronic tophaceous gout.

Mechanism of the acute attack. Good evidence suggests that the central inflammatory event is the phagocytosis of urate crystals by polymorphonuclear leucocytes within the synovial fluid. What triggers the attack is unknown, but it appears likely that the crystals are shed into the synovial fluid from articular cartilage. The crystals, perhaps because they are coated with IgG, are phagocytosed by synovial fluid neutrophils. Once ingested, a crystal causes lysis of the cell, and is thus released to be phagocytosed by another neutrophil. Both the process of phagocytosis and the subsequent cell lysis result in the release of lysosomal enzymes and other inflammatory mediators. Chemotaxins attract further neutrophils. The clinical features point to rapid amplification of the inflammatory process once it has started. What stops it is unknown. Colchicine, which is a drug without influence on uric acid, is thought to act by binding to the cytoplasmic endoskeleton of polymorphonuclear leucocytes and interfering with their participation in the inflammatory reaction.

Chronic tophaceous gout

In the more severe progressive cases of gout, deposits of urate collect in articular cartilage and enlarge to form palpable and visible nodules (tophi) around peripheral limb joints, or attached to bursas or tendons. Another favoured site is the helix of the ear, where they should always be sought. These tophi are generally firm, and the chalky white contents may be visible through the skin. They may soften and discharge urate.

Renal involvement

Some degree of renal failure is common in patients with severe chronic tophaceous gout, and occasionally causes death. In some patients, renal urate calculi are a contributing factor. Most gouty patients do not have calculi, however, and most patients with uric acid calculi do not have gout. A more important cause of renal changes in gout is deposition of urate crystals in the renal parenchyma, which leads to interstitial nephritis. Patients who die of renal failure show at autopsy mixed changes of interstitial nephritis, pyelonephritis and hypertension.

Associated diseases

Amongst gouty subjects there is an increased prevalence of hypertension, atherosclerosis, hypertriglyceridaemia and diabetes. There is no evidence that hyperuricaemia itself is the cause of any of these, apart from the hypertension which may accompany gouty renal failure. Some anti-hypertensive drugs may also cause hyperuricaemia. In some families these traits appear to be inherited together. There is no evidence that lowering plasma urate levels improves cardiovascular status.

The causes of secondary gout have been mentioned on page 234. Table 16.2 is a checklist of conditions which have to be considered.

Table 16.2

Causes of Secondary Gout

Increased purine turnover
Myeloproliferative disorders: polycythaemia rubra
    vera, myeloid leukaemia, myelosclerosis
Other leukaemias
Other neoplasms

Decreased renal urate excretion
Primary renal diseases
Drugs: thiazide diuretics, pyrazinamide, etc.
Lead poisoning
Hypercalcaemia
Myxoedema
Glycogen storage disease

Lesch–Nyhan syndrome

A number of very rare enzyme abnormalities may lead to gout through increased urate formation. The best known is the Lesch–Nyhan syndrome, a fatal X–linked disorder of boys. Affected children develop spasticity, choreo-athetosis, mental retardation, compulsive self-mutilation by biting, gout, urate urolithiasis and renal failure. Plasma and urinary urate levels are high.

Overproduction of urate is due to a deficiency of HGPRT (Fig. 16.1). This interferes with the salvage (reutilisation) pathway, and causes accumulation of PRPP, resulting in accelerated purine synthesis. The pathogenesis of the neurological abnormality is not understood. HGPRT activity can be estimated in red cell lysates. Allopurinol will correct the hyperuricaemia, but not the neurological features.

Investigations

Synovial fluid examination

This is the most positive method of diagnosing gout. The fluid is taken into a plain tube without anticoagulant, and it is important to examine a portion of any clot

that forms, for fibrin enmeshes crystals. A microscope equipped for polarising light is needed. A drop of synovial fluid under a coverslip is examined with the polarising filters ('polars') adjusted so that their planes of transmission are at right angles ('crossed polars'). This gives a dark background against which any urate crystals stand out with bright birefringence. To differentiate from pyrophosphate crystals, a '1st order red compensator' is inserted between the polars. Viewed against a red background, the crystals now take on different colours, depending on their orientation (Fig. 16.3). Many of the crystals lie within synovial neutrophils.

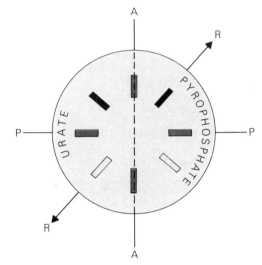

Fig. 16.3 *Differentiation between urate and pyrophosphate crystals by polarised light microscopy. The diagram illustrates the colour changes when rotating crystals between 'crossed polars' and with the first order red compensator in position. PP, plane of polariser; AA, plane of analyser; RR, plane of 'slow component' (γ) of compensator. On the left the colour changes indicate negative birefringence (e.g. urate), on the right positive birefringence (e.g. pyrophosphate). When lying in the planes PP and AA the crystals take on the red background colour.*

Polarising light may also be used to identify crystals in synovial membrane biopsies and in material obtained by scraping with a needle the surface of a possible tophus.

Uric acid determinations

These are satisfactorily performed by autoanalyser. Plasma levels should be interpreted in the light of the many factors, particularly drugs, which may influence them. A persistently normal plasma uric acid level (below about 420 μmol/l, depending on the laboratory) effectively excludes gout, provided the patient is not taking a uric acid-lowering drug. On a low-purine diet, 24-hour urinary urate output should not exceed 3.6 mmol (600 mg). Figures in excess of this indicate increased purine turnover.

Radiology

This is not particularly useful. Tophi invade bone to give juxta-articular 'erosions', but these only appear at a stage when tophi are already apparent clinically. Long-standing tophi may show secondary calcification.

Other investigations

These may be indicated to exclude the various causes of secondary gout (Table 16.2). A standard blood count may point to the need to seek a myeloproliferative disorder such as myeloid leukaemia, polycythaemia rubra vera, or myelofibrosis. Renal function should also be checked.

Diagnosis

Gout enters into the differential diagnosis of any patient with acute episodic arthritis. Every effort should be made to clinch the diagnosis by identifying urate crystals in synovial fluid, in material scraped from a tophus, or from a synovial biopsy. Failing crystal identification, the diagnosis may be made in a man experiencing typical acute attacks in peripheral joints, including podagra, in whom the plasma uric acid is clearly elevated. A positive family history or a clear response of the acute attack to colchicine may lend additional support to the diagnosis. A firm diagnosis of gout cannot be made on lesser criteria.

Two errors in diagnosis are common. One is failure to consider gout in a patient with, for example, a first acute attack in a finger joint. This may result in an incorrect diagnosis of septic arthritis or cellulitis. The other error is to diagnose gout in someone with joint pains which are not characteristic of gout, but in whom plasma uric acid levels are elevated. In these circumstances it is essential to identify urate crystals in order to establish the diagnosis. Contrary to some earlier views, hyperuricaemia is not acceptable as a cause of vague skeletal pains short of true arthritis.

Management

The treatment of gout consists of two separate issues: termination of the individual acute attack, and long-term (interval) management.

The acute attack

The traditional treatment is colchicine by mouth, 1 mg immediately, then 0.5 mg two-hourly until the attack eases. Unfortunately, toxic and therapeutic doses are close, and diarrhoea and vomiting are common. For this reason, one of the NSAIDs is generally used, e.g. indomethacin 50 mg 6-hourly until the pain lessens, then in reducing doses until the attack is over. Other NSAIDs can be used in a similar manner. The patient should carry a supply with which to start treatment at the first sign of an attack.

Interval treatment with a uric acid-lowering drug must never be started during an acute attack: it is liable to worsen and prolong the attack.

Long-term management

Once the treatable causes of secondary gout (Table 16.2) have been excluded, it is necessary to consider how much management is needed. The mildest cases, with infrequent attacks, modest plasma uric acid elevations, and no tophi, may require no more than an adjustment of life style. Reduction of body weight and alcohol intake and avoidance of high-purine food (liver, kidney, etc.) may be sufficient to prevent further attacks. In patients with frequent attacks, chronic joint damage, tophi, renal impairment, or severe hyperuricaemia (above 500 μmol/l), it is necessary to lower the plasma uric acid by drug treatment.

Allopurinol is considered by some as the drug of choice. It competitively inhibits xanthine oxidase (Fig. 16.1) and also suppresses purine synthesis, leading to a reduction of uric acid in both plasma and urine. For reasons which are not understood, rapid lowering of plasma uric acid tends to provoke attacks of acute gout. Allopurinol is therefore started in small doses (100 mg daily), and increased gradually up to 300 mg or more until the plasma uric acid level is normal, which dose is then maintained indefinitely. Prophylactic colchicine, 0.5 mg twice daily, during the period of introducing allopurinol reduces the risk of provoking acute attacks. Occasional patients cannot tolerate allopurinol because of skin rashes.

Allopurinol treatment can reduce the size of tophi (Fig. 16.2). It corrects drug-induced hyperuricaemia, and can be used to treat urate urolithiasis. It can also be used to prevent the acute obstructive urate nephropathy which may occur after cytotoxic or radiation treatment of leukaemia or other proliferative lesions. For most gouty patients allopurinol provides complete control of the disease.

Uricosuric drugs inhibit renal tubular absorption of urate. Probenecid (0.5 to 1.0 g twice daily) or sulphinpyrazone (100 mg 3–4 times daily) provide alternatives to allopurinol. They lose effect if there is renal failure and they may actually increase the hazard of urate urolithiasis.

Asymptomatic hyperuricaemia in itself does not require treatment.

PYROPHOSPHATE ARTHROPATHY (PSEUDOGOUT : CHONDROCALCINOSIS)

Crystals of calcium pyrophosphate dihydrate may be deposited in joint cartilage to produce a characteristic radiological appearance ('chondrocalcinosis'). This is increasingly common with advancing years. It is often asymptomatic, or the crystals may induce episodes of acute synovitis ('pseudogout') or chronic degenerative arthritis. The cause of pyrophosphate deposition is unknown. It occurs in association with certain metabolic diseases, and a familial form affects younger people. Joint damage also may predispose to pyrophosphate deposition.

Clinical Features

Pyrophosphate arthropathy is encountered about as often as urate gout. If affects mainly the middle-aged and elderly of both sexes. A positive family history is uncommon, apart from the rare familial type (see below).

Acute crystal synovitis ('pseudogout')

Acute attacks are similar to those of acute gout, but tend to be somewhat milder and to affect larger limb joints, particularly the knee. Podagra is rare. Untreated attacks may subside within 2–3 weeks to leave a completely normal joint, but occasionally the attack grumbles on in subacute form for many weeks. Attacks may be precipitated by trauma, and a particularly common sequence is for acute synovitis of a knee joint to appear a few days after a major surgical operation. The mechanism of this crystal synovitis is similar to that of acute gout.

Mild systemic features (fever, leucocytosis and raised ESR) may accompany the acute attack.

Chronic degenerative arthritis

Some patients with pyrophosphate deposition develop a chronic degenerative type of arthritis. This may or may not be associated with episodes of acute synovitis (see above). The pathological and clinical features are similar to 'primary' osteoarthritis, and it is assumed that the presence of the crystals in some way predisposes to premature 'degenerative' changes. As with acute attacks, large limb joints are mainly affected, particularly the knee. Wrist involvement sometimes produces median nerve compression (carpal tunnel syndrome). There also appears to be a particular tendency for pyrophosphate arthropathy associated with haemochromatosis (see below) to involve the index and middle finger metacarpophalangeal joints. The tempo of chronic pyrophosphate arthritis varies. It usually resembles osteoarthritis, but occasionally follows a more rapid and destructive course.

Subacute involvement of multiple joints may rarely produce a clinical picture which mimics rheumatoid arthritis.

Assocation with other diseases

Both chondrocalcinosis and pyrophosphate arthropathy appear to occur more commonly amongst patients suffering from certain metabolic disorders, including hypercalcaemia (particularly that due to hyperparathyroidism), haemochromatosis, acromegaly and Wilson's disease. It is also more common in hypermobile patients, and in neuropathic (Charcot) joints. These associations are not understood. It appears as though a variety of factors, including cartilage damage, may predispose to pyrophosphate deposition. A more severe form of pyrophosphate arthropathy, running in families and presenting at a younger age, occurs in certain parts of the world, including Czechoslovakia and Chile. Unlike urate, pyrophosphate deposits appear to result from local synthesis by chondrocytes.

An apparent tendency for chondrocalcinosis to occur in patients with primary (nodal) osteoarthritis has led to speculation about whether pyrophosphate deposition causes osteoarthritis – or vice versa. The available information suggests that pyrophosphate deposition is multifactorial, and that some factor predisposing to osteoarthritis also predisposes to chondrocalcinosis.

Investigations

The key investigations are radiology and examination of synovial fluid for crystals. Polarised light microscopy allows confident differentiation between pleomorphic pyrophosphate crystals, with weak positive birefringence, and urate crystals (Fig. 16.3). The various metabolic conditions with which chrondrocalcinosis may be associated must be excluded by appropriate investigations.

Radiology. Chondrocalcinosis occurs in both fibrocartilage and articular (hyaline) cartilage. In the former it appears as irregular calcification in knee menisci, in the articular disc of the inferior radio-ulnar joint (often known to rheumatologists as the 'triangular ligament'), and in the acetabular labra in the hip. In hyaline cartilage it appears as a stippled line of calcification running close to and parallel with the underlying subchondral bone cortex. Chronic joint changes resemble those in 'primary' osteoarthritis. With destruction of cartilage, chondrocalcinosis may disappear. Occasional cases show markedly destructive changes, with loss of periarticular bone.

Diagnosis

Radiology and polarised-light microscopy of synovial fluid provide the basis for the diagnosis of pyrophosphate arthropathy. The absence of crystals from synovial fluid effectively excludes acute or chronic pyrophosphate arthropathy as the cause of the effusion. However, rare cases of definite pyrophosphate arthropathy do not show chondrocalcinosis.

By far the most useful joints in x-ray screening for chondrocalcinosis are the knees. Chondrocalcinosis may, however, be identified in the wrist, symphysis pubis, elbow, shoulder, hip, metacarpophalangeal or occasionally other joints.

The acute attack has to be differentiated from other causes of acute episodic arthritis, including gout and palindromic rheumatism, and from septic arthritis.

Treatment

Asymptomatic chondrocalcinosis requires no treatment. Acute attacks are managed in a manner similar to acute gout (p. 235), except that colchicine is not known to be effective. Because larger joints are involved, it is more often possible to aspirate the effusion and to inject corticosteroid locally. Chronic joint changes are managed in the same way as osteoarthritis. Associated conditions may require treatment in their own right, but there is no evidence that this influences the pyrophosphate arthropathy. No treatment is known which will lessen the frequency of acute attacks or the advance of chronic changes.

OCHRONOSIS (ALKAPTONURIA)

This rare disorder is inherited as a single autosomal recessive gene. Affected patients lack the liver enzyme homogentisic acid oxidase. This enzyme cleaves the benzene ring in the degradation pathway of the aromatic amino acid tyrosine. Thus homogentisic acid, instead of being converted to maleylaceto-acetic acid, accumulates throughout the body.

The urine turns dark on standing (alkaptonuria), due to oxidation of homogentisic acid. These metabolites also produce pigmentation throughout the connective tissues. Clinically this shows as slate blue discolouration of the ears and sclera.

Accumulation of metabolites in cartilage produces stiffening and secondary degenerative changes. The intervertebral discs are particularly affected, leading to severe spondylosis throughout the spine. Secondary calcification also occurs. Thus x-rays show generalised spondylosis with calcified and narrowed intervertebral disc spaces. Spinal pain and rigidity may resemble ankylosing spondylosis. The condition sometimes extends to produce progressive degenerative changes also in the large proximal joints: shoulders, hips and knees.

HYDROXYAPATITE DEPOSITION

Hydroxyapatite is the mineral of bone. It is also the substance laid down when secondary tissue calcifica-tion occurs. Thus it is found in atheromatous plaques, in calcified costal cartilage, in the subcutaneous calcifica-tion occurring in scleroderma and dermatomyositis, and in calcific supraspinatus tendinitis.

Two recent observations have raised the possibility that hydroxyapatite crystals may play a role in joint disease. The crystals are too small to detect by polarised light microscopy but, through electron mic-roscopy and other techniques, they have been identi-fied in synovial effusions. Further, hydroxyapatite crys-tals have been shown to be capable of inducing synovitis in experimental animals.

The significance of these observations is not yet clear. It remains to be established whether hydroxy-apatite crystals play any part in the pathogenesis of what is at present regarded as 'primary' osteoarthritis. Alternatively, they might be a cause of the 'inflamma-tory' episodes which sometimes punctuate the course of osteoarthritis, and which are generally regarded as being related to disposal of joint debris.

17

Rehabilitation

INTRODUCTION

Rehabilitation has been defined as the process by which one ensures that a patient will make full use of his or her remaining physical, intellectual and social skills. It has also been defined as the process whereby one converts a consumer of welfare services into a tax-payer!

Whatever the definition, it can be seen that we are discussing a patient – but extending the traditional horizons of the doctor and looking at how the individual, in his new (diseased) situation will interact with the surrounding world. We are thus extending into the social sphere, hopefully without losing those parts of the medical model which are of greatest value, i.e. the analysis and treatment of the medical problem.

The diagram below shows the failure of overlap of medical and social models of disease.

It is possible, too, that conclusions drawn on a heterogeneous group of the disabled may have less relevance than an in-depth study of a smaller, more homogeneous population (e.g. those with arthritis).

The traditional medical model deals primarily in diagnostic terms, while the social model (social workers' and sociologists' writings) largely ignores diagnosis and concentrates on functional activity restrictions. Thus, professionals of one discipline do not read what the others write. Perhaps if the models overlapped, or if there were more dialogue between medical and social workers, the whole range of literature would be more widely available.

DEFINITIONS (see diagram below and Table 17.1)

Impairment: Any loss or abnormality of psychological, pysiological or anatomical structure or function.

Disability: Any restriction or lack (resulting from impairment) of ability to perform an activity, in a manner or within the range considered normal for a human being.

Handicap: A disadvantage for a given individual, resulting from an impairment or disability, that limits or prevents the fulfilment of a role that is regarded as normal (taking account of age, sex, and social and cultural factors) for that individual.

Primary prevention: An attempt to prevent disease or impairment before it occurs.

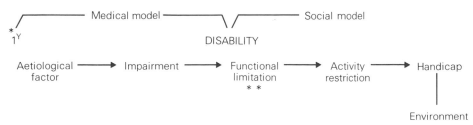

Table 17.1

Index of Self-care

Categories 1–3	Very Severely Handicapped— in need of special care
Category 4	Severely Handicapped— people who either had difficulty with all items of self-care or found most things difficult and some things impossible
Category 5	Severely Handicapped— people who found most items of self-care difficult, or three or four things difficult and some impossible
Category 6	Appreciably Handicapped— people who can do a fair amount for themselves but have difficulty with some items of self-care, or need help with one or two minor items
Category 7	Minor Handicap— people who can do everything for themselves but have difficulty with one or two items of self-care
Category 8	No Apparent Handicap— people to whom physical impairment presents no difficulty in taking care of themselves

This index of self-care (devised by Amelia Harris, 1971), which was used in the National Survey of the Handi-capped, is relatively easy to administer and is used by many Social Service Departments. It is an illustration of the social model of disease.

Secondary prevention: maintenance rehabilitation: The early detection and treatment of disease or impairment with a view to return to normal health.

Tertiary prevention: the avoidance of social handicap: The continuing treatment of a disease or disability to avoid needless progression or complication and the rehabilitation of the individual to minimise any conse-quent handicap. We may indeed ask how many cases of handicap could be prevented by changing the environment. For the 350 million subjects in the Third World, primary prevention is of the greatest impor-tance: i.e. vaccination, immunisation, clean water, and decent housing. For the 100 million in the industrialised world, the causes of disability are different, and secondary and tertiary prevention are of greater significance.

The main causes of chronic disability in adults in the UK are:

Young: mainly congenital impairment and traffic accidents.

Middle-aged: fluctuating disorders such as rheu-matoid arthritis and multiple sclerosis.

Elderly: diseases of degeneration such as cardio-respiratory failure, osteoarthritis, atherosclerosis.

A BRIEF HISTORY OF PROVISION OF CARE FOR THE DISABLED

If we consider the history of care for the chronically ill and disabled in Britain, we find that, in feudal and medieval times, care was provided by the family, the local community and the church. By the 17th century this became formalised in the Poor Law Act which, until overwhelmed by urbanisation and industrialisation, worked tolerably well. Its final breakdown (via the asylum and the workhouse) came in the 1920s, but it was not until the 1940s that the National Health Service was formed. This was perceived mainly as providing acute medical care to cope with reservoirs of curable illness. Many would agree that this has now been admirably accomplished. With the coming of the welfare state, better nutrition and housing, and the economic boom of the 1950s and 1960s, our popula-tion has now become one with a low, stable death rate and a low and slightly less stable fertility rate. Most people can expect five decades in which they are free of physically incapacitating disease. The stereotypes of the crippled child and the wounded soldier seldom apply, and the handicapped person in a wheelchair is not typical. The disabled Westerner is becoming older, is semi-ambulant, and probably suffers from arthritis or has had a stroke.

Health services and social services – particularly the former – have not caught up with these changes. A variety of services is available but individual parts are rarely coordinated. The facilities may thus be hard for the individual to find in a correct sequence, without the help and cooperation of a large number of medical and social workers. Some of these various components of the rehabilitation service are briefly reviewed here.

General Practice

Each general practitioner will have about 300 disabled people on his list. Most of them require infrequent help, though the elderly disabled usually benefit from regular visits. Whilst his patient is adapting to new disability, the general practitioner may require help from other members of the primary care team; the mild stroke, the single joint arthritis, and mild multiple sclerosis are all cases which will be dealt with predominantly at home.

Domiciliary Service

Occupational therapist

Therapists are in short supply, particularly occupational therapists; on the other hand, it has been shown that many new skills (e.g. bathing for an amputee) when taught in hospital, are not carried out efficiently at home because the patient cannot transfer instruction in hospital to the home situation.

If a domiciliary or community occupational therapist (usually based with Social Services) is available, she is invaluable in teaching the patient how to become independent in the real environment. For instance, she can give advice on how a kitchen can be adapted for a wheelchair-bound housewife, or suggest access rails and adaptations to toilet areas, etc.

Physiotherapist

It may take five hours by ambulance to reach a physiotherapy outpatient department for treatment. The benefit to rheumatoid sufferers of this exhausting journey is likely to be minimal, and the diabetic may miss his main meal. On the other hand, domiciliary physiotherapy should probably not be given to, for example, sufferers from cervical spondylosis, where wearing a collar or using analgesics are equally effective. Perhaps the best role for a domiciliary physiotherapist is mainly pedagogic: the family caring for a patient at home after a recent relatively mild stroke will welcome advice on how to move him out of bed, onto a chair or the toilet, and how to dress him and help him to become independent again.

Community nurse

The community nurse will help a patient with bathing, washing and dressing, and give injections, etc.

Support services (Fig. 17.3, p. 247)

The general practitioner is also able to call on a wide range of support services, mostly provided by the Social Services department: home-helps, meals on wheels, street wardens, etc., and local schemes such as Crossroads, Twilighters and Day Care are fairly general.

Twilighters is a local Leeds scheme and Crossroads a national scheme arising from the television series. The helpers in both schemes, who are usually housewives with relevant experience, wash, dress and care for disabled people at the beginning and end of the day. This saves the patient being put to bed early in the afternoon, as may happen when the District Nurse is hard pressed.

Some aids are available from the hospital service, e.g. beds, chairs and commodes; appliances are also available through the hospital appliance officers employed by Social Services, though provision varies in different regions.

FUNCTIONS OF THE TEAM

Team work, both in the primary care team and in hospital, is frequently extolled as the ideal. A case conference, even once weekly, must be felt and seen to be valuable since it takes up a great deal of professional time. In our own Leeds practice we involve the personnel detailed below when we are discussing inpatients: we allow each to contribute to the discussion in an ordered way, give time for an interchange of ideas (patients and families are often seen very differently by the various therapists), set agreed goals, review knowledge and educate ourselves, often by a brief run-down on the disease afflicting the patient under discussion.

The Ward Sister

The ward sister usually has the greatest overall knowledge and experience of the patient. She knows, for example, how he performs when not supervised by the physiotherapist. She will liaise with the occupational therapist so that, for example, the nurses and occupational therapist can help the patient to learn to dress every morning in the same manner. Where work is uncoordinated, it is not unusual to find nurses hurrying a patient to the lavatory, even by wheelchair, when he could be using those skills of standing and walking newly-acquired with great effort in the physiotherapy department.

The Community Nurse

This member of the team may, for the outpatient, take the place of the ward sister. She is usually too busy to come to the case conference. However, functional problems of the patient could be presented on video to her.

The Specialist Health Visitor or Liaison Officer

Some years ago we showed that the rate of readmission of patients, a particular risk during the fortnight immediately after leaving hospital, could be reduced if they could be supported on discharge. Many hospital units (diabetic, children's, etc.) now have their own health visitor as do many general practices. It is our policy to allow the hospital health visitor to hand over care of the discharged patient to his local health visitor when his condition is becoming stable.

Because the hospital environment is so unlike the homes of most patients, it is important for the health visitor to see the home while the patient is in hospital. She will learn about its physical features, as well as the patient's links with neighbours and family, and this will enable the team to be realistic in their aims. Surprisingly, we also found that, if death had occurred, the remaining relative would often turn to the health visitor for comfort in preference to the family doctor. After discharge, she will also assist with practical matters such as which tablets to take and when; how to contact an ambulance service that has failed to take the patient to hospital; and how to call up the aids and appliances that should have arrived but have not come. She thus becomes a trusted friend.

The Physiotherapist

It is often said that the physiotherapist is most skilled in helping the patient to gain mobility. His or her primary task, which is no longer seen as the laying on of hands, the giving of heat and passive therapy, is in reality often a private session of undivided attention to the single and sometimes lonely patient. The physiotherapist's skills must be constructively used. Physiotherapy should not be a placebo to be used when the doctor can think of nothing else to do for his patient; heat or ice or any other physical modality, *alone*, should rarely be prescribed. Group activities should be used at later stages of treatment; they are economical of therapists' time, as long as patients are properly supervised, and the group itself provides stimulation, competition and enjoyment. Work done in the physiotherapy department may be complemented by similar activities masquerading as games or crafts in occupational therapy (e.g. hand exercises could be associated with threading tasks in occupational therapy, or shoulder exercises with printing).

The Occupational Therapist

Occupational therapists are always in short supply and must not be used merely to supply diversional activities for the patient. They are instrumental in helping patients to relearn how to look after themselves. Occupational therapy includes self-care, domestic skills, vocational skills and leisure activities (Fig. 17.1).

The Disablement Resettlement Officer (DRO)

This team member is seconded from the local job centre and, hopefully, is involved with the employed patient from the early days of his illness. It is important for the patient not to lose touch with his own work, wherever there is a possibility of a return to it (even if modified), or at least to retain a connection with his workplace. It is now very difficult to find new employment for older disabled men and women, but their skills may be worth a great deal to their current employers. The DRO liaises with the Employment Rehabilitation Centre, and can arrange for fares to work, can contact

ACTIVITY	DEPENDENT	WITH HELP	INDEPENDENT
Feeding			
Dressing			
Bed			
Chair			
Toilet			
Wash			
Bath			
Householding			
Shopping			
Mobility			

Hopefully with treatment →

Fig. 17.1 *A simple chart of some activities of daily living. This can be further broken down into individual tasks such as brushing teeth, turning key in lock, as necessary, or can be greatly expanded, as required. Some 200 variants exist. (The occupational therapist is largely responsible for teaching the patient these skills.)*

potential employers, and knows of various schemes, aids and adaptations available through the Manpower Services Commission for the working disabled.

The Medical Social Worker

Employed by the Local Authority, she does not like to be thought of as merely the provider of access to benefits even though she is usually most knowledgeable about both contributory and non-contributory benefits (e.g. invalidity benefit, mobility allowance). She is frequently responsible for placement of patients in Part III accommodation, sheltered accommodation, or Cheshire Homes, as appropriate, but she also has counselling skills. She can help both patient and family adapt to the changes that have occurred. Our own medical social worker and therapist run an invaluable Stroke Family Counselling Service, monthly. As with many self-help groups (e.g. Arthritis Care), advice is often most easily taken from those who also suffer.

The Clinical Psychologist

Assessing the patient's current intellectual skills and delineating his previous educational and job history fall to the clinical psychologist, but he can also help in modifying behaviour and in suggesting methods of motivating and engaging the patient in his recovery.

The Speech Therapist

Where there are communication problems to be treated, the speech therapist's skills in analysing such problems overlap with those of the clinical psychologist. Much work remains to be done, both in devising a simple and reproducible method of analysing speech disorders and in evaluating speech therapy techniques in individual diseases. Questions which need to be answered include: what should be the frequency, duration, content and timing of therapy; how far can the professional's work be supplemented by volunteers and group activities; and how could other hospital staff be helping speech-impaired patients?

An expanding range of communicators is becoming available; some are costly (to the NHS and to the patient, in terms of batteries used) but several are potentially of great value.

ASSESSMENT AND GOAL SETTING

The first aims of the doctor examining a patient with a locomotor difficulty must be to take a good history, to examine the patient fully, and to arrive at the correct diagnosis. He then considers the ensuing functional disability, and whether this is static, fluctuant or progressive. Educational, vocational and social histories are also relevant. In order to manage the problem satisfactorily we need to see how patient and disease interact with each other and with the social and physical environment: we need to discuss with our colleagues how we aim to help, in the shorter and longer term, and we have to be able to reassess the situation.

A few situations of increasing complexity will illustrate these points.

Single Joint Arthritis of the Lower Limb

For example, the older man, living with his wife in a council house. Beginning to develop osteoarthritis of the hip, he notices local pain and finds it difficult to negotiate stairs, get into the bath, get off the toilet, put on socks and shoes and cut his toenails. Health permitting, the eventual answer to the problem may be a total hip replacement. The patient may, however, be unsuitable or the disease progress slow. Interim management would then comprise: control of the disease and prevention of further deterioration as far as possible (e.g. by weight reduction) if worthwhile; and reducing the load through the joint by use of a stick or other walking aid. The muscles across the involved joint will also be involved (hip extensors and abductors will have wasted), so physiotherapy designed to improve joint range (e.g. hydrotherapy) will be valuable. Open-ended (unending) physiotherapy is inadvisable; patients and staff are better motivated during short, defined courses of treatment and many patients can maintain improvement with a few simple daily exercises at home.

Pain should always be relieved, as should stiffness: physiotherapy cannot be performed satisfactorily, nor can daily activities be kept up unless both are controlled.

It is unnecessary to hold a case conference about such a relatively simple problem as this and most therapy can be home-based (orchestrated by the general practitioner) or managed in the outpatient department at the district general hospital. A referral to the occupational therapy department for an Activities of Daily Living assessment (Fig. 17.1) should help the patient. The occupational therapist (O.T.) will show the patient how he can rise more easily from a higher chair, will provide a raised lavatory seat, and will arrange for the installation of a rail beside the toilet. Steps and stairs within and outside the house will have to be coped with. Perhaps there could be a downstairs toilet, or ground floor accommodation could be found, with rails installed at the front door. But the O.T. cannot change the design of buses (most of which have a step height of 17 inches, rendering them inaccessible to most of the disabled).

Aids

Prescription of aids should be as precise as drug prescription (Table 17.2). This can be difficult, as aids are not subject to British Standards and are very numerous (there were over 6000 at the last count). The development of Aids Centres in many regions should help practitioners and patients alike: they are resource centres for much information and carry a large stock of aids, which can be tried. The aids most frequently prescribed are ones which assist mobility and those which improve access and safety in the bath. Surgical shoes are costly but extremely helpful to many patients; they are individually made on lasts peculiar to each patient, and can be made in almost any colour and style so that they are usually very acceptable. 'Comfort' and space shoes are also available, which are

---

Table 17.2

Prescription of Aids

1. Diagnosis? Prognosis?
2. Problem(s) arising?
3. Will an aid solve the problem(s)?
4. Other necessary measures?
5. Show patient range of aids (Aids Centre)
6. Patient should *try out* preferred aid (O.T.)
7. Standard equipment preferable
8. Simplest equipment preferable
9. Cheapest effective equipment preferable
10. Be prepared for an aid to have limited life

---

less expensive. Surgical lumbar spine supports can only be prescribed by hospital doctors; they are excellent for backache of many causes, but should be inspected by the doctor to check that they are satisfactory, and in particular to see that the steels are closely apposed to and parallel with the lumbar spine.

Fluctuating Disability

The problems associated with this are illustrated by the adult with chronic inflammatory polyarthritis. Again, we have to consider how we can ameliorate the course of the disease and deal with its interaction with the patient and the environment. The sufferer may well be a woman in the third decade with young children and a house to manage. For the active disease she will need specific antirheumatic drugs, usually anti-inflammatory agents (see p. 198). She will need bed rest in hospital if she cannot rest at home with toddlers, and local rest (with resting splints) to individual joints. Splints at the wrist will improve carrying and gripping. She will also need considerable help in re-ordering her life. First, she will usually welcome education and advice on the nature of the disease and its implications for her. She may need to perform household tasks in alternative ways to prevent damage to the affected joints. Her husband needs to be similarly educated; he could do the heavy shopping and housework, or perhaps a home-help could be employed. Refrigerators and freezers, though expensive, allow for bulk shopping by helpers.

Wheelchairs

If the housewife is in a wheelchair, the kitchen has to be accessible to her, with work surfaces lowered accordingly, and the O.T. may need to visit the house and help make this adjustment. The wheelchair is itself an aid to mobility and, if it is not to restrict the patient, has to be properly prescribed (Table 17.3). Doorways may need

to be widened – or the patient slimmed to fit into a junior chair.

The disabled mother still wishes to look after her children and maintain close contact with them, and she often achieves this very satisfactorily. Her role must not be taken from her; every help and aid must be given to allow her to maintain this function. The O.T. may help greatly, e.g. by discussing the adaptation of clothing or use of disposable nappies, and the health visitor may suggest early use of playgroups and nurseries.

The Arthritic in Employment

Inflammatory polyarthritis is often unpredictable. An arthritic with knee effusions may use crutches to relieve the knees and then find that the shoulders flare up. Gutter crutches, where weight is borne not on hands but on the forearms, may help. Transportation by car to work is often invaluable; many arthritics have insufficient energy to cope with a long bus journey as well as the job. Several of our patients with ankylosing spondylitis were found to have refused promotion because they had found congenial work which they could manage even on bad days.

The Handicapped School-leaver

The loss of mobility throughout childhood has meant that the handicapped school-leaver is less independent than his peers, less able to handle money, and less sure of himself. He may also have multiple handicaps. The adolescent with juvenile chronic arthritis may be of small stature, and will be treated correspondingly, and may have few opportunities to meet young people of the opposite sex. If all these problems are anticipated, the various professionals, parents, and others involved can give help accordingly. The adolescent can be taught to drive (perhaps with an adapted car) and to live independently in a flat or bedsitter.

Progressive Disability

This is exemplified by motor neurone disease. The tempo of the disease is unpredictable but its downward

---

Table 17.3

Prescribing a Wheelchair:
A Few Questions to Ask

1. Is wheelchair for indoors/transit/outdoors?
2. Who propels it:
   a) patient—does he need a powered chair?
   b) relative?
3. What is patient's height, weight and diagnosis?
4. What is narrowest doorway through which chair must pass?
5. Will it go in car?
6. What extras are required?
   e.g. 4-inch latex cushion
   headrest
   desk arms
   attached tray
   mobile arm supports
   detachable arm rests, etc.
   foot rests/straps
7. What modifications are required?
   e.g. is patient an amputee
   or quadriplegic
   or hemiplegic

Wheelchairs can be prescribed by general practitioners on form No. AOFSG.

course is unrelenting. The patient may be able to walk for a long time – precariously balanced above his centre of gravity – but may find he cannot get up when he has fallen to the floor.

Great efforts should be made to help this patient to preserve his ability to transfer from bed to chair and to lavatory or commode within the house (Fig. 17.2).

Later, he may have insufficient power in his arms to dress himself or to raise his arms to his mouth for feeding, and the muscles tire quickly. Ball-bearing arm supports fixed to the wheelchair (if used) may help somewhat (as long as the subject has 90° shoulder abduction) but they are difficult to set up and should, ideally, be used for a single specific function, such as feeding or typing. In hospital, the sunflower limb balancer has counterweights and achieves the same function. Intellect is unimpaired, and the patient with a

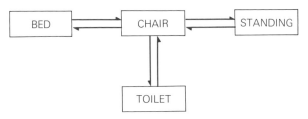

Fig. 17.2 *Transfers. Diagram illustrates the basic moves required of a patient within the home. (The physiotherapist is largely responsible for teaching the patient these skills.)*

helpful and sensitive family can remain at home until the end, pursuing suitable sedentary interests (e.g. ham radio, with adaptation to his radio carried out by the Rehabilitation Engineering Medical Advisory Panel, REMAP). The Royal Association for Disability and Rehabilitation (RADAR, 25 Mortimer Street, London W1N 8AB) has information on sports and other leisure pursuits for the disabled.

It is important to prescribe aids which will remain in use for a substantial period so that the patient's attention is not drawn to his declining function by frequent piecemeal additions. A package of communications aids which anticipate his needs is invaluable.

The rest of the family may also need relief from time to time in the form of holidays and intermittent care and daycare for the disabled member.

Stable Disability

Paraplegia of traumatic onset, quadriplegia and hemiplegia are all characterised by a severe, single neurological incident. The first two should usually be managed, in their early stages, in a specialist unit to which the patient is referred without delay. There are numerous facets to each diagnosis: skin, bowel and genito-urinary care must all be optimal at the time when attention is also paid to the recovery of muscle function, to respiratory and autonomic disturbances, and to the psychological impact of the disease.

Paraplegia

Young paraplegics should usually be able to manage to live independently and many can train, and engage lifelong, in suitable employment. Numerous physical pursuits are possible (as indicated by the success of the paraplegic Olympic Games). The patient may marry. Part of the success of adaptation will be due to the initial meticulous care and teaching of a specialised unit, which provides sufficient support and motivation for the disabled person to grieve and then to plan anew. Continued support is provided by other paraplegics via their self-help group and publications.

An injury to the spinal cord above C4 is incompatible with life because the diaphragm is paralysed. A lesion of C5 renders the patient almost totally dependent even though rhomboid, supraspinatus, infraspinatus and subscapularis muscle functions are preserved. A patient with a C6 lesion may have some hand function and can feed himself with appliances strapped to the wrist. This patient is a good candidate for Possum. Possum is a patient-operated selector mechanism (Latin: 'I am able') which represents a system of environmental controls. The bed-bound patient can control the radio, television and lights, and can operate the door of his home to admit only desired visitors. There are many other adaptations, e.g. to enable the patient to type, and to use the telephone. Used Possum equipment is sometimes available from the Possum Users Association but, if it is required for any length of time, the treating doctor should contact the regional Possum Assessor (a consultant physician, often a neurologist). Many patients with C7 and C8 lesions have a useful hand, and sometimes remarkable independence.

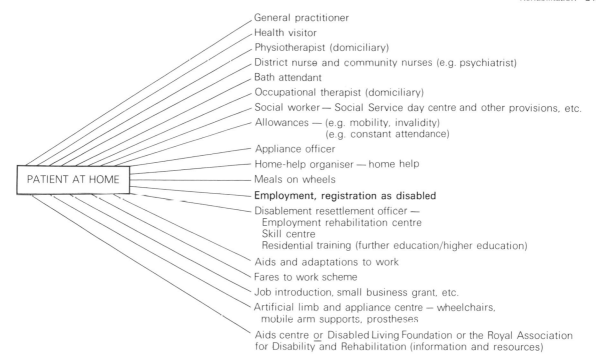

General practitioner
Health visitor
Physiotherapist (domiciliary)
District nurse and community nurses (e.g. psychiatrist)
Bath attendant
Occupational therapist (domiciliary)
Social worker — Social Service day centre and other provisions, etc.
Allowances — (e.g. mobility, invalidity)
(e.g. constant attendance)
Appliance officer
Home-help organiser — home help
Meals on wheels
Employment, registration as disabled
Disablement resettlement officer —
Employment rehabilitation centre
Skill centre
Residential training (further education/higher education)
Aids and adaptations to work
Fares to work scheme
Job introduction, small business grant, etc.
Artificial limb and appliance centre — wheelchairs,
mobile arm supports, prostheses
Aids centre or Disabled Living Foundation or the Royal Association
for Disability and Rehabilitation (information and resources)

PATIENT AT HOME

Fig. 17.3 *The maze of rehabilitation and support services. (The facilities listed are by no means exhaustive.)*

With the development of Prestel and other computer technology it may be possible to provide satisfactory home-based work for quadriplegics. Leisure should also be more pleasurable. Individual patient/computer interfaces may have to be devised.

Hemiplegia

About one-third of those who survive the original acute episode have some return of hand function; two-thirds are able to walk again, in some fashion. One of the most important things to remember about these subjects is that the defect is not of motor power alone, or even of contending with the spasticity of the side consequent on an upper motor neurone lesion. In a right hemiplegia, speech may also be involved, with impairment of reception, synthesis and expression of spoken and/or written language. A left hemiplegia may produce sensory inattention and visuospatial disorganisation. The patient may be further disadvantaged by hypoalgesia, hemianopia, and a variety of psychological problems which require analysis. Since those affected are

usually elderly, they may also suffer from myocardial insufficiency, diabetes mellitus and other disease.

Recovery may be further impeded by poor exercise tolerance; the patient may be unable to hear the physiotherapist's instructions, or perhaps be unable to enunciate as directed by the speech therapist for lack of well-fitting teeth. Attention to such elementary details as well as to finances, the home environment, and the support of ageing and anxious relatives, will make all the difference between failure (with consequent institutionalisation or poor adaptations at home) or a successful return home.

Care of the Chronically Disabled

It is rarely necessary for those disabled by locomotor disorders alone to require institutional care (which is, in any case, in short supply), provided there are adequate support services at home (Fig. 17.3). In sheltered housing, some cover is provided by the warden, but many people will have a network of friends who provide better cover and every effort should be made to keep them in the neighbourhood where they have lived (and developed contacts) for many years. Some people require more help; dining particularly and recreation, food preparation and cooking facilities within the building complex, and this may necessitate admission to a Local Authority home. Others, who have no support at home, may need the shelter of a Cheshire Home or a National Health Service Young Disabled Unit (see Fig. 17.4). When disabled patients live in their own home, relatives often labour for many years under a heavy burden: intermittent relief for them is essential. Day care may enable them to engage in a few hobbies even if they cannot remain at work.

CONCLUSIONS

Facilities for the disabled in the UK are improving, but they have grown in a haphazard fashion. To find the best help, the patient's doctor must know how to contact the relevant services. This can best be achieved by working closely with professional therapists of the rehabilitation team.

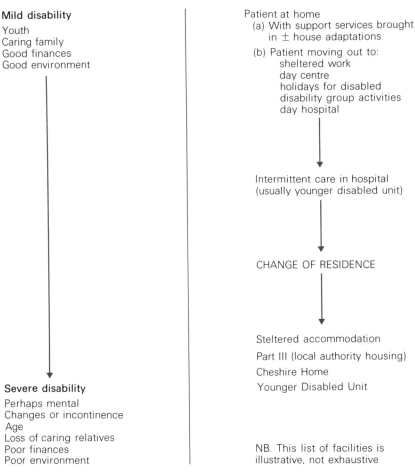

Mild disability
Youth
Caring family
Good finances
Good environment

Severe disability
Perhaps mental
Changes or incontinence
Age
Loss of caring relatives
Poor finances
Poor environment

Patient at home
(a) With support services brought
    in ± house adaptations
(b) Patient moving out to:
    sheltered work
    day centre
    holidays for disabled
    disability group activities
    day hospital

Intermittent care in hospital
(usually younger disabled unit)

CHANGE OF RESIDENCE

Steltered accommodation

Part III (local authority housing)

Cheshire Home

Younger Disabled Unit

NB. This list of facilities is
illustrative, not exhaustive

Fig. 17.4 *Accommodation for disabled people.*

Further Reading

Aids to the Investigation of Peripheral Nerve Injuries (1943). MRC War Memorandum. No. 7 (Reprinted). London: HMSO.

Charnley J. (1970). *The Closed Treatment of Common Fractures*, 3rd edn. London and Edinburgh: Churchill Livingstone.

Dubvowitz V. (1978). *Muscle Disorders in Childhood*. Philadelphia: Saunders.

Duthie R.B., Ferguson A.B. (eds.) (1983). *Mercers Orthopaedic Surgery*, 8th edn. London: Arnold.

Flatt A.E. (1979). *The Care of Minor Hand Injuries*, 4th edn. St. Louis, Toronto and London: Mosby.

Guttmann L. (1973). *Spinal Cord Injuries: Comprehensive Management and Research*. Oxford: Blackwell Scientific Publications.

Jaffe H.L. (1958). *Tumours and Tumorous Conditions of the Bones and Joints*. London: Kimpton.

Keen G. (1975). *Chest Injuries*. Bristol: John Wright & Sons Ltd.

Keim H.A. (1982). *The Adolescent Spine*, 2nd edn. New York: Springer-Verlag.

Lamb D.W., Kuczynski K. (1981). *The Practice of Hand Surgery*. London: Blackwell Scientific Publications.

Menelaus M.B. (1980). *The Orthopaedic Management of Spina Bifida*. London and Edinburgh: Churchill Livingstone.

McGregor I.A. (1980). *Fundamental Techniques of Plastic Surgery*, 7th edn. Edinburgh and London: Churchill Livingstone.

McSweeney T. (1978). Injuries of the spine. In *Operative Surgery*, 3rd edn. Vol. *Accident Surgery*. (London P.S., ed.) pp. 348–73. London: Butterworth.

Rockwood C.A., Green D.P. (1975). *Fractures*. London: Harper and Row.

Salter R.B. (1970). *Textbook of Disorders and Injuries of the Musculo-skeletal System*. Baltimore: Williams & Wilkins.

Sharrard W.J.W. (1979). *Paediatric Orthopaedics and Fractures*, 2nd edn. London: Blackwell Scientific Publications.

Smillie I.S. (1979). *Injuries of the Knee Joint*, 5th edn. London and Edinburgh: Churchill Livingstone.

Smith R. (1979). *Biochemical Disorders of the Skeleton*. London: Butterworth.

Somerville E.W. (1982). *Displacement of the Hip in Childhood*. New York: Springer-Verlag.

Vaughan J. (1981). *The Physiology of Bone*, 3rd edn. Oxford: Clarendon Press.

Williams W.G., Smith R.E. (1977). *Trauma of the Chest. The Coventry Conference*. Bristol: John Wright & Sons Ltd.

Wilson J.N. (ed.) Watson-Jones (1984). *Fractures and Joint Injuries*. Edinburgh and London: Churchill Livingstone.

Wynne-Davies R., Fairbank T.J. (1976). *Fairbanks Atlas of General Affections of the Skeleton*, 2nd edn. London and Edinburgh: Churchill Livingstone.

Index